Neuroendoscopy and Interventional Pain Medicine

(*Volume 1*)

Regenerative Medicine & Peripheral Nerve Endoscopy

Edited by

Kai-Uwe Lewandrowski

Center for Advanced Spine Care of Southern Arizona and Surgical Institute of Tucson, Tucson, AZ, USA

William Omar Contreras López

Clínica Foscal Internacional Autopista Floridablanca - Girón, Km 7, Floridablanca Santander, Colombia

Jorge Felipe Ramírez León

Fundación Universitaria Sanitas Bogotá, D.C., Colombia

Álvaro Dowling

Orthopaedic Spine Surgeon, Director of Endoscopic Spine Clinic Santiago, Chile

&

Morgan P. Lorio

Advanced Orthopedics, 499 East Central Parkway Altamonte Springs, FL 32701, USA

Assistant Editors

Hui-lin Yang

Professor & Chairman of Orthopedic Department
The First Affiliated Hospital of Soochow University
No. 899 Pinghai Road, Suzhou, China

Xifeng Zhang

Department of Orthopedics, Wangjing Hospital
China Academy of Chinese Medical Sciences, Beijing, China

&

Anthony T. Yeung

Desert Institute for Spine Care
Phoenix, AZ, USA

Neuroendoscopy and Interventional Pain Medicines

(Volume 1)

Regenerative Medicine & Peripheral Nerve Endoscopy

Editors: Kai-Uwe Lewandrowski, William Omar Contreras López,

Jorge Felipe Ramírez León, Álvaro Dowling & Morgan P. Lorio

ISBN (Online): 978-981-5274-46-2

ISBN (Print): 978-981-5274-47-9

ISBN (Paperback): 978-981-5274-48-6

need for a court order if at any point you breach any terms of this License Agreement. In no event will any delay or failure by Bentham Science Publishers in enforcing your compliance with this License Agreement constitute a waiver of any of its rights.

3. You acknowledge that you have read this License Agreement, and agree to be bound by its terms and conditions. To the extent that any other terms and conditions presented on any website of Bentham Science Publishers conflict with, or are inconsistent with, the terms and conditions set out in this License Agreement, you acknowledge that the terms and conditions set out in this License Agreement shall prevail.

Bentham Science Publishers Pte. Ltd.
80 Robinson Road #02-00
Singapore 068898
Singapore
Email: subscriptions@benthamscience.net

**BENTHAM
SCIENCE**

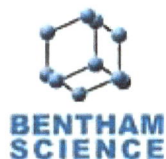

CONTENTS

PREFACE

Welcome to Neuroendoscopy and Interventional Pain Medicine, Vol. 1: Regenerative Medicine & Peripheral Nerve Endoscopy, a comprehensive volume that explores the latest advancements in regenerative medicine and minimally invasive endoscopic techniques. This book brings together the expertise of leading practitioners and researchers at the forefront of these transformative fields.

The growing impact of low back pain on individuals' health and lifespan is a significant concern, and this volume begins by addressing this issue with a focus on future care models that support healthy longevity. The book offers insights into targeted strategies for improving patient outcomes. Advancements in cell-based regeneration are crucial for treating degenerative disc disease. The current concepts and limitations of these strategies, highlighting both the potential and challenges in this evolving field, are discussed in depth. The clinical applications of regenerative strategies are further explored by providing a global perspective on the burden of low back pain and the promise of innovative treatments. Bioengineering strategies for injured or degenerative intervertebral discs are examined, and cutting-edge approaches to disc repair and regeneration are presented. Additionally, an in-depth look at current therapy strategies for vertebral endplates is provided, summarizing valuable information on treatment options for these critical structures. Stem cell therapy holds great promise for spinal cord injury, and the current concepts and advancements in this area are discussed, showcasing the potential for significant breakthroughs in patient recovery and rehabilitation. Minimally invasive and endoscopic techniques continue to revolutionize peripheral nerve decompression, as in ultrasound-guided or single portal endoscopic carpal tunnel release. These innovative approaches offer less invasive solutions for patients suffering from carpal tunnel syndrome. The use of ozone and PRP injections for symptomatic lumbar herniated discs is covered, and the respective chapter provides insights into these emerging treatment modalities and their effectiveness in alleviating pain and improving function. Lastly, the potential of allogeneic stem cell therapy for painful intermediate lumbar degenerative discs is explored, offering a glimpse into the future of regenerative medicine for spinal conditions.

Each chapter in this volume is carefully selected to reflect contemporary trends and innovations in regenerative medicine and endoscopic techniques as they apply to neuroendoscopy and interventional pain management. This book aims to meet the demands of patients, healthcare providers, and policymakers by addressing the need for safer, more efficient, and cost-effective solutions. The editors hope that Vol. 1 of Neuroendoscopy and Interventional Pain Medicine: Regenerative Medicine & Peripheral Nerve Endoscopy serves as an invaluable resource for clinicians and researchers dedicated to advancing the field and improving patient care.

Kai-Uwe Lewandrowski
Center for Advanced Spine Care of Southern Arizona and Surgical
Institute of Tucson
Tucson, AZ, USA

William Omar Contreras López
Clínica Foscal Internacional
Autopista Floridablanca - Girón, Km 7, Floridablanca
Santander, Colombia

Jorge Felipe Ramírez León
Fundación Universitaria Sanitas
Bogotá, D.C., Colombia

Álvaro Dowling
Orthopaedic Spine Surgeon, Director of Endoscopic Spine Clinic
Santiago, Chile

Morgan P. Lorio
Advanced Orthopedics, 499 East Central Parkway
Altamonte Springs, FL 32701, USA

Assistant Editors

Hui-lin Yang
Professor & Chairman of Orthopedic Department
The First Affiliated Hospital of Soochow University
No. 899 Pinghai Road, Suzhou, China

Xifeng Zhang
Department of Orthopedics, Wangjing Hospital
China Academy of Chinese Medical Sciences, Beijing, China

&

Anthony T. Yeung
Desert Institute for Spine Care
Phoenix, AZ, USA

List of Contributors

Álvaro Dowling	Orthopaedic Spine Surgeon, Director of Endoscopic Spine Clinic, Santiago, Chile,
Jaime Moyano	Centro Regional Universitario BarilocheThe institution will open in a new tab, San Carlos de Bariloche, Argentina,
Jorge Felipe Ramírez León	Minimally Invasive Spine Center. Bogotá, D.C., Colombia, Reina Sofía Clinic. Bogotá, D.C., Colombia, Fundación Universitaria Sanitas. Bogotá, D.C., Colombia,
Juan Carlos Vera	Universidad de Chile, Santiago, Chile,
Kai-Uwe Lewandrowski	Center for Advanced Spine Care of Southern Arizona and Surgical Institute of Tucson, Tucson, AZ, USA, Departmemt of Orthopaedics, Fundación Universitaria Sanitas, Bogotá, D.C., Colombia, Department of Neurosurgery in the Video-Endoscopic Postgraduate Program at the Universidade Federal do Estado do Rio de Janeiro - UNIRIO, Rio de Janeiro, Brazil,
Luis Miguel Duchén Rodríguez	Center for Neurological Diseases and Public University of El Alto, La Paz, Bolivia,
Marcelo Molina	Orthopaedic Spine Surgeon, Clínica Las Condes, Instituto Traumatologico, Santiago, Chile, Department of Orthopaedic Surgery, Faculdade de Medicina de Ribeirão Preto - USP (School of Medicine of Ribeirão Preto - University of São Paulo), Ribeirão Preto, SP, Brazil,
Marjan Asefi	University of North Carolina, Greensboro, NC, USA,
Morgan P. Lorio	Advanced Orthopedics, 499 East Central Parkway, Altamonte Springs, FL 32701, USA,
Paul Paterson	Vero Orthopedics, 3955 Indian River Dr, Vero Beach, FL 32960, USA,
Stefan Landgraeber	Universitätsdes Saarlandes, Klinik für Neurochirurgie, Kirrberger Straße 100, 66421 Homburg, Germany,
Stephan Knoll	Biological Therapies Center, La Paz, Bolivia,
Tania Arancibia Baspineiro	Center for Neurological Diseases, La Paz, Bolivia,
William Omar Contreras López	Clínica Foscal Internacional, Autopista Floridablanca - Girón, Km 7, Floridablanca, Santander, Colombia,

CHAPTER 1

The Implications of Low Back Pain on Prolonged Lifespan and Future Targeted Care Models to Support the Pursuit of Healthy Longevity

Álvaro Dowling[1,*] and **Kai-Uwe Lewandrowski**[2,3,4]

[1] *Orthopaedic Spine Surgeon, Director of Endoscopic Spine Clinic, Santiago, Chile*

[2] *Center for Advanced Spine Care of Southern Arizona and Surgical Institute of Tucson, Tucson, AZ, USA*

[3] *Departmemt of Orthopaedics, Fundación Universitaria Sanitas, Bogotá, D.C., Colombia*

[4] *Department of Neurosurgery in the Video-Endoscopic Postgraduate Program at the Universidade Federal do Estado do Rio de Janeiro - UNIRIO, Rio de Janeiro, Brazil*

Abstract: The human desire for everlasting youth and well-being has persisted throughout history. In the modern era, advancements in medicine and the emerging field of longevity have brought this age-old aspiration closer to realization. The remarkable increase in global life expectancy from a mere 30 years in 1870 to an impressive 71 years today, is a monumental healthcare achievement over the past century and a half. This achievement carries profound implications for the economy, necessitating a deeper understanding of the aging process and its influence on economic decision-making. Furthermore, it raises concerns regarding the adjustments required in behavior and lifestyle to adapt to extended lifespans while maintaining a high quality of life. The rise in life expectancy has substantial implications for managing chronic health conditions. Low back pain is nearly ubiquitous, and its global disease burden, particularly in high-socioeconomic standard countries, is high.

The youth and longevity business has carved out a niche from the traditional healthcare industry solely concerned with maintaining a high quality of life while managing the aging process. In this chapter, the authors deliver their perspective on the economic decision-making patterns of an aging population, the demographic changes associated with extended lifespans, and the adaptations in retirement planning and utilization of healthcare systems and social welfare programs. Further, the authors reflect on how aging spine patients adjust their behaviors and lifestyles to align with the demands of prolonged lifespans, prompting considerations of the economic consequences of these adjustments. The pursuit of healthy longevity raises questions about productivity, workforce participation, and the financial implications of supporting extended retire-

---

*** Corresponding author Álvaro Dowling:** Orthopaedic Spine Surgeon, Director of Endoscopic Spine Clinic, Santiago, Chile; E-mail: business@tucsonspine.com

ment periods. Healthy longevity refers to empowering individuals to lead longer lives while maintaining optimal physical, mental, and emotional well-being. Achieving healthy longevity entails making choices that significantly impact long-term health outcomes. The authors describe how the otherwise healthy low back pain patient over 50 should adopt a healthy lifestyle, including regular exercise, balanced nutrition, and stress management, to promote healthy aging while enhancing the quality of life during extended lifespans.

Keywords: Aging patients, Financial implications, Healthy longevity, Low back pain, Productivity, Workforce participation.

INTRODUCTION

For as long as human history has been documented, pursuing the fountain of youth has remained a steadfast endeavor driven by the desire to achieve an extended and healthier lifespan [1]. Today, fueled by remarkable advances in medical science and the exponential growth of the rejuvenation industry, this ancient dream is gradually becoming a reality. An astounding transformation in global life expectancy is a testament to the remarkable progress achieved over the past 150 years in healthcare. From a meager 30 years in 1870 (Fig. **1**), the average lifespan has reached 71 years—an unprecedented milestone [2], leaving a significant health-to-life span gap of 9.2 years [3].

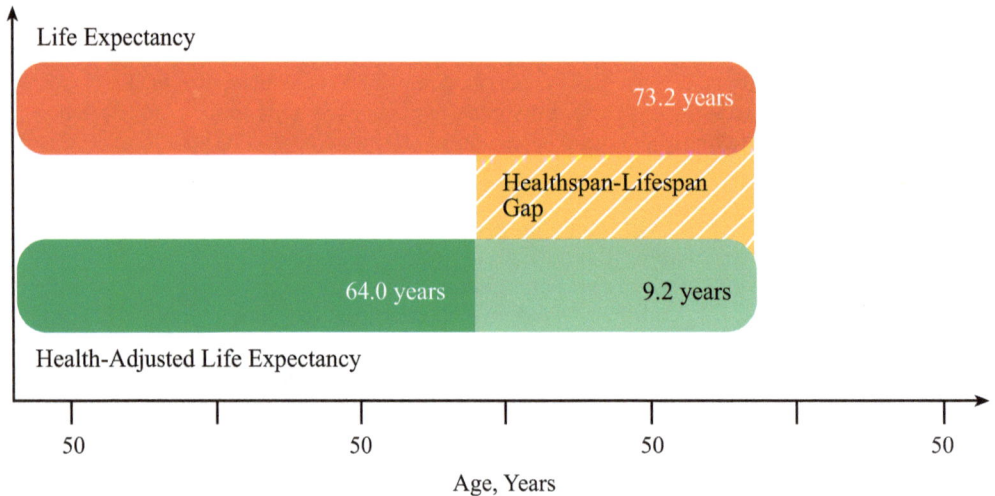

Fig. (1). Illustration of the health span to lifespan gap of 9.2 years [3].

Several considerations regarding longevity and low back pain are of concern [4]. Firstly, the substantial increase in life expectancy necessitates a deeper understanding of the aging process and its implications for economic decision-making. With a population composed of individuals living longer, it becomes imperative to examine the complex dynamics of aging, low back pain, and its associated effects on various economic factors. Demographic shifts, such as an aging workforce and increased retirement periods, call for adaptations in retirement planning, social welfare systems, and healthcare services. Understanding the economic consequences of managing low back pain during a prolonged lifespan should enable patients, their physicians, policymakers, and economists to devise effective strategies that ensure economic stability and sustainability in the face of evolving demographic patterns [5].

Secondly, growing life expectancy raises pressing concerns about the necessary adjustments in behaviors and lifestyle habits to adapt to these long lifespans while preserving a high quality of life despite the burden of degenerative spine disease, which often manifests as low back and neurogenic claudication symptoms. From a practical point of view, it often means that patients need to reassess their choices and habits to navigate the challenges and opportunities presented by healthier longer lives. Associated factors affecting patients' life planning in their later years include financial and career management and healthcare utilization in the context of their overall well-being [1]. Such considerations are essential in enabling individuals to make informed decisions that optimize their well-being throughout their extended lifespans.

The ultimate goal of healthy longevity is to empower individuals to lead longer lives while maintaining optimal physical, mental, and emotional well-being. The key lies in making proactive and sustainable choices that positively impact long-term health outcomes. Engaging in a healthy lifestyle, encompassing regular exercise, a balanced diet, adequate sleep, stress management, and social connectedness, has been repeatedly shown to contribute to healthy aging and high quality of life significantly [1]. These lifestyle choices are fundamental pillars in the pursuit of healthy longevity, providing a robust foundation for individuals to age gracefully and enjoy enhanced well-being [6].

The authors of this chapter have become increasingly aware of a changing outlook in the healthy well-aging patient population and the need to offer treatments commensurate with the patient's goals and functional status. Low back pain is a significant concern for many of the authors' patients over age 50. These types of patients need to be better served by the spine care models running in public health care systems, where image-based criteria are often the foundation of medical necessity criteria for intervention or surgery. Frustrated, they often seek out the private practitioner for help. Hence, the need for a more structured care model for these highly functional patients - a care model that goes beyond the notion that healthy lifestyle choices profoundly impact long-term health outcomes and that regular physical activity has been linked to reduced risks of chronic conditions such as cardiovascular disease, diabetes, and certain cancers.

In this chapter, the authors examine the importance of mental and emotional well-being by highlighting the interplay between psychological health and physical health outcomes. Cultivating practices that foster mental resilience, emotional intelligence, and social support systems contribute to a holistic approach to healthy longevity and are the cornerstone of many business models that revolve around selling the idea of eternal youth.

Commercialization

Investors, entrepreneurs, and established companies have increasingly recognized the vast potential of the longevity market [7]. They actively invest in driving research, development, and commercialization of cutting-edge products and services. The emergent longevity industry is currently at the forefront of efforts to revolutionize healthcare by devising innovative treatments that target aging and aim to extend a healthy lifespan. This industry encompasses diverse sectors, including biotechnology firms, pharmaceutical companies, supplement manufacturers, longevity clinics, and more [8]. The collaborative efforts of these entities are paving the way for groundbreaking advancements in the field.

Moreover, governments and health systems have begun to acknowledge the significance of healthy aging initiatives, acknowledging the opportunity to mitigate the soaring healthcare costs associated with age-related diseases. The impact of the COVID-19 pandemic has further underscored the importance of implementing preventive health measures and addressing the specific vulnerabilities that arise with advancing age. This realization has prompted policymakers and healthcare systems to prioritize initiatives that promote healthy aging and focus on proactive measures to enhance overall well-being in aging populations.

The convergence of investment, entrepreneurial drive, and governmental support signifies a paradigm shift towards prioritizing and harnessing the potential of healthy aging. By fostering collaboration between private and public sectors, we can anticipate accelerated progress in developing effective interventions, therapies, and preventive strategies that address the challenges posed by aging. This concerted effort holds the promise of extending lifespans and ensuring that those extra years are characterized by vitality and well-being.

Strong future growth of the wellness economy has been predicted by the Global Wellness Institute (GWI) with a post-pandemic resurgence, with an average annual growth rate of 9.9%. By 2025, the wellness economy is projected to reach nearly $7.0 trillion [9]. According to the Global Wellness Institute, the wellness economy accounted for 5.1% of global economic output in 2020, underscoring its significant presence and impact. This sector encompasses eleven distinct areas, each contributing to the overall wellness economy (Fig. **2**):

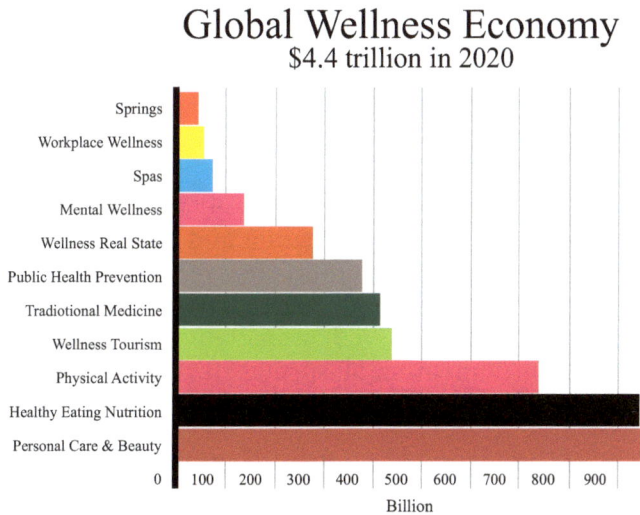

Fig. (2). Graphic illustration of the global wellness economy. Data sourced from the Global Wellness Institute [9].

1. Personal Care & Beauty: Valued at $955 billion, this sector focuses on products and services related to personal grooming and appearance enhancement.

2. Healthy Eating, Nutrition, & Weight Loss: With a value of $946 billion, this sector emphasizes promoting healthy dietary practices, nutrition education, and weight management.

3. Physical Activity: Valued at $738 billion, this sector encompasses various forms of physical exercise, sports, and recreational activities.

4. Wellness Tourism: With a value of $436 billion, wellness tourism involves travel experiences and destinations prioritizing health, relaxation, and well-being.

5. Traditional & Complementary Medicine: This sector, valued at $413 billion, includes practices and therapies beyond conventional medicine, such as herbal remedies, acupuncture, and Ayurveda.

6. Public Health, Prevention, & Personalized Medicine: With a value of $375 billion, this sector promotes public health initiatives, disease prevention, and tailored medical approaches.

7. Wellness Real Estate: Valued at $275 billion, this sector pertains to the development and design of living spaces that prioritize wellness, incorporating features like green buildings, access to nature, and community health amenities.

8. Mental Wellness: With a value of $131 billion, this sector addresses mental health and well-being, encompassing services, therapies, and initiatives that promote emotional balance and psychological well-being.

9. Spas: Valued at $68 billion, the spa industry provides a range of relaxation, beauty, and treatments to enhance physical and mental well-being.

10. Workplace Wellness: With a value of $49 billion, workplace wellness programs aim to improve employee health and well-being through various initiatives, including fitness programs, stress management, and health screenings.

11. Thermal/Mineral Springs: Valued at $39 billion, this sector focuses on utilizing natural thermal and mineral springs for their therapeutic properties, offering opportunities for relaxation and rejuvenation.

These eleven sectors collectively contribute to the growth and dynamism of the wellness economy, shaping a future where well-being and holistic health are central pillars of society and the global economy.

Aging

Aging manifests as a complex process that triggers the progressive functional decline of various tissues and organs. At the molecular, cellular, and physiological levels, aging encompasses many interconnected features, including genome and epigenome alterations, protein homeostasis disruptions, diminished cellular and subcellular functions, and disturbances in immune signaling. As the aging process unfolds, mitochondrial DNA experiences oxidative damage to varying extents, resulting in impaired cellular energy metabolism, cellular dysfunction, and even cell death. The interplay between the antioxidant capacity of mitochondria and age-related changes disrupts physiological cell signaling, compromising cell integrity and hastening aging.

One notable consequence of aging is the emergence of low-grade chronic inflammation, commonly referred to as inflammation. This persistent state of inflammation has been associated with numerous degenerative disorders in human populations. Intriguingly, inflammation induces local tissue inflammation and systemic changes in endocrine, metabolic, and nutritional systems, further exacerbating pro-inflammatory conditions (Fig. **3**).

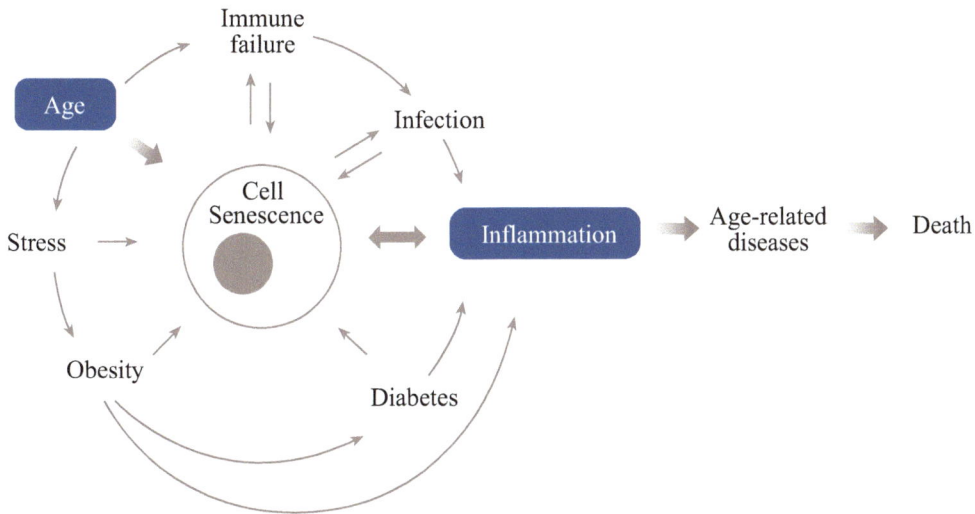

Fig. (3). Graphic illustration of the relationship between aging and inflammation.

Inflammaging assumes a global perspective as it is a common biological denominator underlying a range of seemingly disparate age-related pathologies, including atherosclerosis, cardiovascular diseases, type 2 diabetes, metabolic syndrome, sarcopenia, osteoporosis, cognitive impairment, and frailty [10]. Its role in developing painful disc degeneration, known as degenerative disc disease (DDD), has been particularly emphasized. While localized inflammation within intervertebral disc (IVD) tissue has been extensively investigated in recent years, emerging evidence suggests that systemic inflammation also contributes to DDD (Fig. **4**).

Therefore, interventions targeting the reduction and management of inflammation hold significant promise as powerful tools to modulate and counteract age-related health deterioration, functional decline, and cognitive impairment and ultimately extend the population's lifespan [10]. Researchers and clinicians can unlock novel approaches to enhance overall health and well-being during aging by focusing on strategies that aim to mitigate inflammation.

Degenerative Musculoskeletal Diseases

Degenerative musculoskeletal diseases (DMD), encompassing conditions such as osteoporosis, osteoarthritis, degenerative disc disease, and sarcopenia, pose significant challenges for the aging population. These conditions severely restrict mobility and dexterity, increasing the risk of falls and leading to early retirement, diminished well-being, and reduced social participation. Consequently, they profoundly impact the overall quality of life, causing a significant reduction in well-being [10]. Among these DMDs, intervertebral disc (IVD) degeneration is widely acknowledged as contributing to low back pain. While obesity, genetics, trauma, and sedentary lifestyles have been associated with IVD degeneration, the precise cellular and molecular mechanisms underlying this degeneration are complex and multifactorial.

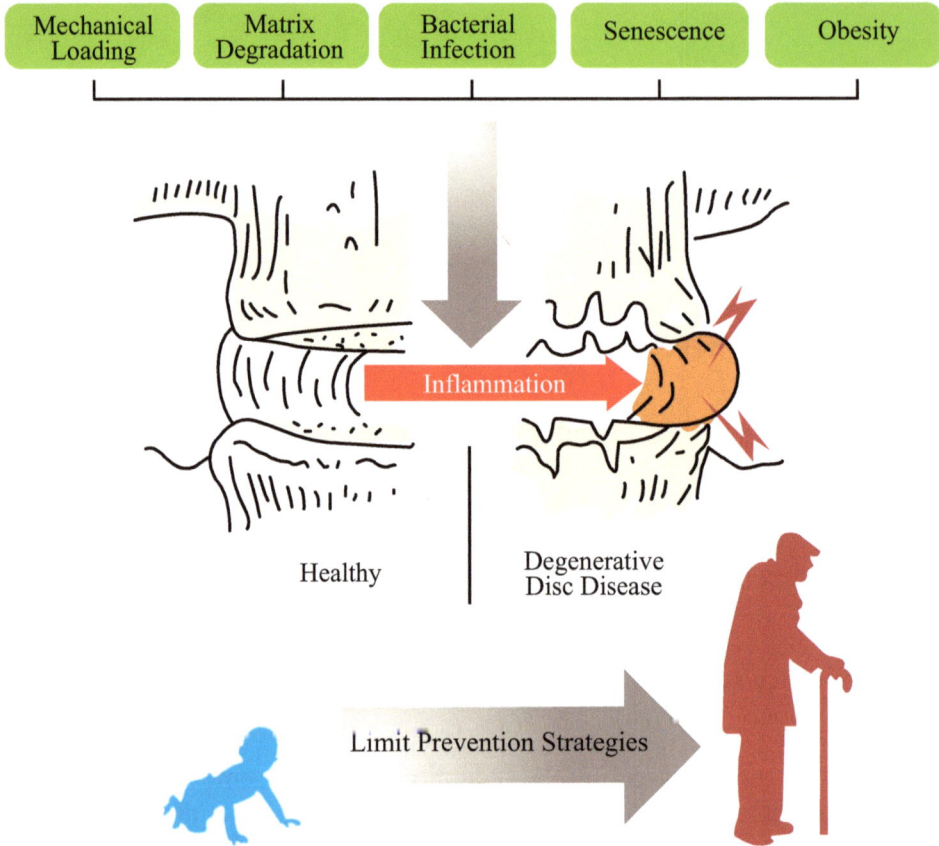

Fig. (4). Graphic illustration of the relationship between localized inflammation within intervertebral disc (IVD) tissue and systemic inflammation which may also contribute to degenerative disc disease.

IVD degeneration is a significant driver of low back pain (LBP), with a lifetime prevalence of 84%. LBP is the primary cause of disability worldwide, affecting most adults at some point in their lives. Since 1990, the number of years lost to disability due to LBP has risen by 54% [11]. Managing low back pain is challenging, as it is often classified as non-specific, with the specific source of pain remaining unidentified. Furthermore, LBP frequently coexists with other medical comorbidities, requiring additional attention and resulting in poorer treatment response. The persistence of low back pain is evident, with approximately two-thirds of patients still experiencing pain after twelve months.

A recent study published in The Lancet highlighted the prevalence of low back pain, one of the most common types of pain reported in healthcare settings drawing upon data from the 2021 Global Burden of Disease Study [12]. In a 2023 Lancet publication, the authors estimated the worldwide prevalence of low back pain between 1990 and 2020 across over 204 countries and territories [13]. The findings revealed that in 2020 alone, low back pain affected a staggering 619 million individuals worldwide, with projections indicating a rise to approximately 843 million by 2050, representing a 36.4% rise. In 2020, the global age-standardized rate of years lived with disability (YLDs) was 832 per 100,000 population, ranging from 578 to 1070. Over the period from 1990 to 2020, there was a decrease in the age-standardized rates of both prevalence and YLDs, amounting to 10.4% (with a range of 10.9 to 10.0) and 10.5% (ranging from 11.1 to 10.0) respectively. Notably, 38.8% (with a range of 28.7 to 47.0) of YLDs were attributed to occupational factors, smoking, and high body mass index (BMI) [13]. The most significant increase is expected in Asia and Africa, primarily driven by population growth. However, aging is anticipated to be the main driver in East Asia, South Asia, Latin America, and the Caribbean. The study, published in The Lancet Rheumatology, is part of the Global Burden of Disease Study 2021. The research highlights that older people face a higher risk as the prevalence of low back pain increases with age, with 85 years being the peak age of impact. The high vulnerability of the elderly population highlights the need for specific clinical guidelines for managing low back pain in this group.

Globally, low back pain accounted for 69 million years lived with disability (YLDs) in 2020, indicating the years spent in suboptimal health. Although there has been a decrease in all-cause YLDs since 1990, low back pain remains the primary driver of YLDs worldwide [13]. The Lancet study identifies several risk factors for low back pain, including smoking, obesity, and occupational ergonomic factors such as repetitive movements and heavy lifting at work [13]. These factors contribute to nearly 40% of the YLDs associated with low back pain. The prevalence of low back pain varies across regions, causes, and age groups. The study analyzes data from 1990 to 2020 in 204 countries and territories. Hungary and the Czech Republic have the highest age-standardized rates of low back pain, while Myanmar and the Maldives have the lowest rates. Population growth and aging are key factors influencing the rankings of different countries in the study [13]. Females exhibited higher global prevalence rates than males across all age groups, with more pronounced differences observed in older age groups, particularly among those over 75 (Fig. **5**). The global age-standardized prevalence rate per 100,000 was also higher in females (9330; 95%

uncertainty interval [UI] 8370–10,500) than in males (5520; 4930–6190). Prevalence and years lived with disability (YLDs) increased with age, reaching peak rates around 85 years. Among all age groups, the 80–84 age group had the highest YLD rate per 100,000 globally (2440; 1470–3490).

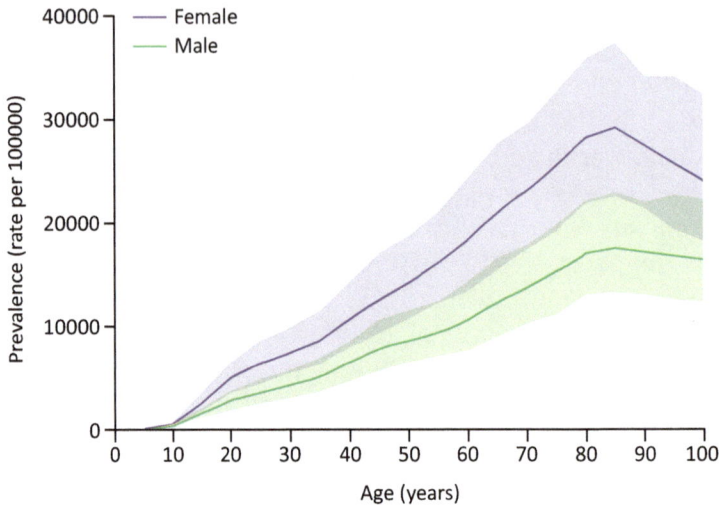

Fig. (5). Global prevalence of low back pain by age and sex in 2020 Shaded areas represent 95% uncertainty intervals. Source: Global Disease Burden Study, 2021.

The study highlights low back pain's enormous societal and economic impact, including productivity loss due to missed workdays and reliance on pain medication and emphasizes the need for public health prevention strategies, particularly for the elderly, and notes that low back pain leads to more people leaving the workforce than any other chronic health condition among working-age populations. Further, research consistently demonstrates a strong correlation between back pain and reduced physical activity [14]. The limitations imposed by back pain often result in a sedentary lifestyle, as individuals avoid movements that exacerbate their discomfort. However, this lack of physical activity can harm overall health, including weight gain, muscle weakness, cardiovascular problems, and an increased risk of chronic conditions such as diabetes and heart disease [14]. Addressing the challenges associated with DMDs and low back pain requires comprehensive approaches that encompass early detection, effective treatment strategies, and a focus on promoting physical activity and overall well-being. By prioritizing research, prevention, and targeted interventions, we can strive to alleviate the burden imposed by these conditions and enhance the quality of life for individuals affected.

Precision Medicine

The emerging paradigm of precision medicine holds immense potential to revolutionize healthcare by customizing interventions to individual needs, ultimately leading to improved patient outcomes and optimized resource utilization. This transformative approach aims to provide more accurate diagnoses, effective treatments, and targeted preventive strategies, resulting in enhanced health outcomes and a higher quality of life for individuals. In low back pain, advancements in diagnostic tools are being harnessed to identify underlying causes and contributing factors, thereby guiding appropriate treatment and prevention strategies. Significant progress has been made in diagnostic imaging technologies, such as magnetic resonance imaging (MRI) [15 - 20], positron emission tomography (PET) [21], and computed tomography (CT) [22]. These state-of-the-art imaging modalities have undergone significant advancements in resolution and diagnostic capabilities. By offering detailed anatomical and functional information, they play a pivotal role in detecting, staging, and following various diseases and conditions.

By leveraging these advanced diagnostic tools, individuals can adopt a proactive approach to their health. Armed with comprehensive information, they can make informed decisions and embrace preventive strategies to maintain optimal wellness and reduce the risk of developing certain diseases or conditions. Precision medicine empowers individuals to understand their unique health profiles and tailor interventions accordingly, promoting early detection, personalized treatment plans, and targeted preventive measures. This individualized approach to healthcare has far-reaching implications [23]. It enables healthcare providers to optimize treatment outcomes by tailoring interventions to each patient's needs, reducing the risk of adverse effects and minimizing healthcare costs associated with trial-and-error approaches [23]. Additionally, precision medicine supports proactive health management, shifting the focus from reactive care to preventive strategies. By identifying risk factors, genetic predispositions, and early disease indicators, interventions can be initiated before symptoms manifest, potentially mitigating the impact of diseases and improving long-term health outcomes.

Precision medicine in pain management and spine care holds the promise for developing novel therapeutics and interventions thereby decreasing the need for opioids. By understanding the intricate molecular and genetic mechanisms underlying pain syndromes, clinicians involved in interventional and surgical pain management can identify specific targets for intervention and design tailored treatments of pain generators that are more effective and potentially less invasive and costly (Fig. **6**).

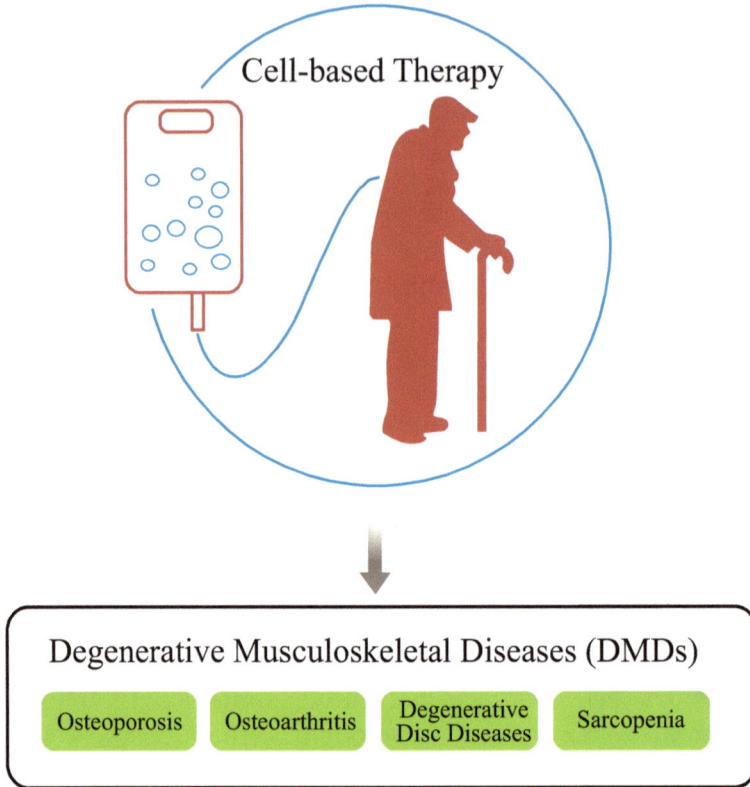

Fig. (6). Graphic illustration of the four disease groups – osteoporosis, osteoarthritis, degenerative disc disease, and sarcopenia that contribute to disease burden in the elderly and the most likely to respond to cell-based anti-aging treatment cards.

Targeted Care Models

As precision medicine continues to evolve, it has the potential to revolutionize healthcare systems, enhancing patient care and fostering a more personalized and proactive approach to well-being. The latter is relevant to aging but a healthy patient who is held back by low back pain-related problems that ultimately impact the physical and emotional outlook on life. By integrating advanced diagnostic tools, genetic profiling, and targeted interventions, targeted precision medicine represents a significant stride toward improving healthcare outcomes and promoting individualized wellness. Many of the chapters are on novel targeted care models based on the improved understanding of the molecular and genetic mechanism of painful conditions affecting the musculoskeletal system and the spine in particular. Patients will increasingly gravitate towards practitioners who address their individual concerns and offer alternatives to the stalemate frequently playing out in public health care systems where red tape and bureaucracy are directing care employing population-based health care models. These systems will likely prove unsustainable because of constant cost overruns, and rationing – nowadays already seen in many healthcare systems - would be the only way to control cost [24 - 26]. Here lies the opportunity for those businesses to address the increasingly unmet needs of patients left without help by the traditional care models (Fig. **7**).

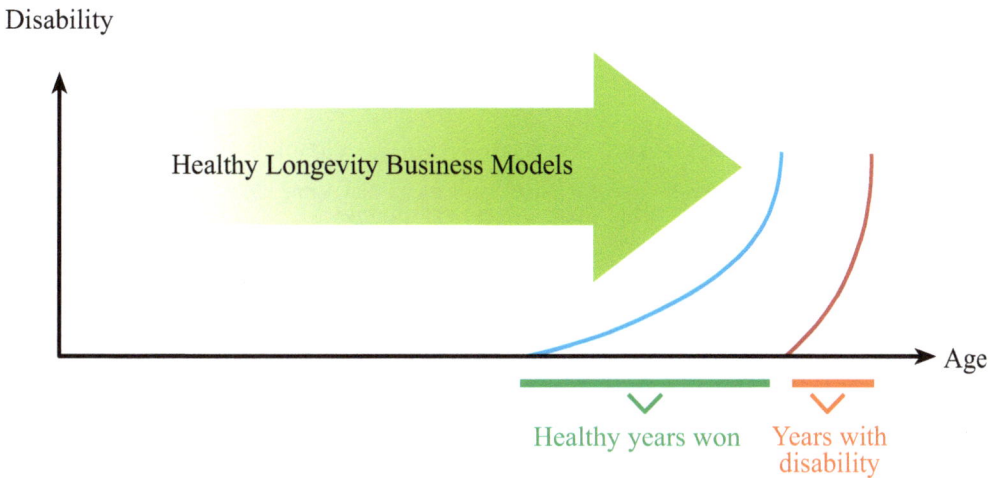

Disability

Healthy Longevity Business Models

Age

Healthy years won   Years with disability

Fig. (7). Graphic illustration of longevity business model aimed at increasing the lifespan in good health.

CONCLUSION

The health longevity market is expected to grow as the world's population ages, and people continue to adopt healthy lifestyles to promote longevity. This includes regular exercise, stress management techniques, sleep optimization, and healthy eating. The marketplace offers various services, products, and experiences intended to support these lifestyle choices. As the quest for eternal youth continues, it is essential to maintain a realistic perspective and focus on promoting healthy lifestyles, preventative care, and advances in medical science. These approaches can significantly improve the quality of life, extend healthy years, and support the overall goal of aging gracefully and maintaining well-being as we age. The intersection of regenerative medicine, stem cells, and intervertebral disc regeneration presents a unique opportunity to promote healthy longevity. By harnessing the regenerative potential of stem cells, clinician-researchers are paving the way for innovative therapies that can restore damaged intervertebral discs, relieve back pain, and improve mobility. The potential preventative effects of these therapies offer the potential to maintain spinal health as people age, contributing to a longer, healthier life with a better quality of life.

REFERENCES

[1]   Woods Ba Biol Mba T, Manson Brown S, Page B. Living longer better. Plast Reconstr Surg 2021; 148(6S): 7S-13S.
        [http://dx.doi.org/10.1097/PRS.0000000000008780] [PMID: 34847092]

[2]   Scott AJ. The longevity society. Lancet Healthy Longev 2021; 2(12): e820-7.
        [http://dx.doi.org/10.1016/S2666-7568(21)00247-6] [PMID: 36098038]

[3]   Garmany A, Yamada S, Terzic A. Longevity leap: mind the healthspan gap. NPJ Regen Med 2021; 6(1): 57.
        [http://dx.doi.org/10.1038/s41536-021-00169-5] [PMID: 34556664]

[4]   Khullar D, Fisher J, Chandra A. Trickle-down innovation and the longevity of nations. Lancet 2019; 393(10187): 2272-4.
        [http://dx.doi.org/10.1016/S0140-6736(19)30345-9] [PMID: 31060799]

[5]   Scott AJ. Achieving a three-dimensional longevity dividend. Nat Aging 2021; 1(6): 500-5.
        [http://dx.doi.org/10.1038/s43587-021-00074-y] [PMID: 37117832]

[6]   Tziraki-Segal C, De Luca V, Santana S, *et al.* Creating a Culture of Health in Planning and Implementing Innovative Strategies Addressing Non-communicable Chronic Diseases. Front Sociol 2019; 4: 9.
        [http://dx.doi.org/10.3389/fsoc.2019.00009] [PMID: 33869336]

[7]   de Magalhães JP, Stevens M, Thornton D. The Business of Anti-Aging Science. Trends Biotechnol 2017; 35(11): 1062-73.
        [http://dx.doi.org/10.1016/j.tibtech.2017.07.004] [PMID: 28778607]

[8]   Scott AJ. The longevity economy. Lancet Healthy Longev 2021; 2(12): e828-35.
        [http://dx.doi.org/10.1016/S2666-7568(21)00250-6] [PMID: 36098039]

[9]   WELLNESS ECONOMY STATISTICS and FACTS: The Global Wellness Institute; 2023 [Available from: https://globalwellnessinstituteorg/press-room/statistics-and-facts/ 2023.

[10]   Lv X, Li W, Ma Y, *et al.* Cognitive decline and mortality among community-dwelling Chinese older people. BMC Med 2019; 17(1): 63.
        [http://dx.doi.org/10.1186/s12916-019-1295-8] [PMID: 30871536]

[11]   Wu PH, Kim HS, Jang IT. Intervertebral Disc Diseases PART 2: A Review of the Current Diagnostic and Treatment Strategies for Intervertebral Disc Disease. Int J Mol Sci 2020; 21(6): 2135.
        [http://dx.doi.org/10.3390/ijms21062135] [PMID: 32244936]

[12]   Vos T, Lim SS, Abbafati C, *et al.* Global burden of 369 diseases and injuries in 204 countries and territories, 1990–2019: a systematic analysis for the Global Burden of Disease Study 2019. Lancet 2020; 396(10258): 1204-22.
        [http://dx.doi.org/10.1016/S0140-6736(20)30925-9] [PMID: 33069326]

[13]   Ferreira ML, de Luca K, Haile LM, *et al.* Global, regional, and national burden of low back pain, 1990–2020, its attributable risk factors, and projections to 2050: a systematic analysis of the Global Burden of Disease Study 2021. Lancet Rheumatol 2023; 5(6): e316-29.
        [http://dx.doi.org/10.1016/S2665-9913(23)00098-X] [PMID: 37273833]

[14]   Min S, Masanovic B, Bu T, *et al.* The Association Between Regular Physical Exercise, Sleep Patterns, Fasting, and Autophagy for Healthy Longevity and Well-Being: A Narrative Review. Front Psychol 2021; 12803421
        [http://dx.doi.org/10.3389/fpsyg.2021.803421] [PMID: 34925198]

[15]   Lewandrowski KU, Yeung A, Lorio MP, *et al.* Personalized Interventional Surgery of the Lumbar Spine: A Perspective on Minimally Invasive and Neuroendoscopic Decompression for Spinal Stenosis. J Pers Med 2023; 13(5): 710.
        [http://dx.doi.org/10.3390/jpm13050710] [PMID: 37240880]

[16]   Lewandrowski KU, Abraham I, Ramírez León JF, *et al.* A Proposed Personalized Spine Care Protocol (SpineScreen) to Treat Visualized Pain Generators: An Illustrative Study Comparing Clinical Outcomes and Postoperative Reoperations between Targeted Endoscopic Lumbar Decompression Surgery, Minimally Invasive TLIF and Open Laminectomy. J Pers Med 2022; 12(7): 1065.
[http://dx.doi.org/10.3390/jpm12071065] [PMID: 35887562]

[17]   Lewandrowski KU, Muraleedharan N, Eddy SA, *et al.* Reliability Analysis of Deep Learning Algorithms for Reporting of Routine Lumbar MRI Scans. Int J Spine Surg 2020; 14(s3): S98-S107.
[http://dx.doi.org/10.14444/7131] [PMID: 33122182]

[18]   Lewandrowski KU, Muraleedharan N, Eddy SA, *et al.* Artificial Intelligence Comparison of the Radiologist Report With Endoscopic Predictors of Successful Transforaminal Decompression for Painful Conditions of the Lumber Spine: Application of Deep Learning Algorithm Interpretation of Routine Lumbar Magnetic Resonance Imaging Scan. Int J Spine Surg 2020; 14(s3): S75-85.
[http://dx.doi.org/10.14444/7130] [PMID: 33208388]

[19]   LewandrowskI KU, Muraleedharan N, Eddy SA, *et al.* Feasibility of Deep Learning Algorithms for Reporting in Routine Spine Magnetic Resonance Imaging. Int J Spine Surg 2020; 14(s3): S86-97.
[http://dx.doi.org/10.14444/7131] [PMID: 33298549]

[20]   Lewandrowski KU. Retrospective analysis of accuracy and positive predictive value of preoperative lumbar MRI grading after successful outcome following outpatient endoscopic decompression for lumbar foraminal and lateral recess stenosis. Clin Neurol Neurosurg 2019; 179: 74-80.
[http://dx.doi.org/10.1016/j.clineuro.2019.02.019] [PMID: 30870712]

[21]   Nusbaum F, Redouté J, Le Bars D, *et al.* Chronic low-back pain modulation is enhanced by hypnotic analgesic suggestion by recruiting an emotional network: a PET imaging study. Int J Clin Exp Hypn 2010; 59(1): 27-44.
[http://dx.doi.org/10.1080/00207144.2011.522874] [PMID: 21104483]

[22]   Ly DP. Evaluation and treatment patterns of new low back pain episodes for elderly adults in the United States, 2011-2014. Med Care 2020; 58(2): 108-13.
[http://dx.doi.org/10.1097/MLR.0000000000001244] [PMID: 31934957]

[23]   Deutsch JE, Gill-Body KM, Schenkman M. Updated Integrated Framework for Making Clinical Decisions Across the Lifespan and Health Conditions. Phys Ther 2022; 102(3)pzab281
[http://dx.doi.org/10.1093/ptj/pzab281] [PMID: 35079823]

[24]   Cheng L, Liu H, Zhang Y, Shen K, Zeng Y. The impact of health insurance on health outcomes and spending of the elderly: evidence from China's New Cooperative Medical Scheme. Health Econ 2015; 24(6): 672-91.
[http://dx.doi.org/10.1002/hec.3053] [PMID: 24777657]

[25]   Dragos SL, Mare C, Dragos CM, Muresan GM, Purcel AA. Does voluntary health insurance improve health and longevity? Evidence from European OECD countries. Eur J Health Econ 2022; 23(8): 1397-411.
[http://dx.doi.org/10.1007/s10198-022-01439-9] [PMID: 35124741]

[26]   Zhang Z, Dong S, Zhang X. Effects of government cash subsidies on health risk behaviors of the rural elderly: Evidence from social pension expansions in China. Tob Induc Dis 2021; 19(March): 1-9.
[http://dx.doi.org/10.18332/tid/132859] [PMID: 33679283]

CHAPTER 2

Current Concepts and Limits of Cell-Based Regeneration Strategies for Degenerative Disc Disease

Alvaro Dowling[1], Marcelo Molina[2], William Omar Contreras López[3,*], Morgan P. Lorio[4], Stefan Landgraeber[5], Jorge Felipe Ramírez León[6,7,8] and Kai-Uwe Lewandrowski[9,10,11]

[1] *Orthopaedic Spine Surgeon, Director of Endoscopic Spine Clinic, Santiago, Chile*

[2] *Orthopaedic Spine Surgeon, Clínica Las Condes, Instituto Traumatologico, Santiago, Chile*

[3] *Clínica Foscal Internacional, Autopista Floridablanca - Girón, Km 7, Floridablanca, Santander, Colombia*

[4] *Advanced Orthopedics, 499 East Central Parkway, Altamonte Springs, FL 32701, USA*

[5] *Universitätsdes Saarlandes, Klinik für Neurochirurgie, Kirrberger Straße 100, 66421 Homburg, Germany*

[6] *Minimally Invasive Spine Center. Bogotá, D.C., Colombia*

[7] *Reina Sofía Clinic. Bogotá, D.C., Colombia*

[8] *Fundación Universitaria Sanitas. Bogotá, D.C., Colombia*

[9] *Center for Advanced Spine Care of Southern Arizona and Surgical Institute of Tucson, Tucson, AZ, USA*

[10] *Departmemt of Orthopaedics, Fundación Universitaria Sanitas, Bogotá, D.C., Colombia*

[11] *Department of Neurosurgery in the Video-Endoscopic Postgraduate Program at the Universidade Federal do Estado do Rio de Janeiro - UNIRIO, Rio de Janeiro, Brazil*

Abstract: Degenerative disc disease stands as the predominant etiological factor behind low back pain. In recent years, the therapeutic modality of mesenchymal stem cell (MSC) infusion directly into the nucleus pulposus of the deteriorating disc has gained prominence. The intricacies of the intervertebral disc, a biomechanically robust tissue, span its components - the annulus fibrosus, nucleus pulposus, and cartilaginous endplates. Compromising the integrity of these elements can precipitate advanced disc degeneration due to biomechanical disruption. Animal models have demonstrated the therapeutic potential of MSCs. Particularly, adipose-derived stem cells (ASCs), a subset of MSCs originating from adipose tissue, possess attributes akin to their bone marrow-derived counterparts, metamorphosing into mesodermal structures, encompassing bone, cartilage, muscle, and fat. Their abundance in the human system,

* **Corresponding author William Omar Contreras López:** Clínica Foscal Internacional, Autopista Floridablanca - Girón, Km 7, Floridablanca, Santander, Colombia; Tel: +573112957003; E-mail: wyllcon@gmail.com

coupled with minimally invasive extraction methods, makes them appealing for regenerative medicine applications. A comprehensive literature assessment presented in this chapter delineates the therapeutic paradigm of MSCs in addressing degenerative disc disease (DDD) pain. To date, research predominantly centered on the nucleus pulposus, while neglecting the annulus fibrosus and cartilaginous endplates. Notably, clinical manifestations like annular ruptures, Modic alterations, or Schmorl's nodal formations typically hint at pathologies within these overlooked structures. The prospects of successful regenerative interventions within the annulus, endplates, or nucleus pulposus remain controversial, considering the hostile, nutrient-deprived milieu of the deteriorating intervertebral disc often culminating in the swift demise of the introduced MSCs. Singularly targeting the compromised nucleus pulposus *via* existing MSC-centric regenerative modalities may not achieve disc restoration. Therefore, MSC-based theurapeutic strategies should not just include the nucleus pulposus but also the affected annulus fibrosus and cartilaginous endplates.

Keywords: Intervertebral disc degeneration, Low back pain, Mesenchymal stem cells, Nucleus pulposus, Regenerative medicine.

INTRODUCTION

Low back pain, which plagues nearly 40% of the global populace, stands as a primary driver of muskuloskeletal disability [1]. This affliction predominantly stems from degenerative disc disease (DDD), an insidious condition marked by the degradation of the extracellular matrix and the decline in cellular viability, especially within the nucleus pulposus [2]. As a potential countermeasure, the *In vivo* reintroduction of live cells into the nucleus pulposus, sourced either from the patient or external donors, is gaining traction as a viable avenue for disc regeneration [3]. The spectrum of cellular candidates under investigation for therapeutic interventions in disc degeneration includes notochordal cells, nucleus pulposus cells, annulus fibrosus cells, chondrocytes, mesenchymal stem cells (MSCs), embryonic stem cells, and induced pluripotent stem cells, among others [4 - 18]. Of particular interest are the MSCs, residing in assorted stem tissues. These cells encapsulate a diverse cohort comprising pluripotent stem cells, progenitors, and mature cells [20]. Their prolific origin, coupled with their innate potential for self-renewal and versatile differentiation, has elevated MSCs as a favored contender for revitalizing the intervertebral disc *via* transplantation. Contemporary clinical explorations have elucidated the utility of MSCs, either autonomously or synergistically with biomaterial frameworks, to rejuvenate compromised discs [2, 3]. While these strides are commendable, the MSC-therapies are not covered by most health insurance carriers.

Normal Structures and Natural Healing

The annulus fibrosus (AF) repair mechanism is hampered, in part, due to the scant cell populations' struggle to metabolize and renew extensive collagen fiber aggregations, an obstacle further exacerbated by a constricted vascular supply [19]. The sophisticated constitution of the AF poses considerable obstacles to tissue regeneration endeavors [20]. Contemporary knowledge offers a modest understanding of the AF's foundational cellular biology, notably concerning the origins and functional capacities of specific cell clusters, and their phenotypic transformations post-trauma or in disease states. The viability of regenerative modalities that can surmount the demanding mechanical stresses and austere intra-disc milieu to realize effective AF regeneration remains unanswered [21].

Architecturally, the AF is layered into 15-25 concentric laminae, with slanting collagen fibers organized parallelly within each lamina. These fibers' angle-ply orientation (θ) diminishes progressively from $\pm$ 62° to $\pm$ 45° relative to the vertical axis, transitioning from the disc's periphery towards its center [22]. Glycosaminoglycan proportions amplify from 3% to 8% per wet weight as one traverses from the AF's external to internal sectors, concurrent with a declining type I to type II collagen ratio. The inner AF predominantly hosts spherical fibrocartilaginous cells, while its exterior is rich in elongated fibroblast-resembling cells. The AF environment also nurtures diverse cell types, including peripheral, interlamellar, and stem/progenitor cells.

The cartilaginous endplate, a svelte hyaline cartilage layer, bears resemblances with articular cartilage. Despite comprehensive studies on articular cartilage restoration, the nuances of endplate repair remain comparatively less explored [22]. Past endeavors in cartilage regeneration often culminated in the emergence of fibrocartilage as opposed to reinstating the native collagen lattice, resulting in functional inadequacy. Consequently, the rejuvenation of pristine cartilaginous endplate structures becomes paramount in addressing back pain and preserving disc nutrient supply. However, the poorly understood mechanisms of endplate restoration, compounded by gaps in comprehension regarding its cellular biology and biomechanics, have stymied the formulation of efficacious therapeutic approaches targeting cartilaginous endplates in the context of low back pain.

Normal Structure of the Intervertebral Disc

The IVD is a fibrocartilage structure that connects the vertebral bodies, contributing to spine mobility and acting as a shock absorber. It consists of three main structures: the nucleus pulposus (NP), the annulus fibrosus (AF), and the cartilaginous endplates (CEPs). The NP, located at the core of the IVD, contains NP stem/progenitor cells, notochordal cells, chondrocyte-like cells, water, and extracellular matrix (ECM) [23]. The ECM of NP comprises proteoglycans and collagen type II, providing hydration and pressure resistance. The AF surrounds the NP and primarily comprises collagen type I arranged concentrically. It has inner and outer regions, with the inner AF containing more collagen type II and proteoglycans, while the outer AF predominates collagen type I [10]. The CEPs, avascular organs, border the vertebral bodies and facilitate nutrient supply through diffusion.

The nucleus pulposus (NP) serves as the central component of the intervertebral disc (IVD) structure. It consists of various cell types, including NP stem/progenitor cells (NPPCs), notochordal cells, chondrocyte-like cells, water, and extracellular matrix (ECM) [24, 25]. The ECM of the NP is primarily composed of proteoglycans and collagen type II, with proteoglycans attracting water and contributing to the high hydration level of the NP. This hydrated state enables the NP to withstand the pressure exerted on the spinal structure and fulfill its role in resisting compression [25, 26].

Surrounding the NP is the annulus fibrosus (AF), with cartilaginous endplates (CEPs) bordering the vertebral bodies on the outer side [23, 26, 27]. The AF predominantly consists of concentrically arranged collagen type I [25, 26]. It can be divided into two parts: the inner AF, adjacent to the NP, which contains a higher proportion of collagen type II and proteoglycans, and the outer AF, where collagen type I is more predominant [23, 28]. Compared to the NP, the AF contains less collagen type II. The CEPs, the other hand, are avascular structures with a network of capillaries in the center, which facilitates vascularization of the vertebral bodies [24]. The CEPs serve as a gateway for nutritional supply through a diffusion mechanism [28].

Pathophysiology

The onset of this degenerative cascade is marked by the calcification of the cartilage endplate (CEP) coupled with the attrition of notochordal cells in the IVD [29]. Such calcification impairs the diffusion process, hindering the transport of oxygen and vital nutrients to the IVD [30, 31]. This disruption catalyzes an upsurge in lactic acid concentration, inducing an acidic milieu within the IVD. This acidic ambience not only undermines nutrient supply but also instigates cellular apoptosis, accelerating the degeneration process [26, 32]. Subsequently, there is a downtrend in the extracellular matrix (ECM) synthesis, whereas matrix metalloproteinases (MMPs) – the catalysts of ECM catabolism – either maintain their activity or intensify [31]. Proinflammatory agents, namely interleukin (IL) and tumor necrosis factor (TNF)-α, amplify this catabolic drive. They inhibit proteoglycan and collagen synthesis, accentuate MMP operations, and incite inflammation. The collaborative effects of TNF-α, IL, and nerve fibers play a pivotal role in pain genesis associated with IVD degeneration. As degeneration progresses, the IVD's sensory innervation increases, encompassing the CEPs, which is believed to be influenced by the release of neurotrophic factors by deteriorating IVD cells and vascular tissues, thereby intensifying the pathophysiological pain response [31, 33, 34].

Both physiologically aged and pathologically compromised intervertebral discs manifest diminished signal intensity in T2-weighted magnetic resonance imaging, leading to the appearance of "black discs" [19]. Disc degeneration due to aging arises from diminished nucleus pulposus cellular activity or numbers, subsequently causing a reduction in ECM, especially proteoglycans, synthesis [19]. Contrastingly, painful degenerative discs are typified by structural breaches and the emergence of vascularized granulation tissue, which originates from annulus fibrosus tears or flawed endplates, permeating into the nucleus pulposus, paired with pronounced nociceptive innervation [35, 36]. Any breach, be it in the annulus fibrosus or endplate, instantaneously modifies the disc's biomechanical dynamics, inducing nucleus pulposus decompression and magnified annulus fibrosus strain [19]. Animal degeneration models have underscored that disruptions in the annulus or endplate invariably precipitate degenerative transformations throughout the disc [37]. As degeneration ensues, the nucleus pulposus contracts and its intrinsic hydrostatic pressure diminishes, shifting a higher mechanical burden onto the annulus fibrosus [19]. In such a biomechanical context, reparative strategies at the cellular level within the annulus fibrosus or nucleus pulposus are rendered impractical, not due to cellular inadequacies but owing to the transformed local biomechanical millieu.

Mesenchymal Stem Cells

Stem cells are classified into several categories, notably embryonic, fetal, adult, and induced pluripotent stem cells [38]. Among this spectrum, MSCs stand out, drawing substantial global research interest. These cells are a subset of adult stem cells [39], offering both ethical advantages and genomic stability [40]. Impressively, MSCs boast the capacity to metamorphose into diverse connective tissue cell types [38, 39]. Their versatility has been harnessed in fields like wound repair, dermatological restoration, hair rejuvenation, sweat gland recuperation, corneal regeneration, and neural differentiation, leveraging their ectodermal differentiation prowess [39, 41]. Under tailored *In vitro* settings, MSCs can differentiate into mesodermal, ectodermal, and endodermal lineages. Their transition to mesodermal tissues, for instance, adipocytes, osteoblasts, and chondrocytes, is intuitive given their shared embryological roots [42]. Additionally, through meticulously crafted protocols, MSCs can be guided to evolve into endodermal tissues, inclusive of hepatic and pancreatic varieties [43].

Adipose-Derived Stem Cells

Adipose-derived stem cells (ASCs) necessitate precise classification, ensuring they are differentiated from progenitor cells and other stem cell variants. Whereas progenitor cells are demarcated by their finite proliferative capacity and specialization into distinct cell entities, stem cells are characterized by their intrinsic capability for self-regeneration and aptitude to differentiate across a more extensive cellular spectrum, emphasizing their multipotency [45]. Within this cellular continuum, MSCs, encapsulating ASCs, are a subset of multipotent cells endowed with the versatility to metamorphose into adipocytes, osteoblasts, and chondrocytes [46]. ASCs, with their origins rooted in adipose compartments [44, 46], have garnered significant interest for their potential therapeutic interventions, predominantly within musculoskeletal pathologies. These cells, reminiscent of their stem cell counterparts, are endowed with the ability for robust proliferation and expansive differentiation.

A notable distinction of ASCs vis-à-vis MSCs from alternative provenances is the copiousness of their origin coupled with a diminutive associated risk [47 - 49]. Adipose matrices, ubiquitously distributed across human anatomy, become facile sources. The therapeutic efficacy of surgically procured subcutaneous adipose tissue, upon transplantation to lesioned locales, has been empirically affirmed [50, 51]. Such tissues stand as fecund repositories of multipotent stemmatic entities [52]. Anatomically, the human system predominantly delineates its adipose repositories into two quintessential types: the brown and white adipose tissues [53, 54].

The Difference between White and Brown Adipose Tissue

Adipose tissue, comprising approximately 20-30% of the body constitution in typical individuals, presents a multifaceted distribution pattern contingent on factors like body mass index, gender, and muscular composition. The adipose tissue proportion can escalate in obesity, culminating in detrimental health outcomes [51]. Notwithstanding these negative aspects, adipose tissue has been earmarked as a promising reservoir for adipose-derived stem cells (ASCs). These cells offer a more favorable and minimally invasive alternative to bone marrow-derived mesenchymal stem cells (BMSCs) [46, 48]. Adipose tissue is woven with brown and white adipose fibers, each manifesting unique characteristics and functions [53 - 55].

White adipocytes, or white fat cells, stand in contrast to their brown counterparts. Brown adipocytes are typified by their multilocular structure, minuscule lipid vesicles, and pronounced oxygen dependency, as evidenced by their rich vascular networks [56]. Predominantly localized in areas like the neck, mediastinum, and interscapular spaces, brown fat is ubiquitous in neonates but wanes with advancing age [51]. Its characteristic ruddy hue is attributed to a high mitochondrial count and iron concentration. Moreover, brown fat is punctuated with an intricate web of unmyelinated nerves, facilitating sympathetic stimulation to the adipocytes [54, 55].

Acting as a thermogenic dynamo, brown adipose tissue is instrumental in energy expenditure, forestalling obesity. The thermogenic prowess originates from its mitochondrial content [54, 55]. The thermogenic pathway within brown adipose tissue entails glucose and fat oxidation, engendering heat, under the aegis of uncoupling protein (UCP) 1. This mitochondrial protein disrupts adenosine triphosphate generation during oxidative phosphorylation by modulating the mitochondrial membrane gradient [56]. UCP1, exclusive to brown adipose tissue, is subject to adrenergic modulation *via* its sympathetic nexus, orchestrating thermogenesis [51, 55].

Conversely, white adipocytes, characterized by their unilocular morphology and expansive lipid vacuoles, punctuate the subcutaneous and visceral terrains, exuding a pale yellow hue [56]. Dubbed the "maligned fat," white adipose tissue can skew metabolism, symbolizing an overindulgence in caloric assimilation. In stark contrast to the UCP1-laden brown adipose tissue, white fat predominantly expresses the UCP2 isoform [56]. Its metabolism involves lipolysis, transmuting triglycerides into free fatty acids. Overbearing white adipose tissue and rampant lipolysis can set the stage for insulin unresponsiveness [51]. Recent scientific discoveries have highlighted the existence of beige adipocytes nestled within the white adipose milieu, especially in regions like the inguinal area [56]. Beige adipocytes, while bearing semblance to white fat cells in energy storage, resonate with brown fat cells' thermogenic capabilities [57].

Harvesting

Intriguingly, ASCs sourced from white adipose tissue exhibit distinct characteristics compared to their counterparts from brown adipose tissue [56]. Furthermore, the anatomical origin of these cells introduces subtle variations. Yet, the viability of cells derived from subcutaneous fat remains consistent across diverse anatomical locales [58]. The extraction methodology is commendably non-invasive and ensures a prolific yield of stromal and stem cells. The abundant reservoir of abdominal fat emerges as the preeminent source of adipose tissue [47,

48]. There are two avenues for adipose tissue retrieval: as a solid mass or as a lipoaspirate. While surgical resection is employed to acquire solid adipose tissue, techniques such as power-assisted liposuction (PAL) and laser-assisted liposuction (LAL) are preferred for obtaining lipoaspirates [59]. Lipoaspiration presents a facile means to access subcutaneous deposits. Remarkably, the choice of liposuction modality remains inconsequential to the functional integrity of ASCs. However, PAL is especially preferred for its therapeutic efficacy, given its augmented cellular proliferation capabilities and diminished cellular degradation [58].

A range of enzymatic agents, spanning collagenase, dispase, trypsin, and more, are deployed for the meticulous digestion of segmented adipose tissue. Nonetheless, the medical community awaits the establishment of a gold-standard protocol [45]. Recommended parameters for digestion encompass a consistent 37°C temperature, a variable digestion duration ranging from 30 minutes to beyond an hour, and specific tissue mass-to-volume ratios [45, 58]. Protease concentrations exhibit considerable heterogeneity across protocols. Once isolated, ASCs are typically cultivated in monolayer configurations on conventional tissue culture dishes, nurtured by a basal medium fortified with 10% fetal bovine serum. An aspirated adipose sample, on average, furnishes an impressive yield of approximately 3.5×10^5 to 1×10^6 ASCs for every gram [60].

Stem Cell Formation and Identification

In the regenerative milieu, ASCs, a subset of stem cells, exemplify their prowess by augmenting tissue wound repair, primarily *via* endothelial differentiation and the amplification of Vascular Endothelial Growth Factor (VEGF). Mesenchymal stem cells (MSCs), contingent upon environmental and physiological cues, harbor the potential to embark upon diverse differentiation trajectories, encompassing osteogenesis, chondrogenesis, myogenesis, marrow stroma, tendogenesis, lipogenesis, and beyond. Within the adipose paradigm, MSCs exhibit plasticity, differentiating into endothelial cells, smooth myocytes, and both white and brown adipocytes. This process ensues from adipoblasts metamorphosing into preadipocytes, culminating in mature adipocytes. The fate of MSC differentiation into either brown or white adipose variants hinges on the inherent stem cell precursors, particularly the dichotomy of Myf5-positive and Myf5-negative cellular entities.

Clinical research is increasingly interested in secretome derived from ASCs, specifically the purified exosomes, having potential in regenerative therapeutics. A secretome is a mosaic of microvesicles and exosomes laden with a spectrum of biologically dynamic proteins, lipids, and nucleic constituents. While a codified modus operandi for ASC secretome production remains elusive, the virtues of exosomes, such as resilience, uncomplicated storage dynamics, cost-effectiveness, and attenuated immunological rejection propensity post-transplantation, are indisputable. Proteomic explorations primarily decode the secretomic blueprint of ASCs, though the ramifications of ASC procurement and propagation on the secretome's constitution warrant more profound insights [58].

To authenticate ASC attributes, flow cytometric scrutinization of cellular surface markers remains the gold standard. The International Society for Cellular Therapy (ISCT) in tandem with the International Federation for Adipose Therapeutics and Science (IFATS) have delineated a triad of quintessential criteria for ASCs: propensity for plastic adherence, the expression manifold encompassing CD73, CD90, and CD105—simultaneously eschewing markers like CD14, CD11b, CD45, CD19, CD79, and HLA-DR—and the intrinsic capacity to differentiate into preadipocytes, chondrocytes, or osteoblasts. Nuanced markers such as CD36 (GPIIIb) and CD106 (VCAM-1) further demarcate ASCs from their bone marrow MSC counterparts. Though CD117 and CD34 expressions are typically absent in MSCs, instances of CD34 expression in ASCs have been documented [45, 58, 60].

For meticulous identification, a synergistic analysis employing both positive and negative markers for ASCs is advocated. Empirical evidence suggests that the modality of sample acquisition exerts negligible influence on the expression of surface markers. Moreover, ASCs, even under extended culture, showcase a remarkable phenotype stability, consistently expressing markers including CD90, CD44, CD34, and CD45, further corroborating the stable nature of ASC surface marker expressions across culture phases [61].

Mesenchymal Stem Cell Injection for DDD

The nucleus pulposus, an intricate gelatinous core enriched with proteoglycans, is encased within the protective embrace of the annulus fibrosus and the cartilaginous endplates. Its physiologic prowess is contingent upon the integrity of these surrounding structures. Contemporary therapeutic interventions employing MSCs for disc degenerative diseases (DDD) predominantly direct their efforts towards the nucleus pulposus, with aspirations to replenish its cellular constituents or attenuate the degenerative milieu [2, 3].

Is this therapeutic approach justified? A detailed understanding of the issue requires several clarifications. Initially, one must be clear that MSC-based interventions are curated for painful discs rather than the asymptomatic disc transformations inherent to aging. Painful discs consistently exhibit structural defects, either in the annulus fibrosus or the cartilaginous endplates, whereas discs with intact annulus fibrosus and cartilaginous endplates tend to be painless. Structural defects initiate disc degeneration throughout the entire disc, including the nucleus pulposus, which becomes secondary. Thus, even in scenarios where MSC administration augments proteoglycan production within the nucleus pulposus, the biomechanical equilibrium remains jeopardized until the aberrations in the annulus fibrosus or the cartilaginous endplates are rectified. Inevitably, a nucleus pulposus, even if partially rejuvenated, is predisposed to subsequent degenerative episodes if the overarching structural defects persist. This underscores the imperative to not singularly focus on the degenerated nucleus pulposus but also to address anomalies in the annulus fibrosus or the cartilaginous endplates in therapeutic regimens.

Mechanism of Action of MSCs for DDD

Originally, the therapeutic paradigm posited that introducing MSCs into the degenerated nucleus pulposus might prompt them to adopt the phenotype of nucleus pulposus cells, thereby replenishing the disc. However, subsequent studies mandated a recalibration of this hypothesis [62]. Investigations employing tagged MSCs in animal knee joints unveiled a swift decline in the injected cell population. In a matter of weeks, their presence became undetectable. Analogously, the majority of introduced MSCs either succumbed or experienced apoptosis within a mere four days post-injection, a consequence attributed to the disc's ischemic microenvironment [63].

A thorough appreciation of MSCs' therapeutic attributes requires a detailed understanding of the molecular pathways they orchestrate, synthesizing insights from existing literature yields three cardinal mechanisms: (1) Paracrine-mediated activities through soluble mediators and extracellular vesicles (EVs); (2) Mesodermal differentiation; and (3) Efferocytosis [62 - 64]. Exosomes and microvesicles, subsets of MSC-sourced EVs, have emerged as indispensable agents in cellular dialogue, eliciting physiological transformations in recipient tissues [65]. Furthermore, efferocytosis—the act of resident tissue macrophages engulfing compromised or moribund MSCs—initiates the release of mediators like interleukin-10 and transforming growth factor-β, orchestrating immune modulation [66].

Despite modest engraftment rates, typically below 3%, MSC's beneficial effects are primarily attributed to these aforementioned mechanisms. Extracellular vesicles, especially, have garnered significant interest. These membrane-bound nanostructures are adept at ferrying an array of biomolecules, from proteins to non-coding RNAs. Exosomes, diminutive lipid membrane vesicles sized between 30 and 150 nm, function as molecular couriers, liberated from a progenitor cell and assimilated by proximate cells, often *via* ligand-receptor associations. Pioneering studies on MSC-derived exosomes (MSC-Exos) reveal their comparable functionality to MSCs but with attributes like enhanced penetrative potential and superior storage stability [66, 67]. Ectosomes, or microvesicles, span from 50 to 1000 nm and are intrinsic to myriad processes, from cellular communication to organ remodeling. When MSCs face functional impairments or cell demise, efferocytosis ensues. This uptake culminates in the evolution of macrophages toward an anti-inflammatory signature and the secretion of soluble immunomodulatory agents, inducing immunosuppression or tolerance [63, 64].

MSC Clinical Trials

For several decades, the therapeutic potential of MSCs has been a focal point of clinical investigations. Yet, the outcomes from advanced clinical studies did produce benefits projected by preliminary preclinical experiments in diverse disease paradigms [63]. Discrepancies have surfaced between the outcomes derived from MSCs cultivated in industrial versus academic settings, adding layers of complexity to the MSC therapy debate. Numerous variables, such as donor variability, *Ex vivo* cultivation, cellular senescence, immunogenicity, and preservation strategies, significantly influence the therapeutic yield of MSCs [68].

Human MSCs in culture exhibit pronounced inhibitory actions on immune cells, notably T cells, B cells, and dendritic cells. This immunosuppressive prowess can be attributed to the synthesis of indoleamine 2,3-dioxygenase (IDO) and related effector molecules, with their effects being amplified upon interferon (IFN)-γ exposure [68]. However, the amplitude of the IDO-mediated response isn't uniform across MSC samples harvested from various healthy donors, even when the MSCs appear phenotypically identical and are activated by IFN-γ in a similar fashion [69]. Contemporary understanding suggests that IFN-γ-primed human MSCs wield enhanced immunosuppressive capabilities in vitro, and their *In vivo* potency is intrinsically tied to their IFN-γ responsiveness.

This brings forth a consequential therapeutic implication: Patients endowed with MSCs from donors demonstrating tepid IFN-γ responses might not reap as much benefit as those benefitting from donors characterized by robust IFN-γ responses. Moreover, prolonged cultivation of human MSCs has been linked with phenotypical aberrations such as telomere attrition, which could potentially impinge upon their regenerative and immunosuppressive faculties [63, 70, 71]. Thus, elucidating a definitive immunophenotypic blueprint for MSCs could streamline the selection of altruistic donors, ensuring that MSC contributions are optimally immunomodulatory. Such a strategy could mitigate the pitfalls of introducing suboptimal cellular therapies in pivotal clinical settings [63].

Functional *versus* Structural Improvements

Clinical studies examining MSC therapy for low back pain predominantly indicate its efficacy in ameliorating pain and enhancing functional outcomes. Yet, there remains a paucity of evidence supporting tangible structural ameliorations within intervertebral discs [2]. The abbreviated survival span of infused MSCs, precipitated by immune responses and nutrient and oxygen deprivation, poses challenges. While the therapeutic potency of MSCs is largely conferred by their paracrine actions, the evanescent existence of the paracrine-derived solutes hinders enduring therapeutic impacts on intervertebral disc degeneration (IDD).

The unique physiological architecture of intervertebral discs, characterized by their avascularity and sparse cellular density, intimates that disc repair in humans, inclusive of disc height restoration, might proceed at a more languid pace than observed in animal counterparts. For context, the half-life of proteoglycans within human intervertebral discs spans 3-6 years. In stark contrast, fibrous proteins, including collagen and elastin, tout half-lives exceeding 50 years, underscoring the deliberate tempo of matrix production and breakdown within this tissue [72].

Efficacious cell therapeutic regimens should encompass interventions for both the nucleus pulposus and the surrounding annulus fibrosus or cartilaginous endplates. Contrarily, extant cell-centric clinical investigations have myopically targeted the nucleus pulposus, marking a palpable oversight in regenerative tactics. The zenith of success for any cellular intervention is conceivably attainable only after the biomechanical rejuvenation of the compromised disc [73].

The Ethics of MSC Therapies

In several nations, a multitude of clinics operate beyond regulatory oversight, providing services driven by profit rather than evidence-based outcomes. Such establishments often overstate the therapeutic outcomes, yet their assertions remain unsubstantiated by empirical data [64]. Moreover, the lead on advanced phase III trials for the majority of MSC therapies has been taken by industrial sponsors, eliciting skepticism regarding the field's perhaps premature enthusiasm. This skepticism frequently finds its roots in the questionable practices of these unregulated stem cell clinics on a global scale, which exploit the yet unconfirmed promise of regenerative treatments, MSCs included, as panaceas [63].

CONCLUSION

The intervertebral disc, with its intricate assembly of three distinct cartilaginous elements, demands a multifaceted approach to restoration. Rather than exclusively addressing the compromised nucleus pulposus, strategies should encompass the annulus fibrosus and cartilaginous endplates. Despite their link to low back pain, these regions have seen a paucity of detailed biological research. Singularly aiming regenerative efforts, especially those based on MSCs, at the deteriorated nucleus pulposus may prove ineffectual. A holistic grasp of the disc's cellular dynamics, biomechanical shifts, and pathophysiological nuances post-injury or during degeneration is pivotal, paving the way for regenerative interventions that resembles pristine native tissue.

REFERENCES

[1]   Vlaeyen JWS, Maher CG, Wiech K, *et al.* Low back pain. Nat Rev Dis Primers 2018; 4(1): 52.
        [http://dx.doi.org/10.1038/s41572-018-0052-1] [PMID: 30546064]

[2]   Binch ALA, Fitzgerald JC, Growney EA, Barry F. Cell-based strategies for IVD repair: clinical progress and translational obstacles. Nat Rev Rheumatol 2021; 17(3): 158-75.
        [http://dx.doi.org/10.1038/s41584-020-00568-w] [PMID: 33526926]

[3]   Williams RJ, Tryfonidou MA, Snuggs JW, Le Maitre CL. Cell sources proposed for nucleus pulposus regeneration. JOR Spine 2021; 4(4)e1175
        [http://dx.doi.org/10.1002/jsp2.1175] [PMID: 35005441]

[4]   Acosta FL Jr, Metz L, Adkisson HD IV, *et al.* Porcine intervertebral disc repair using allogeneic juvenile articular chondrocytes or mesenchymal stem cells. Tissue Eng Part A 2011; 17(23-24): 3045-55.
        [http://dx.doi.org/10.1089/ten.tea.2011.0229] [PMID: 21910592]

[5]   Bach FC, Tellegen AR, Beukers M, *et al.* Biologic canine and human intervertebral disc repair by notochordal cell-derived matrix: from bench towards bedside. Oncotarget 2018; 9(41): 26507-26.
        [http://dx.doi.org/10.18632/oncotarget.25476] [PMID: 29899873]

[6]   Ganey T, Libera J, Moos V, *et al.* Disc chondrocyte transplantation in a canine model: A treatment for degenerated or damaged intervertebral disc. Spine 2003; 28(23): 2609-20.
        [http://dx.doi.org/10.1097/01.BRS.0000097891.63063.78] [PMID: 14652478]

[7]   Gao C, Ning D, Sang C, Zhang Y. Rapamycin prevents the intervertebral disc degeneration *via* inhibiting differentiation and senescence of annulus fibrosus cells. Aging (Albany NY) 2018; 10(1): 131-43.
        [http://dx.doi.org/10.18632/aging.101364] [PMID: 29348392]

[8]   Gorensek M, Jaksimović C, Kregar-Velikonja N, *et al.* Nucleus pulposus repair with cultured autologous elastic cartilage derived chondrocytes. Cell Mol Biol Lett 2004; 9(2): 363-73.
        [PMID: 15213815]

[9]   Iwashina T, Mochida J, Sakai D, *et al.* Feasibility of using a human nucleus pulposus cell line as a cell source in cell transplantation therapy for intervertebral disc degeneration. Spine 2006; 31(11): 1177-86.
        [http://dx.doi.org/10.1097/01.brs.0000217687.36874.c4] [PMID: 16688029]

[10]   Hoogendoorn RJW, Lu ZF, Kroeze RJ, Bank RA, Wuisman PI, Helder MN. Adipose stem cells for intervertebral disc regeneration: Current status and concepts for the future. J Cell Mol Med 2008; 12(6a): 2205-16.
        [http://dx.doi.org/10.1111/j.1582-4934.2008.00291.x] [PMID: 18298653]

[11]   Ma W, Tavakoli T, Derby E, Serebryakova Y, Rao MS, Mattson MP. Cell-extracellular matrix interactions regulate neural differentiation of human embryonic stem cells. BMC Dev Biol 2008; 8(1): 90.
        [http://dx.doi.org/10.1186/1471-213X-8-90] [PMID: 18808690]

[12]   Noriega DC, Ardura F, Hernández-Ramajo R, *et al.* Intervertebral disc repair by allogeneic
       mesenchymal bone marrow cells. Transplantation 2017; 101(8): 1945-51.
       [http://dx.doi.org/10.1097/TP.0000000000001484] [PMID: 27661661]

[13]   Omlor GW, Lorenz S, Nerlich AG, Guehring T, Richter W. Disc cell therapy with bone-marro-
       -derived autologous mesenchymal stromal cells in a large porcine disc degeneration model. Eur Spine
       J 2018; 27(10): 2639-49.
       [http://dx.doi.org/10.1007/s00586-018-5728-4] [PMID: 30141058]

[14]   Peng B, Yang H, Peng B. Human umbilical cord mesenchymal stem cell transplantation for the
       treatment of chronic discogenic low back pain. Pain Physician 2014; 4(17): E525-30.
       [http://dx.doi.org/10.36076/ppj.2014/17/E525] [PMID: 25054402]

[15]   Sheyn D, Ben-David S, Tawackoli W, *et al.* Human iPSCs can be differentiated into notochordal cells
       that reduce intervertebral disc degeneration in a porcine model. Theranostics 2019; 9(25): 7506-24.
       [http://dx.doi.org/10.7150/thno.34898] [PMID: 31695783]

[16]   Vadalà G, Russo F, Ambrosio L, Loppini M, Denaro V. Stem cells sources for intervertebral disc
       regeneration. World J Stem Cells 2016; 8(5): 185-201.
       [http://dx.doi.org/10.4252/wjsc.v8.i5.185] [PMID: 27247704]

[17]   Xia K, Zhu J, Hua J, *et al.* Intradiscal injection of induced pluripotent stem cell-derived nucleus
       pulposus-Like cell-seeded polymeric microspheres promotes rat disc regeneration. Stem Cells Int
       2019; 2019: 1-14.
       [http://dx.doi.org/10.1155/2019/6806540] [PMID: 31191679]

[18]   Zhu Y, Liang Y, Zhu H, *et al.* The generation and functional characterization of induced pluripotent
       stem cells from human intervertebral disc nucleus pulposus cells. Oncotarget 2017; 8(26): 42700-11.
       [http://dx.doi.org/10.18632/oncotarget.17446] [PMID: 28498811]

[19]   Adams MA, Roughley PJ. What is intervertebral disc degeneration, and what causes it? Spine 2006;
       31(18): 2151-61.
       [http://dx.doi.org/10.1097/01.brs.0000231761.73859.2c] [PMID: 16915105]

[20]   Peredo AP, Gullbrand SE, Smith HE, Mauck RL. Putting the pieces in place: Mobilizing cellular
       players to improve annulus fibrosus repair. Tissue Eng Part B Rev 2021; 27(4): 295-312.
       [http://dx.doi.org/10.1089/ten.teb.2020.0196] [PMID: 32907498]

[21]   Torre OM, Mroz V, Bartelstein MK, Huang AH, Iatridis JC. Annulus fibrosus cell phenotypes in
       homeostasis and injury: implications for regenerative strategies. Ann N Y Acad Sci 2019; 1442(1): 61-
       78.
       [http://dx.doi.org/10.1111/nyas.13964] [PMID: 30604562]

[22]   Peng BG, Yan XJ. Barriers to mesenchymal stromal cells for low back pain. World J Stem Cells 2022;
       14(12): 815-21.
       [http://dx.doi.org/10.4252/wjsc.v14.i12.815] [PMID: 36619693]

[23]   Rustenburg CME, Emanuel KS, Peeters M, Lems WF, Vergroesen PPA, Smit TH. Osteoarthritis and
       intervertebral disc degeneration: Quite different, quite similar. JOR Spine 2018; 1(4)e1033
       [http://dx.doi.org/10.1002/jsp2.1033] [PMID: 31463450]

[24]   Erwin WM, Hood KE. The cellular and molecular biology of the intervertebral disc: A clinician's
       primer. J Can Chiropr Assoc 2014; 58(3): 246-57.
       [PMID: 25202152]

[25]   Ohtori S, Inoue G, Miyagi M, Takahashi K. Pathomechanisms of discogenic low back pain in humans
       and animal models. Spine J 2015; 15(6): 1347-55.
       [http://dx.doi.org/10.1016/j.spinee.2013.07.490] [PMID: 24657737]

[26]   Kepler CK, Ponnappan RK, Tannoury CA, Risbud MV, Anderson DG. The molecular basis of
       intervertebral disc degeneration. Spine J 2013; 13(3): 318-30.
       [http://dx.doi.org/10.1016/j.spinee.2012.12.003] [PMID: 23537454]

[27]   Iatridis JC, Nicoll SB, Michalek AJ, Walter BA, Gupta MS. Role of biomechanics in intervertebral disc degeneration and regenerative therapies: What needs repairing in the disc and what are promising biomaterials for its repair? Spine J 2013; 13(3): 243-62.
[http://dx.doi.org/10.1016/j.spinee.2012.12.002] [PMID: 23369494]

[28]   Oichi T, Taniguchi Y, Oshima Y, Tanaka S, Saito T. Pathomechanism of intervertebral disc degeneration. JOR Spine 2020; 3(1)e1076
[http://dx.doi.org/10.1002/jsp2.1076] [PMID: 32211588]

[29]   Kos N, Gradisnik L, Velnar T. A brief review of the degenerative intervertebral disc disease. Med Arh 2019; 73(6): 421-4.
[http://dx.doi.org/10.5455/medarh.2019.73.421-424] [PMID: 32082013]

[30]   Rodrigues-Pinto R, Richardson SM, Hoyland JA. An understanding of intervertebral disc development, maturation and cell phenotype provides clues to direct cell-based tissue regeneration therapies for disc degeneration. Eur Spine J 2014; 23(9): 1803-14.
[http://dx.doi.org/10.1007/s00586-014-3305-z] [PMID: 24777668]

[31]   Wuertz K, Haglund L. Inflammatory mediators in intervertebral disk degeneration and discogenic pain. Global Spine J 2013; 3(3): 175-84.
[http://dx.doi.org/10.1055/s-0033-1347299] [PMID: 24436868]

[32]   Loibl M, Wuertz-Kozak K, Vadala G, Lang S, Fairbank J, Urban JP. Controversies in regenerative medicine: Should intervertebral disc degeneration be treated with mesenchymal stem cells? JOR Spine 2019; 2(1)e1043
[http://dx.doi.org/10.1002/jsp2.1043] [PMID: 31463457]

[33]   Lyu FJ, Cui H, Pan H, *et al.* Painful intervertebral disc degeneration and inflammation: From laboratory evidence to clinical interventions. Bone Res 2021; 9(1): 7.
[http://dx.doi.org/10.1038/s41413-020-00125-x] [PMID: 33514693]

[34]   Feng C, Liu H, Yang M, Zhang Y, Huang B, Zhou Y. Disc cell senescence in intervertebral disc degeneration: Causes and molecular pathways. Cell Cycle 2016; 15(13): 1674-84.
[http://dx.doi.org/10.1080/15384101.2016.1152433] [PMID: 27192096]

[35]   Peng B, Hao J, Hou S, *et al.* Possible pathogenesis of painful intervertebral disc degeneration. Spine 2006; 31(5): 560-6.
[http://dx.doi.org/10.1097/01.brs.0000201324.45537.46] [PMID: 16508552]

[36]   Freemont AJ, Watkins A, Le Maitre C, *et al.* Nerve growth factor expression and innervation of the painful intervertebral disc. J Pathol 2002; 197(3): 286-92.
[http://dx.doi.org/10.1002/path.1108] [PMID: 12115873]

[37]   Daly C, Ghosh P, Jenkin G, Oehme D, Goldschlager T. A review of animal models of intervertebral disc degeneration: Pathophysiology, regeneration, and translation to the clinic. BioMed Res Int 2016; 2016: 1-14.
[http://dx.doi.org/10.1155/2016/5952165] [PMID: 27314030]

[38]   Ding DC, Shyu WC, Lin SZ. Mesenchymal stem cells. Cell Transplant 2011; 20(1): 5-14.
[http://dx.doi.org/10.3727/096368910X] [PMID: 21396235]

[39]   Richardson SM, Hoyland JA, Mobasheri R, Csaki C, Shakibaei M, Mobasheri A. Mesenchymal stem cells in regenerative medicine: Opportunities and challenges for articular cartilage and intervertebral disc tissue engineering. J Cell Physiol 2010; 222(1): 23-32.
[http://dx.doi.org/10.1002/jcp.21915] [PMID: 19725073]

[40]   Wei X, Yang X, Han Z, Qu F, Shao L, Shi Y. Mesenchymal stem cells: A new trend for cell therapy. Acta Pharmacol Sin 2013; 34(6): 747-54.
[http://dx.doi.org/10.1038/aps.2013.50] [PMID: 23736003]

[41]   Jadalannagari S, Aljitawi OS. Ectodermal differentiation of wharton's jelly mesenchymal stem cells for tissue engineering and regenerative medicine applications. Tissue Eng Part B Rev 2015; 21(3):

314-22.
[http://dx.doi.org/10.1089/ten.teb.2014.0404] [PMID: 25517045]

[42]   Miana VV, Prieto González EA. Adipose tissue stem cells in regenerative medicine. Ecancermedicalscience 2018; 12: 822.
[http://dx.doi.org/10.3332/ecancer.2018.822] [PMID: 29662535]

[43]   Azandeh S, Gharravi AM, Orazizadeh M, Khodadi A, Hashemi Tabar M. Improvement of mesenchymal stem cell differentiation into the endoderm lineage by four step sequential method in biocompatible biomaterial. Bioimpacts 2016; 6(1): 9-13.
[http://dx.doi.org/10.15171/bi.2016.02] [PMID: 27340619]

[44]   Pittenger MF, Discher DE, Péault BM, Phinney DG, Hare JM, Caplan AI. Mesenchymal stem cell perspective: cell biology to clinical progress. NPJ Regen Med 2019; 4(1): 22.
[http://dx.doi.org/10.1038/s41536-019-0083-6] [PMID: 31815001]

[45]   Bourin P, Bunnell BA, Casteilla L, *et al.* Stromal cells from the adipose tissue-derived stromal vascular fraction and culture expanded adipose tissue-derived stromal/stem cells: A joint statement of the International Federation for Adipose Therapeutics and Science (IFATS) and the International Society for Cellular Therapy (ISCT). Cytotherapy 2013; 15(6): 641-8.
[http://dx.doi.org/10.1016/j.jcyt.2013.02.006] [PMID: 23570660]

[46]   Feisst V, Meidinger S, Locke MB. From bench to bedside: Use of human adipose-derived stem cells. Stem Cells Cloning 2015; 8: 149-62.
[PMID: 26586955]

[47]   Francis SL, Duchi S, Onofrillo C, Di Bella C, Choong PFM. Adipose-derived mesenchymal stem cells in the use of cartilage tissue engineering: The need for a rapid isolation procedure. Stem Cells Int 2018; 2018: 1-9.
[http://dx.doi.org/10.1155/2018/8947548] [PMID: 29765427]

[48]   Huri PY, Hamsici S, Ergene E, Huri G, Doral MN. Infrapatellar fat pad-derived stem cell-based regenerative strategies in orthopedic surgery. Knee Surg Relat Res 2018; 30(3): 179-86.
[http://dx.doi.org/10.5792/ksrr.17.061] [PMID: 29554720]

[49]   Hye Kim J, Gyu Park S, Kim WK, Song SU, Sung JH. Functional regulation of adipose-derived stem cells by PDGF-D. Stem Cells 2015; 33(2): 542-56.
[http://dx.doi.org/10.1002/stem.1865] [PMID: 25332166]

[50]   Caplan AI. Mesenchymal stem cells: Time to change the name! Stem Cells Transl Med 2017; 6(6): 1445-51.
[http://dx.doi.org/10.1002/sctm.17-0051] [PMID: 28452204]

[51]   Hutchings G, Janowicz K, Moncrieff L, *et al.* The proliferation and differentiation of adipose-derived stem cells in neovascularization and angiogenesis. Int J Mol Sci 2020; 21(11): 3790.
[http://dx.doi.org/10.3390/ijms21113790] [PMID: 32471255]

[52]   Baer P, Overath J, Urbschat A, *et al.* Effect of different preconditioning regimens on the expression profile of murine adipose-derived stromal/stem cells. Int J Mol Sci 2018; 19(6): 1719.
[http://dx.doi.org/10.3390/ijms19061719] [PMID: 29890767]

[53]   Wald D, Teucher B, Dinkel J, *et al.* Automatic quantification of subcutaneous and visceral adipose tissue from whole body magnetic resonance images suitable for large cohort studies. J Magn Reson Imaging 2012; 36(6): 1421-34.
[http://dx.doi.org/10.1002/jmri.23775] [PMID: 22911921]

[54]   Peng XG, Ju S, Fang F, *et al.* Comparison of brown and white adipose tissue fat fractions in *ob, seipin*, and *Fsp27* gene knockout mice by chemical shift-selective imaging and ^{1}H-MR spectroscopy. Am J Physiol Endocrinol Metab 2013; 304(2): E160-7.
[http://dx.doi.org/10.1152/ajpendo.00401.2012] [PMID: 23149622]

[55]   Rosell M, Kaforou M, Frontini A, *et al.* Brown and white adipose tissues: intrinsic differences in gene

expression and response to cold exposure in mice. Am J Physiol Endocrinol Metab 2014; 306(8): E945-64.
[http://dx.doi.org/10.1152/ajpendo.00473.2013] [PMID: 24549398]

[56]   Tsuji W, Rubin JP, Marra KG. Adipose-derived stem cells: Implications in tissue regeneration. World J Stem Cells 2014; 6(3): 312-21.
[http://dx.doi.org/10.4252/wjsc.v6.i3.312] [PMID: 25126381]

[57]   Wang QA, Tao C, Jiang L, *et al.* Distinct regulatory mechanisms governing embryonic versus adult adipocyte maturation. Nat Cell Biol 2015; 17(9): 1099-111.
[http://dx.doi.org/10.1038/ncb3217] [PMID: 26280538]

[58]   Palumbo P, Lombardi F, Siragusa G, Cifone M, Cinque B, Giuliani M. Methods of isolation, characterization and expansion of human adipose-derived stem cells (ASCs): An overview. Int J Mol Sci 2018; 19(7): 1897.
[http://dx.doi.org/10.3390/ijms19071897] [PMID: 29958391]

[59]   Bajek A, Gurtowska N, Olkowska J, *et al.* Does the harvesting technique affect the properties of adipose☐derived stem cells?—the comparative biological characterization. J Cell Biochem 2017; 118(5): 1097-107.
[http://dx.doi.org/10.1002/jcb.25724] [PMID: 27608167]

[60]   Frese L, Dijkman PE, Hoerstrup SP. Adipose tissue-derived stem cells in regenerative medicine. Transfus Med Hemother 2016; 43(4): 268-74.
[http://dx.doi.org/10.1159/000448180] [PMID: 27721702]

[61]   Bajek A, Gurtowska N, Gackowska L, *et al.* Does the liposuction method influence the phenotypic characteristic of human adipose-derived stem cells? Biosci Rep 2015; 35(3)e00212
[http://dx.doi.org/10.1042/BSR20150067] [PMID: 26182374]

[62]   Barry F. MSC therapy for osteoarthritis: An unfinished story. J Orthop Res 2019; 37(6): 1229-35.
[http://dx.doi.org/10.1002/jor.24343] [PMID: 31081558]

[63]   Galipeau J, Sensébé L. Mesenchymal stromal cells: Clinical challenges and therapeutic opportunities. Cell Stem Cell 2018; 22(6): 824-33.
[http://dx.doi.org/10.1016/j.stem.2018.05.004] [PMID: 29859173]

[64]   Krampera M, Le Blanc K. Mesenchymal stromal cells: Putative microenvironmental modulators become cell therapy. Cell Stem Cell 2021; 28(10): 1708-25.
[http://dx.doi.org/10.1016/j.stem.2021.09.006] [PMID: 34624232]

[65]   Seo Y, Kim HS, Hong IS. Stem cell-derived extracellular vesicles as immunomodulatory therapeutics. Stem Cells Int 2019; 2019: 1-10.
[http://dx.doi.org/10.1155/2019/5126156] [PMID: 30936922]

[66]   Chang X, Ma Z, Zhu G, Lu Y, Yang J. New perspective into mesenchymal stem cells: Molecular mechanisms regulating osteosarcoma. J Bone Oncol 2021; 29100372
[http://dx.doi.org/10.1016/j.jbo.2021.100372] [PMID: 34258182]

[67]   Du T, Ju G, Zhou J, *et al.* Microvesicles derived from human umbilical cord mesenchyme promote M2 macrophage polarization and ameliorate renal fibrosis following partial nephrectomy *via* hepatocyte growth factor. Hum Cell 2021; 34(4): 1103-13.
[http://dx.doi.org/10.1007/s13577-021-00525-z] [PMID: 33860459]

[68]   Galipeau J. The mesenchymal stromal cells dilemma—does a negative phase III trial of random donor mesenchymal stromal cells in steroid-resistant graft-versus-host disease represent a death knell or a bump in the road? Cytotherapy 2013; 15(1): 2-8.
[http://dx.doi.org/10.1016/j.jcyt.2012.10.002] [PMID: 23260081]

[69]   François M, Romieu-Mourez R, Li M, Galipeau J. Human MSC suppression correlates with cytokine induction of indoleamine 2,3-dioxygenase and bystander M2 macrophage differentiation. Mol Ther 2012; 20(1): 187-95.

[http://dx.doi.org/10.1038/mt.2011.189] [PMID: 21934657]

[70]   DiGirolamo CM, Stokes D, Colter D, Phinney DG, Class R, Prockop DJ. Propagation and senescence of human marrow stromal cells in culture: a simple colony☐forming assay identifies samples with the greatest potential to propagate and differentiate. Br J Haematol 1999; 107(2): 275-81.
[http://dx.doi.org/10.1046/j.1365-2141.1999.01715.x] [PMID: 10583212]

[71]   Bork S, Pfister S, Witt H, *et al.* DNA methylation pattern changes upon long☐term culture and aging of human mesenchymal stromal cells. Aging Cell 2010; 9(1): 54-63.
[http://dx.doi.org/10.1111/j.1474-9726.2009.00535.x] [PMID: 19895632]

[72]   Sivan SS, Hayes AJ, Wachtel E, *et al.* Biochemical composition and turnover of the extracellular matrix of the normal and degenerate intervertebral disc. Eur Spine J 2014; 23(S3) (Suppl. 3): 344-53.
[http://dx.doi.org/10.1007/s00586-013-2767-8] [PMID: 23591805]

[73]   Vergroesen PPA, Kingma I, Emanuel KS, *et al.* Mechanics and biology in intervertebral disc degeneration: a vicious circle. Osteoarthritis Cartilage 2015; 23(7): 1057-70.
[http://dx.doi.org/10.1016/j.joca.2015.03.028] [PMID: 25827971]

CHAPTER 3

Current Clinical Applications of Regenerative Strategies for Lumbar Degenerative Disc Disease and Global Disease Burden Due to Low Back Pain

Álvaro Dowling[1], Marjan Asefi[2], Jaime Moyano[3], Jorge Felipe Ramírez León[4,5,6], Kai-Uwe Lewandrowski[7,8,9] and William Omar Contreras López[10,*]

[1] *Orthopaedic Spine Surgeon, Director of Endoscopic Spine Clinic, Santiago, Chile*

[2] *University of North Carolina, Greensboro, NC, USA*

[3] *Centro Regional Universitario BarilocheThe institution will open in a new tab, San Carlos de Bariloche, Argentina*

[4] *Minimally Invasive Spine Center. Bogotá, D.C., Colombia*

[5] *Reina Sofía Clinic. Bogotá, D.C., Colombia*

[6] *Fundación Universitaria Sanitas. Bogotá, D.C., Colombia*

[7] *Center for Advanced Spine Care of Southern Arizona and Surgical Institute of Tucson, Tucson, AZ, USA*

[8] *Departmemt of Orthopaedics, Fundación Universitaria Sanitas, Bogotá, D.C., Colombia*

[9] *Department of Neurosurgery in the Video-Endoscopic Postgraduate Program at the Universidade Federal do Estado do Rio de Janeiro - UNIRIO, Rio de Janeiro, Brazil*

[10] *Clínica Foscal Internacional, Autopista Floridablanca - Girón, Km 7, Floridablanca, Santander, Colombia*

Abstract: Degenerative disc disease, coupled with its consequential low back pain, presents a profound global health challenge, with efficacious clinical interventions still being subject to controversy. Cutting-edge strategies are being developed, targeting both pain mitigation and tissue regeneration. Both concentrated bone marrow aspirate and mesenchymal stem cells (MSCs) have displayed clinical potential in alleviating pain associated with degenerative disc disease. By harnessing molecular and genetic techniques, the utilization of growth factors, cytokines, and the modulation of autophagy and apoptosis processes offers hope in arresting disease progression, fostering tissue recuperation, and tempering inflammatory cascades. This chapter furnishes readers with a contemporary overview of therapeutic and regenerative modalities in clinical use and succinctly delineates the grading of the extant pinnacle clinical evidence.

* **Corresponding author William Omar Contreras López:** Clínica Foscal Internacional, Autopista Floridablanca - Girón, Km 7, Floridablanca, Santander, Colombia; Tel: +573112957003; E-mail: wyllcon@gmail.com

Keywords: Autologous platelet-rich plasma, Autologous mesenchymal stem cells, Low back pain.

INTRODUCTION

Defined succinctly, low back pain is characterized by discomfort in the posterior region, spanning from the twelfth rib's lower margin to the lower gluteal folds, potentially extending into one or both lower extremities, persisting for a minimum of one day [1].

As global demographics trend older, the prevalence of low back pain intensifies, becoming a ubiquitous health concern. This ailment exerts considerable morbidity and places an economic strain on numerous healthcare systems internationally. Its genesis is multifaceted; while a fraction can be attributed to genetic predispositions [2], psychological etiologies are also implicated [3]. Traumatic events may exacerbate disc degeneration [4]. Predominantly, age-induced disc degeneration is identified as the primary precursor to debilitating low back pain, commonly initiated by intervertebral disc degeneration. Consequently, afflictions of the facet joints can result in restricted mobility, often accompanied by radiculopathy, or sciatica [5 - 7]. In extreme scenarios, the compression of the cauda equina can lead to nerve root damage, intense pain, paralysis, and urinary or fecal incontinence [8 - 10]. Predominantly, surgical interventions, either decompression alone or in combination with fusion, are the foremost treatments for discogenic low back pain arising from advanced degenerative disc disease [11 - 14]. Notably, artificial disc replacements [15, 16] and other innovative interventions [17 - 24] are frequently deemed unsuitable for advanced disease stages or have not met the rigorous criteria of the FDA's approval process.

Traditional surgical interventions, like laminectomy and fusion, frequently mandate hospital stays, especially among older adults [25, 26]. They may be fraught with complications: blood loss [27], dural tears [28], postoperative pain, infections [29, 30], and a myriad of other post-surgical challenges [25, 31 - 42] often necessitating unplanned post-operative care [43]. Additionally, these procedures carry a substantial risk of reoperation [44 - 46], commonly attributable to hardware malfunctions, degeneration escalation, spinal instability, or deformities [47 - 52]. The functional deterioration ensuing from such procedures underlines the imperative for alternative methodologies. The paradigm is gradually shifting towards early-stage, minimally invasive [53], and regenerative interventions [54 - 59], opposing the historical predilection for extensive late-stage surgical reconstructions.

Recent empirical evidence underscores the efficacy of minimal interventions, employing direct visualization for patients grappling with degenerative spinal stenosis, potentially with concomitant disc herniation [43, 60 - 62]. Preservation of the intervertebral disc's innate shock-absorbing functionality in compromised spinal movement scenarios has been advocated and tested by several experts [63]. Given the limitations intrinsic to the conventional surgical approach for spinal ailments, burgeoning research is centered on pioneering interventional modalities. The expanding research corpus substantiates this trend [64]. This chapter endeavors to encapsulate the contemporary zenith in regenerative therapies for intervertebral disc degeneration, acknowledging that the scope might not be exhaustive, and myriad validated restorative methodologies might emerge in the future.

Global Disease Burden

Globally, degenerative spinal conditions are ubiquitously observed and are an escalating concern with advancing age. Such maladies exert profound strain on both individuals and the overarching healthcare infrastructure. Specifically, intervertebral disc degeneration stands out as a noteworthy contributor to this worldwide health challenge, often culminating in prolonged disabilities among the affected.

The esteemed Global Disease Burden (GBD) study characterizes low back pain as discomfort manifesting in the posterior torso, ranging from the twelfth rib's base to the lower gluteal contours, potentially radiating into the lower extremities, and persisting for at least a day. This ailment's global impact is profound: in 2019 alone, low back pain emerged as the predominant Level 3 contributor to years lived with disability (YLDs), accounting for an estimated 63.7 million (95% UI 45.0–85.2) YLDs or approximately 7.4% (6.2–8.7) of the global total (as illustrated in Fig. **1**).

The GBD investigation encompassed a comprehensive assortment of studies on low back pain, including four centered on its incidence, 446 on prevalence, three on remission, and 15 others directly related to this ailment, with a conspicuous absence of studies focusing on its causes of death [65 - 68]. The 2019 iteration of the GBD study [67] diverged from its 2010 predecessor by omitting studies rooted in lifetime recall surveys, due to the variability in recall durations of lifelong back pain experiences exceeding the scope of a singular adjustment factor. Moreover, insurance data from Taiwan was disregarded due to its paucity. Corrections for potential biases were meticulously executed using meta-regression network analysis, specifically the Bayesian, regularized, trimmed approach (MR-BRT) [67, 69]. Adjustments accommodated studies that delineated overly extensive anatomical regions, episodes surpassing three months, varying recall periods, and constraints like pain that hampered activities. The analysis also accounted for surveys targeting school-aged children and insurance data originating from the USA. The resultant data vividly underscores the heightened disease burden, particularly from musculoskeletal disorders, predominantly observed in individuals aged between 35 and 65 (refer to Figs. **2** and **3**). A detailed breakdown of the incidence and prevalence data concerning low back pain disorders for the year 2019 is systematically presented in Table **1**.

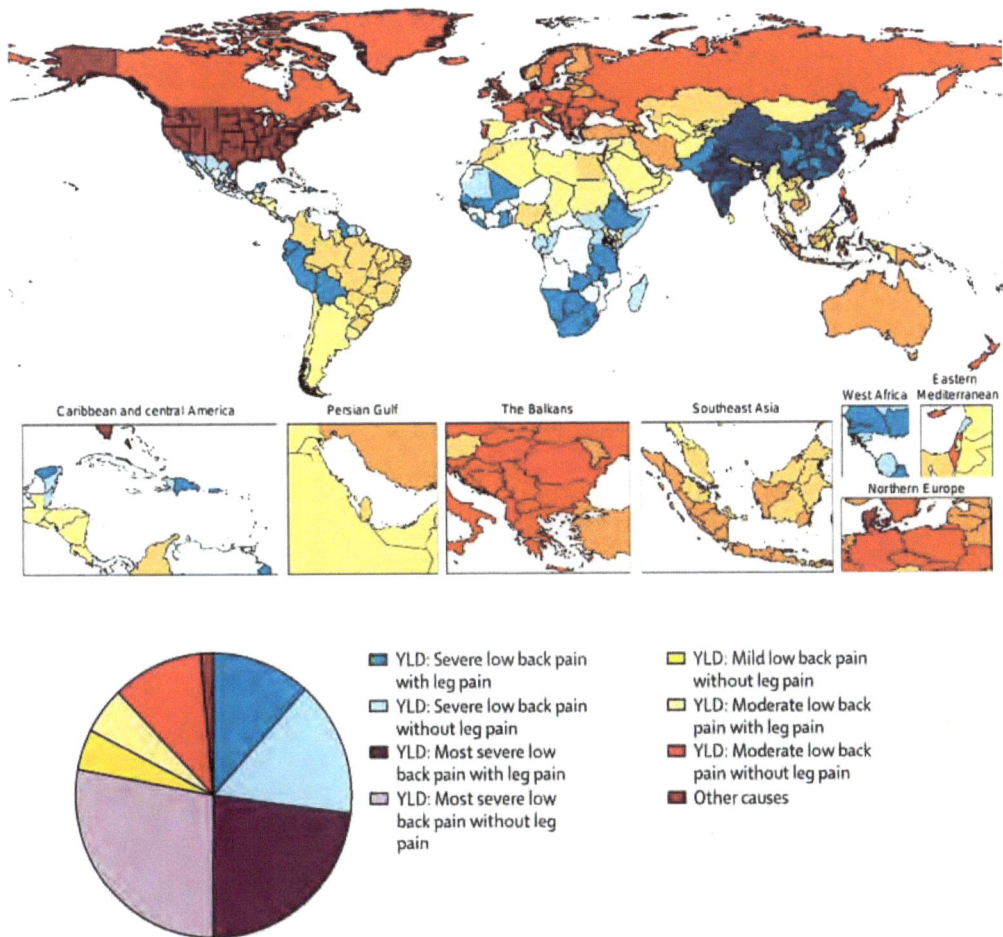

Fig. (1). Top panel: Age-standardized DALY rates (per 100 000) by location, both sexes, 2019. Bottom Panel: Composition of DALYs by constituent sequelae YLDs for both sexes combined, 2019. <u>Source</u>: Institute for Health Metrics Evaluation. Used with permission. All rights reserved.

Low back pain consistently emerged as a significant Level 3 contributor to worldwide mortality and morbidity metrics, including years of life lost (YLLs), years lived with disability (YLDs), and the disability-adjusted life year (DALYs) in the years 1990, 2010, and 2019, encompassing both genders. It is worth noting that Level 3 designations also cover conditions such as tuberculosis, stroke, and vehicular accident-induced injuries. Tracing the trajectory from 1990 to 2019, low back pain steadfastly stood out as a primary determinant for YLDs. When evaluating DALYs, it ascended the ranks from 13th in 1990, to 12th in 2010, and further advanced to 9th in 2019 [67, 70].

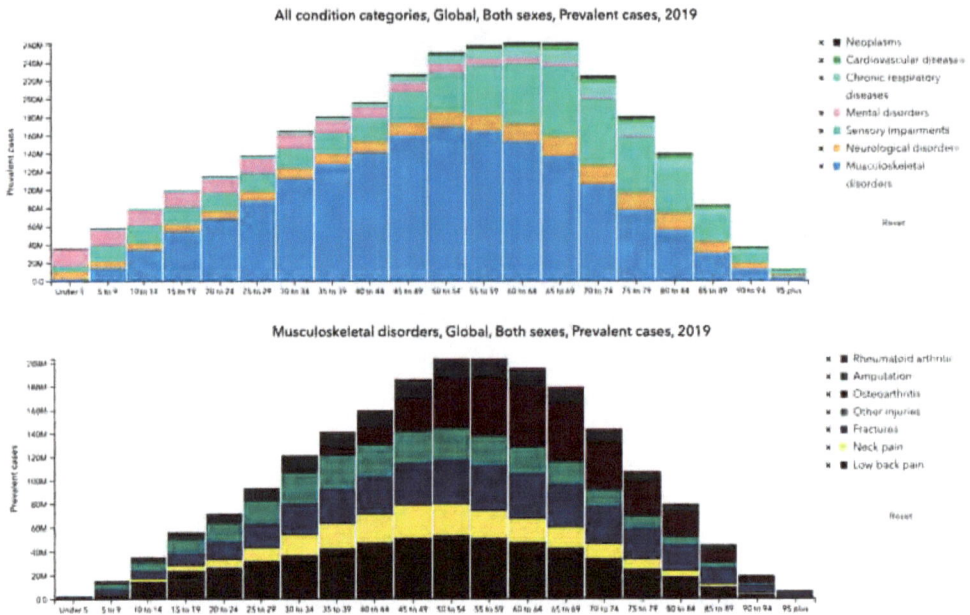

Fig. (2). Top panel: Disease burden of prevalent cases for all conditions for both sexes by age 2019. Bottom Panel: Disease burden for musculoskeletal disorders for both sexes by age, 2019, showing a disproportionally higher disease burden from spinal disorders including neck and back pain between the ages of 35 and 65. <u>Source</u>: Institute for Health Metrics Evaluation. Used with permission. All rights reserved. Source: Institute for Health Metrics Evaluation. Used with permission. All rights reserved.

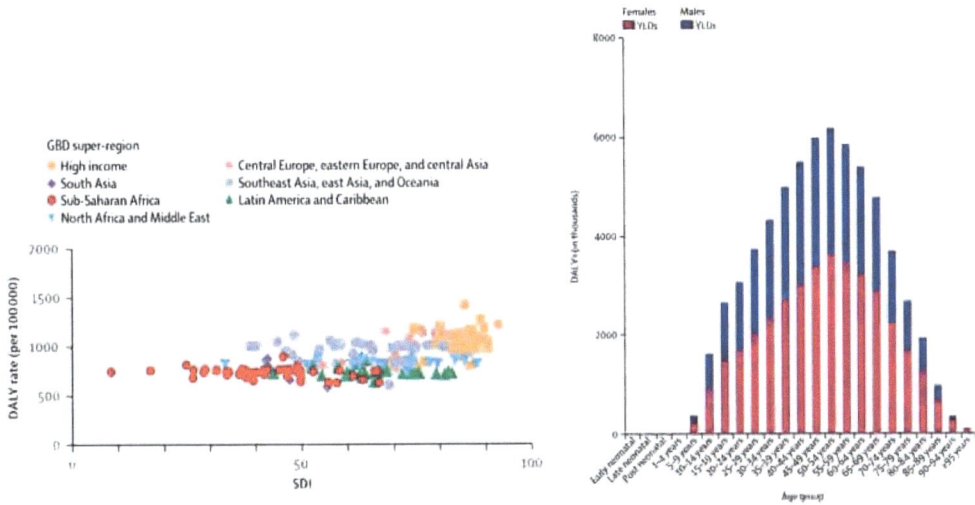

Fig. (3). Left panel: The socio-demographic Index (SDI) is plotted versus DALYs as a summary measure of spectrum development by countries or other geographic areas. Right panel: Composition of YLDs by age group and sex, 2019. <u>Source</u>: Institute for Health Metrics Evaluation. Used with permission. All rights reserved.

Table 1. Global prevalence, incidence, deaths, YLLs, YLDs, and DALYs in counts and age-standardized rates for both sexes, females, and males, 2019, with percentage change between 2010 and 2019.

	Prevalence		Incidence		Deaths		YLLs		YLDs		DALYs		-
-	Cases (millions)	Rate (per 100 000)	Cases (millions)	Rate (per 100 000)	Deaths (millions)	Rate (per 100 000)	YLLs (millions)	Rate (per 100 000)	YLDs (millions)	Rate (per 100 000)	DALYs (millions)	Rate (per 100 000)
2019													
Both Sexes	568 (505 to 641)	6972·5 (6190·5 to 7860·5)	223 (198 to 253)	2748·9 (2425·8 to 3106·9)	—	—	—	—	63·7 (45·0 to 85·2)	780·2 (549·3 to 1046·1)	63·7 (45·0 to 85·2)	780·2 (549·3 to 1046·1)
Females	332 (295 to 374)	7949·0 (7067·8 to 8967·5)	128 (114 to 145)	3094·1 (2740·8 to 3491·2)	—	—	—	—	36·8 (26·1 to 49·5)	884·0 (625·1 to 1186·9)	36·8 (26·1 to 49·5)	884·0 (625·1 to 1186·9)
Males	237 (210 to 266)	5941·6 (5280·3 to 6671·8)	95·3 (83·9 to 108)	2386·4 (2105·6 to 2707·7)	—	—	—	—	26·8 (18·9 to 35·9)	670·9 (471·2 to 897·5)	26·8 (18·9 to 35·9)	670·9 (471·2 to 897·5)
Percentage change 2010-19													
Both Sexes	13·5% (12·2 to 14·8)	−4·1% (−4·7 to −3·5)	14·6% (13·3 to 15·9)	−2·4% (−2·8 to −2·0)	—	—	—	—	13·1% (11·8 to 14·5)	−4·1% (−4·8 to −3·5)	13·1% (11·8 to 14·5)	−4·1% (−4·8 to −3·5)

(Table 1) cont.....

-	Prevalence		Incidence		Deaths		YLLs		YLDs		DALYs	-
-	Cases (millions)	Rate (per 100 000)	Cases (millions)	Rate (per 100 000)	Deaths (millions)	Rate (per 100 000)	YLLs (millions)	Rate (per 100 000)	YLDs (millions)	Rate (per 100 000)	DALYs (millions)	Rate (per 100 000)
2019												
Females	14·6% (13·2 to 16·0)	−3·4% (−4·1 to −2·9)	16·2% (14·7 to 17·6)	−1·4% (−1·8 to −0·9)	—	—	—	—	14·2% (12·9 to 15·7)	−3·5% (−4·2 to −2·9)	14·2% (12·9 to 15·7)	−3·5% (−4·2 to −2·9)
Males	12·0% (10·7 to 13·4)	−4·9% (−5·7 to −4·1)	12·5% (11·2 to 13·7)	−3·8% (−4·3 to −3·2)	—	—	—	—	11·6% (10·4 to 13·1)	−5·0% (−5·7 to −4·2)	11·6% (10·4 to 13·1)	−5·0% (−5·7 to −4·2)
Numbers in parentheses are 95% uncertainty intervals.												

The Socio-Demographic Index (SDI) offers a consolidated gauge reflecting the developmental status of nations or specific geographical zones. With a scaling range from 0 to 1, the SDI amalgamates the per capita income rankings, average educational achievements, and fertility statistics of all regions covered by the GBD analysis [67]. The 2019 global survey discerned a rehabilitation requisite spanning 2.4 billion individuals across all health conditions, of which 570 million instances were attributed to low back pain. This corresponded to an escalatory surge of 69.4% in YLDs from 1990 to 2019, as illustrated in Fig. (4).

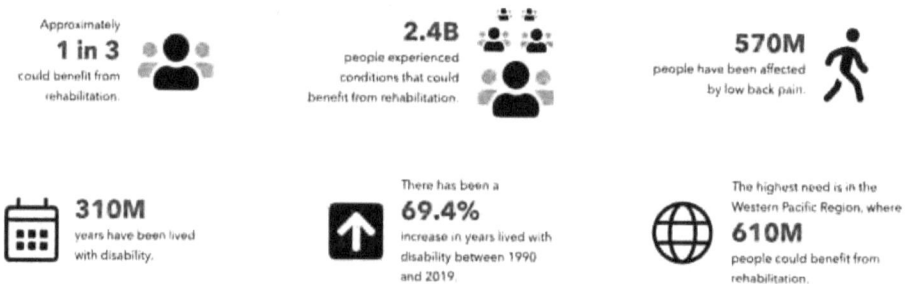

Global key findings, 2019

Approximately **1 in 3** could benefit from rehabilitation.

2.4B people experienced conditions that could benefit from rehabilitation.

570M people have been affected by low back pain.

310M years have been lived with disability.

There has been a **69.4%** increase in years lived with disability between 1990 and 2019.

The highest need is in the Western Pacific Region, where **610M** people could benefit from rehabilitation.

Fig. (4). Global need for rehabilitation: 2.4 Billion people experienced conditions that could benefit from rehabilitation including 570 Million that suffered from low back pain. Source: Institute for Health Metrics Evaluation. Used with permission. All rights reserved.

Degenerative Disc Disease

The intervertebral disc, is composed of the central nucleus pulposus (NP), the encircling annulus fibrosus (AF), and cartilaginous endplates. Notably, the AF is derived from the mesenchyme, while the NP hails from the notochord. It is conjectured that the vanishing of notochordal cells during adolescence within the NP is a precursory signal of degeneration; this is in tandem with the commencement of morphological and biochemical alterations seen in the disc from a young age [71]. These discs, situated within the spine, are acclaimed as the most substantial avascular structures in the human body. Their blood supply, sourced from the segmental and intracanal vessels, is exceedingly delicate, especially within the AF and NP [72-74]. Such a paucity of nutrients in this hypoxic milieu is postulated to instigate early cellular apoptosis and subsequent demise [75]. Culminating the degenerative spectrum [76, 77], the NP might undergo total dissolution. In many deteriorated spinal motion segments — where the intervertebral disc has approached its functional terminus — these structures are often vacuous or laden with inanimate tissue exhibiting fissures, cavities, and delamination from the endplates [78, 79]. The concurrent inflammatory cascade is hypothesized to stimulate endplate innervation through nociceptive receptors [80] that link to the basivertebral nerve [81]. Recent pain management modalities have considered ablating this particular structure as a therapeutic strategy [82-87].

The Molecular Basis of Disc Degeneration

A myriad of molecular pathways are implicated in the deterioration of lumbar intervertebral discs. Prominently, matrix metalloproteinases (MMPs), a family of enzymes, orchestrate the disintegration of the extracellular matrix. Specifically, MMP-3 or stromelysin-1 has a pivotal role in undermining proteoglycans and collagen within afflicted discs [88]. Concomitantly, pro-inflammatory mediators, including interleukin-1β (IL-1β) and tumor necrosis factor-alpha (TNF-α), exacerbate disc degeneration by skewing the equilibrium between matrix production and its subsequent degradation, culminating in tissue compromise [89]. Oxidative stress is another malefactor, producing reactive oxygen species (ROS) that instigate DNA lesions, cellular apoptosis, and additional matrix deterioration, further fuelling disc degeneration.

In a thorough literature examination by Kim JW *et al.* [75], compelling evidence illuminated the instrumental role of hypoxia-inducible factor-1alpha (HIF-1α) in disc degeneration. As an integral transcriptional regulator, HIF-1α mediates adaptive responses under hypoxic conditions, vital for the sustenance of the disc's nucleus pulposus (NP). Thus, its prospective utility as a precocious diagnostic marker and a therapeutic target in degenerative disc pathology is intriguing.

Autophagy, as discerned within the intervertebral disc, emerges as an influential mechanism potentially elucidating the terminal stages of the degenerative cascade, typified by the attenuation or obliteration of the nucleus pulposus. An investigative foray by Yurube *et al.* aimed at formulating therapeutic strategies targeting this molecular mechanism [90]. Recent scientific discoveries into the nexus between polymorphisms in collagen-encoding genes and the inception of disc degeneration were made. Evident candidates encompass genes like COL1A1, COL2A1, COL9A2, COL9A3, COL11A1, and COL11A2, anchoring the genetic framework for collagen disintegration within both the annulus fibrosus and nucleus pulposus, with burgeoning research probing the roles of genes such as COL1A2 and COL9A1 [91]. An encompassing review [92] meticulously amalgamates insights into the genetic determinants modulating collagen dynamics within intervertebral discs, emphasizing the diverse collagen types' functionality. Augmented comprehension of the pathogenesis of defective collagen synthesis may empower clinicians to implement treatments rooted in pathogenic rationale, optimizing therapeutic outcomes.

Regenerative Strategies

In a vivo investigation utilizing rat tails, a discernible disruption in autophagy of the nucleus pulposus' (NP) notochordal cells coupled with the initiation of apoptosis in its non-notochordal cells was observed following mechanically-induced disc degeneration. This highlighted autophagy's paramountcy in stabilizing notochordal cell equilibrium by mitigating apoptosis within the NP of intervertebral discs.

Ito and his colleagues spearheaded an *In vitro* exploration with human degenerative disc cells harvested surgically, probing the repressive impact of autophagy. Utilizing RNA interference of the autophagy-related gene 5 (ATG5) initially, and later augmenting with chloroquine, they investigated the repercussions of autophagy inhibition on cellular dynamics, inclusive of apoptosis, senescence, and matrix degradation. Their findings underscored autophagy's protective shield against apoptosis and senescence in human disc cells without any direct influence on matrix breakdown [93].

With bovine intervertebral discs bearing phenotypic parallels to humans, Calio M *et al.* [91] leveraged them as a robust model to decrypt the pathophysiological intricacies of disc degeneration. Employing a dual strategy of single-cell and bulk RNA sequencing on pristine bovine tail discs, they pinpointed 27 NP-specific and 24 AF-specific genes. Their research unveiled the cellular makeup of bovine discs, highlighting the coexistence of notochordal-like and progenitor cells in the NP, and a melange of stem, fibroblast-like, and endothelial progenitor cells in the annulus fibrosus (AF).

Takeoka *et al.* [94], with a distinctive modus operandi, cultivated bovine tail disc NP cells under the influence of chondroitin sulfate proteoglycan or hyaluronan, while concurrently mimicking spinal kinetics through the hydrostatic pressure.

Their observations proposed the synergistic anabolic influence of chondroitin sulfate proteoglycan and hydrostatic pressure, earmarking chondroitin sulfate proteoglycan as a potential therapeutic bedrock for degenerative disc maladies.

In an exhaustive review helmed by Croft AS *et al.* [95], the efficacy of therapies centered around mesenchymal stromal cells (MSCs) for disc degeneration was scrutinized. Preliminary studies spotlighted MSCs that mirrored disc cell characteristics. Further, the incorporation of MSCs within hydrogel matrices was explored. Clinical trials echoed favorable results post intradiscal MSC deployment, epitomized by symptomatic relief and MRI-enhanced disc morphology. Furthermore, the targeted MSC homing capability is the cutting edge in intradiscal cell therapy.

Friedmann A *et al.* [96] embarked on an evaluation of a hydrogel, imbued with autologous adipose-derived stem cells, aiming to fathom its restorative prowess. Utilizing a sheep model with nucleotomy-induced disc anomalies and following a longitudinal assessment spanning a year, their methodology, albeit without significant histological or radiological contrasts, showcased a propitious avenue for combating degenerative disc afflictions.

Platelet-Rich Plasma (PRP)

In orthopaedic surgery, a surge of interest in autologous biological therapies is occuring. Central to these advances is platelet-rich plasma (PRP), but a plethora of commercial PRP preparation systems has raised doubts about PRP quality and uniformity. These uncertainties have led to inconsistent results in orthopedic and spinal procedures, creating ambiguity around PRP preparation and formulation standardization for distinct clinical scenarios. A limited number of systematic literature reviews on PRP technology exist, leaving several dimensions of personalized therapeutic protocols, including bioformulation, platelet dosage, angiogenesis, antimicrobial characteristics, and PRP's analgesic properties, unsettled in orthopedic surgery. Nonetheless, PRP has shown potential in arenas like tendon repair, bone restoration, spinal fusion augmentation [97], and enhanced results in major joint replacement procedures [98].

In vitro investigations into PRP's influence on osteoblasts (OB) and fibroblasts (FB) employed various PRP concentrations. Grazlami [99] examined primary human oral FBs and OBs under both activated and non-activated plasma conditions with PRP concentrations from 2.5-fold up to 4.2-5.5-fold. Cell proliferation was notably observed at the 24 and 72-hour marks. Increased secretion of osteocalcin (OCN), osteoprotegerin (OPG), and transforming growth factor beta1 (TGF-beta1) was also evident. Surprisingly, a 2.5-fold concentration was most effective, with higher levels diminishing cell growth. Additionally, PRP concentration hikes led to elevated OCN but reduced OPG levels at both observation points. The findings highlighted PRP's dose-dependent influence on oral FBs and OBs, emphasizing PRP's prospective *In vivo* role.

Recent clinical research by pain management and spinal surgery specialists has indicated PRP's potential utility alongside epidural steroid injections [100] and when combined with transforaminal endoscopic discectomy [101, 102]. A comprehensive literature search [103] emphasized PRP and epidural steroid injections in musculoskeletal and spinal ailments, revealing their synergistic anti-inflammatory and regenerative capabilities, extended pain relief durations, and potentially diminished requirements for recurring epidural steroid injections. Additionally, PRP's growth factors and cytokines have demonstrated abilities in tissue healing, fostering cellular growth, angiogenesis, and extracellular matrix development, ultimately contributing to heightened tissue recuperation. Moreover, PRP, in combination with epidural steroid injections, has indicated the potential for disc rejuvenation, alleviating pain, and enhancing functional recovery. Comprehensive reviews have indicated a favorable safety record for the combined treatment, suggesting a need for more extensive randomized trials to refine treatment protocols and elucidate underlying action mechanisms.

Utilizing PRISMA guidelines, a systematic review assessed intradiscal PRP injections' merit for degenerative discs, revealing significant clinical improvement [104]. An analysis of five articles (90 participants) indicated notable pain reduc-

tion post-lumbar intradiscal PRP injection, though the evidence's level (mainly level IV) precludes conclusive determinations on efficacy.

A subsequent meta-analysis [103] involving 13 studies (319 patients) highlighted PRP's analgesic potential for lumbar disc ailments. However, no evidence supported structural or functional improvements, suggesting a need for superior clinical studies.

After transforaminal endoscopic lumbar discectomy (TELD) for lumbar disc herniation (LDH), recurrences, often due to annulus fibrosus defects, are seldom. A case-control observational study evaluated PRP injections post-TELD in relation to disc remodeling and LDH recurrence rates. Of 108 patients, 51 received PRP injections, revealing marked improvements in pain scores and functional outcomes. MRI data also indicated greater disc recuperation and fewer LDH recurrences in the PRP cohort. This study underscores PRP's potential as an adjunct to TELD in mitigating LDH recurrence.

Autologous Bone Marrow Mesenchymal Stem Cells

The therapeutic efficacy and safety of bone marrow mesenchymal stem cells (BM-MSCs) in treating severe chronic low back pain and their anti-inflammatory, immunomodulatory, and regenerative properties have not been established through controlled studies. Other applications of BM-MSCs were tried in spinal fusion applications [105, 106]. However, spinal fusion applications of BM-MSCs are beyond the focus of this chapter on regenerative medicine applications for painful degenerative disc disease. A specific study aimed to assess the effectiveness of autologous BM-MSCs in patients with painful lumbar degenerative disc disease involving pain from adjacent structures [107]. This prospective, open-label, nonrandomized, parallel-controlled, 2-arm exploratory study conducted at an interventional pain management and regenerative medicine clinic involved administering a one-time injection of bone marrow concentrate into spinal structures, including discs, facets, spinal nerves, and sacroiliac joints, in addition to conventional treatment. The control group received standard treatment consisting of nonsteroidal anti-inflammatory drugs, over-the-counter drugs, structured exercise programs, physical therapy, spinal injections, and opioids. Oswestry Disability Index (ODI), Numeric Rating Scale (NRS-11), EuroQOL 5-Dimensional Questionnaire (EQ-5D-3L), Global Mental Health (GMH), and Global Physical Health (GPH) were used as primary outcome measures. In the study group, total nucleated cells, colony-forming units-fibroblast, CD34-positive cell numbers, and platelets were also recorded, along with post-procedure magnetic resonance imaging changes. Outcomes at 1, 3, 6, and 12 months showed significant improvement in functional status measured by ODI, pain relief measured by NRS-11, and other parameters measured by EQ-5-3L, GMH, and GPH, in the study group relative to the control group at all periods. The results showed significant improvements at 12-month follow-up, with 67% of the patients in the study group achieving minimal clinically significant difference (MCID) utilizing ODI compared to 8% in the control group. Greater than 2-point pain reduction was seen in 74% of the patients at three months, 66% at six months, and 56% at 12 months. Both MCID and pain relief of 2 points were significantly different compared to the control group. Opioid use decreased in the investigational group, whereas there was a slight increase in the control group. Age, gender, opioid use, and body mass index did not affect the outcomes in the stem cell group. While this study was limited by its execution in a single center, nonrandomized study with a risk of bias. The authors concluded that this first available controlled study, the simultaneous injection of BM-MSCs into multiple structures, including disc, facet joints, nerve roots, and sacroiliac joints based on clinical presentation, demonstrated the feasibility of the approach in patients with end-stage painful degenerative disc disease.

Another study also looked at using concentrated bone marrow aspirate (cBMA) to treat patients with painful degenerative disc disease. Wolf *et al.* injected cBMA intradiscally in 37 patients [108]. The pain was rated using the VAS, ODI, and SF-36 scores. Patients were dichotomized into two groups: 1) Group 1- pre-injection NRS > 5, and Group 2 - Pre-injection NRS ≤ 5. Significant VAS reductions were observed at the final one-year follow-up of 38.9%. Comparison between group 1 to group 2 patients showed a 44.4% VAS reduction in high-baseline-pain patients and 33.3% in low-baseline-pain patients. There were also significant ODI and SF-36 at a similar level. This study and earlier studies [109, 110] also corroborated the conclusion that intradiscal cBMA injections may be effective in reducing pain and improving function, particularly in patients with relatively higher initial pain may have the potential for the most significant improvement.

Current Evidence for Biologics in Clinical Management of Low Back Pain

Amid a myriad of experimental regenerative therapies examined *In vitro* at cellular, molecular, and genetic dimensions, substantial clinical corroboration advocating their utility in managing painful spinal conditions remains scarce. A pivotal systematic review by Navani *et al.* on behalf of the American Society of Interventional Pain Physicians (ASIPP) delineated guiding principles for the judicious application of such avant-garde technologies [57]. The investigatory methodology encompassed establishing explicit objectives and germane queries. A multidisciplinary expert consortium, hailing from diverse medical niches and geographical precincts, participated in sculpting crafting these guidelines, ensuring rigorous disclosure of potential conflicts of interest. The authors thoroughly reviewed the regenerative medicine literature, evaluating the potency, safety profile, and potential adverse events, culminating in a comprehensive synthesis of existing literature. The grading methodology utilized the criteria delineated by the Agency for Healthcare Research and Quality (AHRQ). In essence, the literature surrounding platelet-rich plasma (PRP) utilization, which encompasses a superior-grade randomized controlled trial (RCT), several intermediate-grade observational studies, a singular-arm meta-analysis, and systematic review data, is rated at Level III evidence. Concurrently, the evidence encompassing medicinal signaling/mesenchymal stem cell (MSCs) interventions, armed with a top-tier RCT, multiple mid-tier observational studies, a single-arm meta-analysis, and dual systematic reviews, is likewise classified as Level III. For lumbar epidural injections, the evidence caliber is pegged at Level IV, rooted in an elite RCT, several pertinent mid-level observational studies, and a singular-arm meta-analysis. Lumbar facet joint interventions, underpinned by an exemplary RCT and two intermediate observational studies, are accorded a Level IV evidence ranking. Sacroiliac joint interventions, fortified by a premier RCT, midgrade observational data, and a baseline case narrative, are also situated at Level IV evidence. The 2019 ASIPP directive underscores that prevailing clinical proof for intradiscal PRP and MSC injections nestles at Level III, whereas PRP injections into lumbar facet joints, lumbar epidurals, and sacroiliac joints are demarcated at Level IV.

The ASIPP advocates that before embarking on regenerative therapeutic avenues, there should be diagnostic substantiation underscoring the biological treatment's necessity. This should be predicated upon a profound discourse about patient aspirations, coupled with comprehensive patient education about the biological modalities, whilst meticulously evaluating the patient's holistic medical chronicle. Regenerative treatments can be orchestrated as standalone interventions or synergistically with other modalities, encompassing structured physiotherapeutic regimens, cognitive behavioral therapy, and conventional medical treatments, as mandated. Such therapies ought to augment entrenched conventional protocols, not supplant them. Physicians should be persistently cognizant of new developments, recalls, and directives disseminated by the Food and Drug Administration (FDA) and other regulatory bodies, ensuring a judicious approach to biological treatments, and recognizing inherent limitations.

CONCLUSION

Degenerative disc disease and the associated low back pain symptoms rank high on the priority list of conditions causing a global disease burden. However, clinical implementation for treating low back pain is limited. Several molecular, genetic, and cellular regenerative strategies are under investigation at a preclinical benchtop level. These innovative approaches aim to address the underlying causes of low back pain and promote tissue regeneration. Cellular therapies, including concentrated bone marrow aspirate (cBMA) or mesenchymal stem cells (MSCs), can potentially improve functional outcomes and reduce pain in patients with degenerative disc disease. Molecular interventions, such as growth factors or cytokines, are being explored to enhance tissue repair and modulate inflammatory responses. Advancements in genetic research have opened new avenues for personalized medicine, allowing targeted interventions based on an individual's genetic profile. Gene therapy approaches, including the delivery of therapeutic genes or gene editing techniques, offer exciting possibilities for promoting tissue regeneration and alleviating low back pain. While these regenerative strategies are still evolving, they provide a promising direction for developing effective and tailored treatments for low back pain. Continued research and clinical trials will further refine and optimize these strategies, ultimately improving patient outcomes and quality of life in individuals suffering from this debilitating condition.

REFERENCES

[1]   Mayer HM. Discogenic low back pain and degenerative lumbar spinal stenosis – how appropriate is surgical treatment? Schmerz 2001; 15(6): 484-91.
[http://dx.doi.org/10.1007/s004820100036] [PMID: 11793155]

[2]   Urban JPG, Fairbank JCT. Current perspectives on the role of biomechanical loading and genetics in development of disc degeneration and low back pain; a narrative review. J Biomech 2020; 102109573
[http://dx.doi.org/10.1016/j.jbiomech.2019.109573] [PMID: 32000991]

[3]   MacGregor AJ, Andrew T, Sambrook PN, Spector TD. Structural, psychological, and genetic influences on low back and neck pain: A study of adult female twins. Arthritis Care Res 2004; 51(2): 160-7.
[http://dx.doi.org/10.1002/art.20236] [PMID: 15077255]

[4]   Cooke PM, Lutz GE. Internal disc disruption and axial back pain in the athlete. Phys Med Rehabil Clin N Am 2000; 11(4): 837-65.
[http://dx.doi.org/10.1016/S1047-9651(18)30104-9] [PMID: 11092021]

[5]   Dreyer SJ, Dreyfuss PH. Low back pain and the zygapophysial (facet) joints. Arch Phys Med Rehabil 1996; 77(3): 290-300.
[http://dx.doi.org/10.1016/S0003-9993(96)90115-X] [PMID: 8600875]

[6]   Prescod K, Bedaysie H, Mahadeo S, Capildeo K. Lumbar spine synovial cysts. A case report and review of the literature. West Indian Med J 2002; 51(3): 181-3.
[PMID: 12501549]

[7]   Bydon M, Alvi MA, Goyal A. Degenerative Lumbar Spondylolisthesis. Neurosurg Clin N Am 2019; 30(3): 299-304.
[http://dx.doi.org/10.1016/j.nec.2019.02.003] [PMID: 31078230]

[8]   Germon T, Ahuja S, Casey ATH, Todd NV, Rai A. British Association of Spine Surgeons standards of care for cauda equina syndrome. Spine J 2015; 15(3) (Suppl.): S2-4.
[http://dx.doi.org/10.1016/j.spinee.2015.01.006] [PMID: 25708139]

[9]   Srikandarajah N, Boissaud-Cooke MA, Clark S, Wilby MJ. Does early surgical decompression in cauda equina syndrome improve bladder outcome? Spine 2015; 40(8): 580-3.
[http://dx.doi.org/10.1097/BRS.0000000000000813] [PMID: 25646751]

[10]   Li X, Dou Q, Hu S, *et al.* Treatment of cauda equina syndrome caused by lumbar disc herniation with percutaneous endoscopic lumbar discectomy. Acta Neurol Belg 2016; 116(2): 185-90.
[http://dx.doi.org/10.1007/s13760-015-0530-0] [PMID: 26292929]

[11]   Raad M, Donaldson CJ, El Dafrawy MH, *et al.* Trends in isolated lumbar spinal stenosis surgery among working US adults aged 40–64 years, 2010–2014. J Neurosurg Spine 2018; 29(2): 169-75.
[http://dx.doi.org/10.3171/2018.1.SPINE17964] [PMID: 29799337]

[12]   Ziino C, Mertz K, Hu S, Kamal R. Decompression With or Without Fusion for Lumbar Stenosis. Spine 2020; 45(5): 325-32.
[http://dx.doi.org/10.1097/BRS.0000000000003250] [PMID: 32045402]

[13]   Bouknaitir JB, Carreon LY, Brorson S, Pedersen CF, Andersen MØ. Wide Laminectomy, Segmental Bilateral Laminotomies, or Unilateral Hemi-Laminectomy for Lumbar Spinal Stenosis. Spine 2021; 46(21): 1509-15.
[http://dx.doi.org/10.1097/BRS.0000000000004043] [PMID: 34618710]

[14]   Katz JN, Zimmerman ZE, Mass H, Makhni MC. Diagnosis and Management of Lumbar Spinal Stenosis. JAMA 2022; 327(17): 1688-99.
[http://dx.doi.org/10.1001/jama.2022.5921] [PMID: 35503342]

[15]   Blumenthal S, McAfee PC, Guyer RD, *et al.* A prospective, randomized, multicenter Food and Drug Administration investigational device exemptions study of lumbar total disc replacement with the CHARITE artificial disc versus lumbar fusion: part I: evaluation of clinical outcomes. Spine 2005;

30(14): 1565-75.
[http://dx.doi.org/10.1097/01.brs.0000170587.32676.0e] [PMID: 16025024]

[16]   Delamarter R, Zigler JE, Balderston RA, Cammisa FP, Goldstein JA, Spivak JM. Prospective, randomized, multicenter Food and Drug Administration investigational device exemption study of the ProDisc-L total disc replacement compared with circumferential arthrodesis for the treatment of two-level lumbar degenerative disc disease: results at twenty-four months. J Bone Joint Surg Am 2011; 93(8): 705-15.
[http://dx.doi.org/10.2106/JBJS.I.00680] [PMID: 21398574]

[17]   Jin D, Qu D, Zhao L, Chen J, Jiang J. Prosthetic disc nucleus (PDN) replacement for lumbar disc herniation: preliminary report with six months' follow-up. J Spinal Disord Tech 2003; 16(4): 331-7.
[http://dx.doi.org/10.1097/00024720-200308000-00004] [PMID: 12902948]

[18]   Shim CS, Lee SH, Park CW, *et al*. Partial disc replacement with the PDN prosthetic disc nucleus device: early clinical results. J Spinal Disord Tech 2003; 16(4): 324-30.
[http://dx.doi.org/10.1097/00024720-200308000-00003] [PMID: 12902947]

[19]   Wilke HJ, Heuer F, Neidlinger-Wilke C, Claes L. Is a collagen scaffold for a tissue engineered nucleus replacement capable of restoring disc height and stability in an animal model? Eur Spine J 2006; 15(Suppl 3): S433-8.
[http://dx.doi.org/10.1007/s00586-006-0177-x]

[20]   Ahrens M, Tsantrizos A, Donkersloot P, *et al*. Nucleus replacement with the DASCOR disc arthroplasty device: interim two-year efficacy and safety results from two prospective, non-randomized multicenter European studies. Spine 2009; 34(13): 1376-84.
[http://dx.doi.org/10.1097/BRS.0b013e3181a3967f] [PMID: 19440167]

[21]   Zhang Z, Zhao L, Qu D, Jin D. Artificial nucleus replacement: surgical and clinical experience. Orthop Surg 2009; 1(1): 52-7.
[http://dx.doi.org/10.1111/j.1757-7861.2008.00010.x] [PMID: 22009782]

[22]   Reitmaier S, Wolfram U, Ignatius A, *et al*. Hydrogels for nucleus replacement—Facing the biomechanical challenge. J Mech Behav Biomed Mater 2012; 14: 67-77.
[http://dx.doi.org/10.1016/j.jmbbm.2012.05.010] [PMID: 22963748]

[23]   Pimenta L, Marchi L, Oliveira L, Nogueira-Neto J, Coutinho E, Amaral R. Elastomeric Lumbar Total Disc Replacement: Clinical and Radiological Results With Minimum 84 Months Follow-Up. Int J Spine Surg 2018; 12(1): 49-57.
[http://dx.doi.org/10.14444/5009] [PMID: 30280083]

[24]   Zengerle L, Köhler A, Debout E, Hackenbroch C, Wilke HJ. Nucleus replacement could get a new chance with annulus closure. Eur Spine J 2020; 29(7): 1733-41.
[http://dx.doi.org/10.1007/s00586-020-06419-2] [PMID: 32333186]

[25]   Deyo RA, Mirza SK, Martin BI, Kreuter W, Goodman DC, Jarvik JG. Trends, major medical complications, and charges associated with surgery for lumbar spinal stenosis in older adults. JAMA 2010; 303(13): 1259-65.
[http://dx.doi.org/10.1001/jama.2010.338] [PMID: 20371784]

[26]   Wang MY, Cummock MD, Yu Y, Trivedi RA. An analysis of the differences in the acute hospitalization charges following minimally invasive versus open posterior lumbar interbody fusion. J Neurosurg Spine 2010; 12(6): 694-9.
[http://dx.doi.org/10.3171/2009.12.SPINE09621] [PMID: 20515357]

[27]   Patel AA, Zfass-Mendez M, Lebwohl NH, *et al*. Minimally Invasive Versus Open Lumbar Fusion: A Comparison of Blood Loss, Surgical Complications, and Hospital Course. Iowa Orthop J 2015; 35: 130-4.
[PMID: 26361455]

[28]   Costa F, Alves OL, Anania CD, Zileli M, Fornari M. Decompressive Surgery for Lumbar Spinal Stenosis: WFNS Spine Committee Recommendations. World Neurosurg X 2020; 7100076

[http://dx.doi.org/10.1016/j.wnsx.2020.100076] [PMID: 32613189]

[29] O'Toole JE, Eichholz KM, Fessler RG. Surgical site infection rates after minimally invasive spinal surgery. J Neurosurg Spine 2009; 11(4): 471-6.
[http://dx.doi.org/10.3171/2009.5.SPINE08633] [PMID: 19929344]

[30] Smith JS, Shaffrey CI, Sansur CA, *et al.* Rates of infection after spine surgery based on 108,419 procedures: a report from the Scoliosis Research Society Morbidity and Mortality Committee. Spine 2011; 36(7): 556-63.
[http://dx.doi.org/10.1097/BRS.0b013e3181eadd41] [PMID: 21192288]

[31] Ramirez LF, Thisted R. Complications and demographic characteristics of patients undergoing lumbar discectomy in community hospitals. Neurosurgery 1989; 25(2): 226-31.
[http://dx.doi.org/10.1227/00006123-198908000-00012] [PMID: 2770987]

[32] Samudrala S, Khoo LT, Rhim SC, Fessler RG. Complications during anterior surgery of the lumbar spine: an anatomically based study and review. Neurosurg Focus 1999; 7(6)E11
[http://dx.doi.org/10.3171/foc.1999.7.6.12] [PMID: 16918208]

[33] Tay BBK, Berven S, Pascuzzi RM, Roos KL, Engstrom JW. Indications, techniques, and complications of lumbar interbody fusion. Semin Neurol 2002; 22(2): 221-30.
[http://dx.doi.org/10.1055/s-2002-36545] [PMID: 12524567]

[34] Kraemer R, Wild A, Haak H, Herdmann J, Krauspe R, Kraemer J. Classification and management of early complications in open lumbar microdiscectomy. Eur Spine J 2003; 12(3): 239-46.
[http://dx.doi.org/10.1007/s00586-002-0466-y] [PMID: 12799998]

[35] McLain RF, Bell GR, Kalfas I, Tetzlaff JE, Yoon HJ. Complications associated with lumbar laminectomy: a comparison of spinal versus general anesthesia. Spine 2004; 29(22): 2542-7.
[http://dx.doi.org/10.1097/01.brs.0000144834.43115.38] [PMID: 15543071]

[36] Ahn Y, Lee HY, Lee SH, Lee JH. Dural tears in percutaneous endoscopic lumbar discectomy. Eur Spine J 2011; 20(1): 58-64.
[http://dx.doi.org/10.1007/s00586-010-1493-8] [PMID: 20582555]

[37] Phan K, Maharaj M, Assem Y, Mobbs RJ. Review of early clinical results and complications associated with oblique lumbar interbody fusion (OLIF). J Clin Neurosci 2016; 31: 23-9.
[http://dx.doi.org/10.1016/j.jocn.2016.02.030] [PMID: 27349468]

[38] Imajo Y, Taguchi T, Neo M, *et al.* Complications of spinal surgery for elderly patients with lumbar spinal stenosis in a super-aging country: An analysis of 8033 patients. J Orthop Sci 2017; 22(1): 10-5.
[http://dx.doi.org/10.1016/j.jos.2016.08.014] [PMID: 27646205]

[39] Machado GC, Maher CG, Ferreira PH, *et al.* Trends, Complications, and Costs for Hospital Admission and Surgery for Lumbar Spinal Stenosis. Spine 2017; 42(22): 1737-43.
[http://dx.doi.org/10.1097/BRS.0000000000002207] [PMID: 28441309]

[40] Lewandrowski KU. Incidence, Management, and Cost of Complications After Transforaminal Endoscopic Decompression Surgery for Lumbar Foraminal and Lateral Recess Stenosis: A Value Proposition for Outpatient Ambulatory Surgery. Int J Spine Surg 2019; 13(1): 53-67.
[http://dx.doi.org/10.14444/6008] [PMID: 30805287]

[41] Strömqvist F, Sigmundsson FG, Strömqvist B, Jönsson B, Karlsson MK. Incidental durotomy in degenerative lumbar spine surgery – a register study of 64,431 operations. Spine J 2019; 19(4): 624-30.
[http://dx.doi.org/10.1016/j.spinee.2018.08.012] [PMID: 30172899]

[42] Rosas S, Knio ZO, Gowd AK, Luo TD, Emory CL, O'Gara TJ. Cost and Complications of Single-Level Lumbar Decompression in Those Over and Under 75. Spine 2021; 46(1): 29-34.
[http://dx.doi.org/10.1097/BRS.0000000000003686] [PMID: 32925688]

[43] Yeung A, Roberts A, Zhu L, Qi L, Zhang J, Lewandrowski KU. Treatment of Soft Tissue and Bony Spinal Stenosis by a Visualized Endoscopic Transforaminal Technique Under Local Anesthesia.

Neurospine 2019; 16(1): 52-62.
[http://dx.doi.org/10.14245/ns.1938038.019] [PMID: 30943707]

[44]   Kim CH, Chung CK, Park CS, Choi B, Kim MJ, Park BJ. Reoperation rate after surgery for lumbar herniated intervertebral disc disease: nationwide cohort study. Spine 2013; 38(7): 581-90.
[http://dx.doi.org/10.1097/BRS.0b013e318274f9a7] [PMID: 23023591]

[45]   Heindel P, Tuchman A, Hsieh PC, *et al.* Reoperation Rates After Single-level Lumbar Discectomy. Spine 2017; 42(8): E496-501.
[http://dx.doi.org/10.1097/BRS.0000000000001855] [PMID: 27548580]

[46]   Fjeld OR, Grøvle L, Helgeland J, *et al.* Complications, reoperations, readmissions, and length of hospital stay in 34 639 surgical cases of lumbar disc herniation. Bone Joint J 2019; 101-B(4): 470-7.
[http://dx.doi.org/10.1302/0301-620X.101B4.BJJ-2018-1184.R1] [PMID: 30929479]

[47]   Lee CS, Hwang CJ, Lee SW, *et al.* Risk factors for adjacent segment disease after lumbar fusion. Eur Spine J 2009; 18(11): 1637-43.
[http://dx.doi.org/10.1007/s00586-009-1060-3] [PMID: 19533182]

[48]   Yee TJ, Terman SW, La Marca F, Park P. Comparison of adjacent segment disease after minimally invasive or open transforaminal lumbar interbody fusion. J Clin Neurosci 2014; 21(10): 1796-801.
[http://dx.doi.org/10.1016/j.jocn.2014.03.010] [PMID: 24880486]

[49]   Li XC, Huang CM, Zhong CF, Liang RW, Luo SJ. Minimally invasive procedure reduces adjacent segment degeneration and disease: New benefit-based global meta-analysis. PLoS One 2017; 12(2)e0171546
[http://dx.doi.org/10.1371/journal.pone.0171546] [PMID: 28207762]

[50]   Sakti YM, Mafaza A, Lanodiyu ZA, Sakadewa GP, Magetsari R. Management of distal adjacent segment disease due to central subsidence of PLIF using local anesthetic transforaminal foraminotomy and lumbar discectomy. Int J Surg Case Rep 2020; 77: 269-75.
[http://dx.doi.org/10.1016/j.ijscr.2020.10.089] [PMID: 33189009]

[51]   Mullin BB, Rea GL, Irsik R, Catton M, Miner ME. The effect of postlaminectomy spinal instability on the outcome of lumbar spinal stenosis patients. J Spinal Disord 1996; 9(2): 107-16.
[http://dx.doi.org/10.1097/00002517-199604000-00004] [PMID: 8793776]

[52]   Olivares OB, Carrasco MV, Pinto GI, Tonda FN, Riera Martínez JA, González AS. Preoperative and Postoperative Sagittal Alignment and Compensatory Mechanisms in Patients With Posttraumatic Thoracolumbar Deformities Who Undergo Corrective Surgeries. Int J Spine Surg 2021; 15(3): 585-90.
[http://dx.doi.org/10.14444/8079] [PMID: 33963023]

[53]   Yeung A, Lewandrowski KU. Early and staged endoscopic management of common pain generators in the spine. J Spine Surg 2020; 6(S1) (Suppl. 1): S1-5.
[http://dx.doi.org/10.21037/jss.2019.09.03] [PMID: 32195407]

[54]   Gou S, Oxentenko SC, Eldrige JS, *et al.* Stem cell therapy for intervertebral disk regeneration. Am J Phys Med Rehabil 2014; 93(11) (Suppl. 3): S122-31.
[http://dx.doi.org/10.1097/PHM.0000000000000152] [PMID: 25122106]

[55]   Pettine KA, Suzuki RK, Sand TT, Murphy MB. Autologous bone marrow concentrate intradiscal injection for the treatment of degenerative disc disease with three-year follow-up. Int Orthop 2017; 41(10): 2097-103.
[http://dx.doi.org/10.1007/s00264-017-3560-9] [PMID: 28748380]

[56]   Sanapati J, Manchikanti L, Atluri S, *et al.* Do Regenerative Medicine Therapies Provide Long-Term Relief in Chronic Low Back Pain: A Systematic Review and Metaanalysis. Pain Physician 2018; 21(6): 515-40.
[PMID: 30508983]

[57]   Navani A, Manchikanti L, Albers SL, *et al.* Responsible, Safe, and Effective Use of Biologics in the Management of Low Back Pain: American Society of Interventional Pain Physicians (ASIPP)

Guidelines. Pain Physician 2019; 22(1S): S1-S74.
[PMID: 30717500]

[58]   Tavakoli J, Diwan AD, Tipper JL. Advanced Strategies for the Regeneration of Lumbar Disc Annulus Fibrosus. Int J Mol Sci 2020; 21(14): 4889.
[http://dx.doi.org/10.3390/ijms21144889] [PMID: 32664453]

[59]   Lutz C, Cheng J, Prysak M, Zukofsky T, Rothman R, Lutz G. Clinical outcomes following intradiscal injections of higher-concentration platelet-rich plasma in patients with chronic lumbar discogenic pain. Int Orthop 2022; 46(6): 1381-5.
[http://dx.doi.org/10.1007/s00264-022-05389-y] [PMID: 35344055]

[60]   Lewandrowski KU, Ransom NA. Five-year clinical outcomes with endoscopic transforaminal outside-in foraminoplasty techniques for symptomatic degenerative conditions of the lumbar spine. J Spine Surg 2020; 6(S1) (Suppl. 1): S54-65.
[http://dx.doi.org/10.21037/jss.2019.07.03] [PMID: 32195416]

[61]   Yeung A, Lewandrowski KU. Five-year clinical outcomes with endoscopic transforaminal foraminoplasty for symptomatic degenerative conditions of the lumbar spine: a comparative study of *inside-out* versus *outside-in* techniques. J Spine Surg 2020; 6(S1) (Suppl. 1): S66-83.
[http://dx.doi.org/10.21037/jss.2019.06.08] [PMID: 32195417]

[62]   Jarebi M, Awaf A, Lefranc M, Peltier J. A matched comparison of outcomes between percutaneous endoscopic lumbar discectomy and open lumbar microdiscectomy for the treatment of lumbar disc herniation: a 2-year retrospective cohort study. Spine J 2021; 21(1): 114-21.
[http://dx.doi.org/10.1016/j.spinee.2020.07.005] [PMID: 32683107]

[63]   Wu PH, Kim HS, Jang IT. Intervertebral Disc Diseases PART 2: A Review of the Current Diagnostic and Treatment Strategies for Intervertebral Disc Disease. Int J Mol Sci 2020; 21(6): 2135.
[http://dx.doi.org/10.3390/ijms21062135] [PMID: 32244936]

[64]   Paliwal S, Chaudhuri R, Agrawal A, Mohanty S. Regenerative abilities of mesenchymal stem cells through mitochondrial transfer. J Biomed Sci 2018; 25(1): 31.
[http://dx.doi.org/10.1186/s12929-018-0429-1] [PMID: 29602309]

[65]   Driscoll T, Jacklyn G, Orchard J, *et al.* The global burden of occupationally related low back pain: estimates from the Global Burden of Disease 2010 study. Ann Rheum Dis 2014; 73(6): 975-81.
[http://dx.doi.org/10.1136/annrheumdis-2013-204631] [PMID: 24665117]

[66]   Hoy D, March L, Brooks P, *et al.* The global burden of low back pain: estimates from the Global Burden of Disease 2010 study. Ann Rheum Dis 2014; 73(6): 968-74.
[http://dx.doi.org/10.1136/annrheumdis-2013-204428] [PMID: 24665116]

[67]   Vos T, Lim SS, Abbafati C, *et al.* Global burden of 369 diseases and injuries in 204 countries and territories, 1990–2019: a systematic analysis for the Global Burden of Disease Study 2019. Lancet 2020; 396(10258): 1204-22.
[http://dx.doi.org/10.1016/S0140-6736(20)30925-9] [PMID: 33069326]

[68]   Safiri S, Kolahi AA, Smith E, *et al.* Global, regional and national burden of osteoarthritis 1990-2017: a systematic analysis of the Global Burden of Disease Study 2017. Ann Rheum Dis 2020; 79(6): 819-28.
[http://dx.doi.org/10.1136/annrheumdis-2019-216515] [PMID: 32398285]

[69]   Díez FJ, Mira J, Iturralde E, Zubillaga S. DIAVAL, a Bayesian expert system for echocardiography. Artif Intell Med 1997; 10(1): 59-73.
[http://dx.doi.org/10.1016/S0933-3657(97)00384-9] [PMID: 9177816]

[70]   Haagsma JA, Maertens de Noordhout C, Polinder S, *et al.* Assessing disability weights based on the responses of 30,660 people from four European countries. Popul Health Metr 2015; 13(1): 10.
[http://dx.doi.org/10.1186/s12963-015-0042-4] [PMID: 26778920]

[71]   Kim HS, Wu PH, Jang IT. Lumbar Degenerative Disease Part 1: Anatomy and Pathophysiology of Intervertebral Discogenic Pain and Radiofrequency Ablation of Basivertebral and Sinuvertebral Nerve

Treatment for Chronic Discogenic Back Pain: A Prospective Case Series and Review of Literature. Int J Mol Sci 2020; 21(4): 1483.
[http://dx.doi.org/10.3390/ijms21041483] [PMID: 32098249]

[72]   Macnab I, St Louis EL, Grabias SL, Jacob R. Selective ascending lumbosacral venography in the assessment of lumbar-disc herniation. An anatomical study and clinical experience. J Bone Joint Surg Am 1976; 58(8): 1093-8.
[http://dx.doi.org/10.2106/00004623-197658080-00009] [PMID: 794071]

[73]   Griepp RB, Ergin MA, Galla JD, *et al.* Surgery for acquired heart disease looking for the artery of adamkiewicz: A quest to minimize paraplegia after operations for aneurysms of the descending thoracic and thoracoabdominal aorta. J Thorac Cardiovasc Surg 1996; 112(5): 1202-15.
[http://dx.doi.org/10.1016/S0022-5223(96)70133-2] [PMID: 8911316]

[74]   Charles YP, Barbe B, Beaujeux R, Boujan F, Steib JP. Relevance of the anatomical location of the Adamkiewicz artery in spine surgery. Surg Radiol Anat 2011; 33(1): 3-9.
[http://dx.doi.org/10.1007/s00276-010-0654-0] [PMID: 20589376]

[75]   Kim JW, Jeon N, Shin DE, *et al.* Regeneration in Spinal Disease: Therapeutic Role of Hypoxia-Inducible Factor-1 Alpha in Regeneration of Degenerative Intervertebral Disc. Int J Mol Sci 2021; 22(10): 5281.
[http://dx.doi.org/10.3390/ijms22105281] [PMID: 34067899]

[76]   Kirkaldy-Willis WH, Farfan HF. Instability of the lumbar spine. Clin Orthop Relat Res 1982; (165): 110-23.
[PMID: 6210480]

[77]   Keim HA, Kirkaldy-Willis WH. Low back pain. Clin Symp 1987; 39(6): 1-32.
[PMID: 2963721]

[78]   Lewandrowski KU, León JFR, Yeung A. Use of "Inside-Out" Technique for Direct Visualization of a Vacuum Vertically Unstable Intervertebral Disc During Routine Lumbar Endoscopic Transforaminal Decompression—A Correlative Study of Clinical Outcomes and the Prognostic Value of Lumbar Radiographs. Int J Spine Surg 2019; 13(5): 399-414.
[http://dx.doi.org/10.14444/6055] [PMID: 31741829]

[79]   Lewandrowski KU, Zhang X, Ramírez León JF, Teixeira de Carvalho PS, Hellinger S, Yeung A. Lumbar vacuum disc, vertical instability, standalone endoscopic interbody fusion, and other treatments: an opinion based survey among minimally invasive spinal surgeons. J Spine Surg 2020; 6(S1) (Suppl. 1): S165-78.
[http://dx.doi.org/10.21037/jss.2019.11.02] [PMID: 32195425]

[80]   Goudman L, Marinazzo D, Van de Steen F, *et al.* The influence of nociceptive and neuropathic pain states on the processing of acute electrical nociceptive stimulation: A dynamic causal modeling study. Brain Res 2020; 1733146728
[http://dx.doi.org/10.1016/j.brainres.2020.146728] [PMID: 32067965]

[81]   Antonacci MD, Mody DR, Heggeness MH. Innervation of the human vertebral body: a histologic study. J Spinal Disord 1998; 11(6): 526-31.
[http://dx.doi.org/10.1097/00002517-199812000-00013] [PMID: 9884299]

[82]   Becker S, Hadjipavlou A, Heggeness MH. Ablation of the basivertebral nerve for treatment of back pain: a clinical study. Spine J 2017; 17(2): 218-23.
[http://dx.doi.org/10.1016/j.spinee.2016.08.032] [PMID: 27592808]

[83]   Fischgrund JS, Rhyne A, Franke J, *et al.* Intraosseous basivertebral nerve ablation for the treatment of chronic low back pain: a prospective randomized double-blind sham-controlled multi-center study. Eur Spine J 2018; 27(5): 1146-56.
[http://dx.doi.org/10.1007/s00586-018-5496-1] [PMID: 29423885]

[84]   Fischgrund JS, Rhyne A, Franke J, *et al.* Intraosseous Basivertebral Nerve Ablation for the Treatment of Chronic Low Back Pain: 2-Year Results From a Prospective Randomized Double-Blind Sham-

Controlled Multicenter Study. Int J Spine Surg 2019; 13(2): 110-9.
[http://dx.doi.org/10.14444/6015] [PMID: 31131209]

[85] Khalil JG, Smuck M, Koreckij T, *et al.* A prospective, randomized, multicenter study of intraosseous basivertebral nerve ablation for the treatment of chronic low back pain. Spine J 2019; 19(10): 1620-32.
[http://dx.doi.org/10.1016/j.spinee.2019.05.598] [PMID: 31229663]

[86] Wong DA. Basivertebral nerve ablation: does the path followed suggest this technology is ready for adoption into clinical practice?: COMMENTARY ON: Khalil J et al. A prospective, randomized, multicenter study of intraosseous basivertebral nerve ablation for the treatment of chronic low back pain. SpineJ 2019; 10(10): 1620-32.
[http://dx.doi.org/10.1016/j.spinee.2019.05.598]

[87] Lorio M, Clerk-Lamalice O, Rivera M, Lewandrowski KU. ISASS Policy Statement 2022: Literature Review of Intraosseous Basivertebral Nerve Ablation. Int J Spine Surg 2022; 16(6): 1084-94.
[http://dx.doi.org/10.14444/8362] [PMID: 36266051]

[88] Le Maitre CL, Freemont AJ, Hoyland JA. Localization of degradative enzymes and their inhibitors in the degenerate human intervertebral disc. J Pathol 2004; 204(1): 47-54.
[http://dx.doi.org/10.1002/path.1608] [PMID: 15307137]

[89] Kepler CK, Markova DZ, Dibra F, *et al.* Expression and relationship of proinflammatory chemokine RANTES/CCL5 and cytokine IL-1β in painful human intervertebral discs. Spine 2013; 38(11): 873-80.
[http://dx.doi.org/10.1097/BRS.0b013e318285ae08] [PMID: 23660804]

[90] Yurube T, Hirata H, Ito M, *et al.* Involvement of Autophagy in Rat Tail Static Compression-Induced Intervertebral Disc Degeneration and Notochordal Cell Disappearance. Int J Mol Sci 2021; 22(11): 5648.
[http://dx.doi.org/10.3390/ijms22115648] [PMID: 34073333]

[91] Calió M, Gantenbein B, Egli M, Poveda L, Ille F. The Cellular Composition of Bovine Coccygeal Intervertebral Discs: A Comprehensive Single-Cell RNAseq Analysis. Int J Mol Sci 2021; 22(9): 4917.
[http://dx.doi.org/10.3390/ijms22094917] [PMID: 34066404]

[92] Yurube T, Han I, Sakai D. Concepts of Regeneration for Spinal Diseases in 2021. Int J Mol Sci 2021; 22(16): 8356.
[http://dx.doi.org/10.3390/ijms22168356] [PMID: 34445063]

[93] Ito M, Yurube T, Kanda Y, *et al.* Inhibition of Autophagy at Different Stages by ATG5 Knockdown and Chloroquine Supplementation Enhances Consistent Human Disc Cellular Apoptosis and Senescence Induction rather than Extracellular Matrix Catabolism. Int J Mol Sci 2021; 22(8): 3965.
[http://dx.doi.org/10.3390/ijms22083965] [PMID: 33921398]

[94] Takeoka Y, Paladugu P, Kang JD, Mizuno S. Augmented Chondroitin Sulfate Proteoglycan Has Therapeutic Potential for Intervertebral Disc Degeneration by Stimulating Anabolic Turnover in Bovine Nucleus Pulposus Cells under Changes in Hydrostatic Pressure. Int J Mol Sci 2021; 22(11): 6015.
[http://dx.doi.org/10.3390/ijms22116015] [PMID: 34199496]

[95] Croft AS, Illien-Jünger S, Grad S, Guerrero J, Wangler S, Gantenbein B. The Application of Mesenchymal Stromal Cells and Their Homing Capabilities to Regenerate the Intervertebral Disc. Int J Mol Sci 2021; 22(7): 3519.
[http://dx.doi.org/10.3390/ijms22073519] [PMID: 33805356]

[96] Friedmann A, Baertel A, Schmitt C, *et al.* Intervertebral Disc Regeneration Injection of a Cell-Loaded Collagen Hydrogel in a Sheep Model. Int J Mol Sci 2021; 22(8): 4248.
[http://dx.doi.org/10.3390/ijms22084248] [PMID: 33921913]

[97] Shehadi J, Elzein S, Beery P, Spalding MC, Pershing M. Combined administration of platelet rich plasma and autologous bone marrow aspirate concentrate for spinal cord injury: a descriptive case

series. Neural Regen Res 2021; 16(2): 362-6.
[http://dx.doi.org/10.4103/1673-5374.290903] [PMID: 32859799]

[98]   Everts PA, van Erp A, DeSimone A, Cohen DS, Gardner RD. Platelet Rich Plasma in Orthopedic Surgical Medicine. Platelets 2021; 32(2): 163-74.
[http://dx.doi.org/10.1080/09537104.2020.1869717] [PMID: 33400591]

[99]   Graziani F, Ivanovski S, Cei S, Ducci F, Tonetti M, Gabriele M. The *in vitro* effect of different PRP concentrations on osteoblasts and fibroblasts. Clin Oral Implants Res 2006; 17(2): 212-9.
[http://dx.doi.org/10.1111/j.1600-0501.2005.01203.x] [PMID: 16584418]

[100]   Xu Z, Wu S, Li X, Liu C, Fan S, Ma C. Ultrasound-Guided Transforaminal Injections of Platelet-Rich Plasma Compared with Steroid in Lumbar Disc Herniation: A Prospective, Randomized, Controlled Study. Neural Plast 2021; 2021: 1-11.
[http://dx.doi.org/10.1155/2021/5558138] [PMID: 34135954]

[101]   Jiang Y, Zuo R, Yuan S, *et al.* Transforaminal Endoscopic Lumbar Discectomy with versus without Platelet-Rich Plasma Injection for Lumbar Disc Herniation: A Prospective Cohort Study. Pain Res Manag 2022; 2022: 1-9.
[http://dx.doi.org/10.1155/2022/6181478] [PMID: 35296040]

[102]   Le VT, Nguyen Dao LT, Nguyen AM. Transforaminal injection with autologous platelet-rich plasma in lumbar disc herniation: A single-center prospective study in Vietnam. Asian J Surg 2022.
[PMID: 35637114]

[103]   Muthu S, Jeyaraman M, Chellamuthu G, Jeyaraman N, Jain R, Khanna M. Does the Intradiscal Injection of Platelet Rich Plasma Have Any Beneficial Role in the Management of Lumbar Disc Disease? Global Spine J 2022; 12(3): 503-14.
[http://dx.doi.org/10.1177/2192568221998367] [PMID: 33840260]

[104]   Hirase T, Jack RA II, Sochacki KR, Harris JD, Weiner BK. Systemic Review: Is an Intradiscal Injection of Platelet-Rich Plasma for Lumbar Disc Degeneration Effective? Cureus 2020; 12(6)e8831
[http://dx.doi.org/10.7759/cureus.8831] [PMID: 32607308]

[105]   Blanco JF, Villarón EM, Pescador D, *et al.* Autologous mesenchymal stromal cells embedded in tricalcium phosphate for posterolateral spinal fusion: results of a prospective phase I/II clinical trial with long-term follow-up. Stem Cell Res Ther 2019; 10(1): 63.
[http://dx.doi.org/10.1186/s13287-019-1166-4] [PMID: 30795797]

[106]   Ichiyanagi T, Anabuki K, Nishijima Y, Ono H. Isolation of mesenchymal stem cells from bone marrow wastes of spinal fusion procedure (TLIF) for low back pain patients and preparation of bone dusts for transplantable autologous bone graft with a serum glue. Biosci Trends 2010; 4(3): 110-8.
[PMID: 20592461]

[107]   Atluri S, Murphy MB, Dragella R, *et al.* Evaluation of the Effectiveness of Autologous Bone Marrow Mesenchymal Stem Cells in the Treatment of Chronic Low Back Pain Due to Severe Lumbar Spinal Degeneration: A 12-Month, Open-Label, Prospective Controlled Trial. Pain Physician 2022; 25(2): 193-207.
[PMID: 35322978]

[108]   Wolff M, Shillington JM, Rathbone C, Piasecki SK, Barnes B. Injections of concentrated bone marrow aspirate as treatment for Discogenic pain: a retrospective analysis. BMC Musculoskelet Disord 2020; 21(1): 135.
[http://dx.doi.org/10.1186/s12891-020-3126-7] [PMID: 32111220]

[109] Pettine K, Suzuki R, Sand T, Murphy M. Treatment of discogenic back pain with autologous bone marrow concentrate injection with minimum two year follow-up. Int Orthop 2016; 40(1): 135-40.
[http://dx.doi.org/10.1007/s00264-015-2886-4] [PMID: 26156727]

[110] Pettine KA, Murphy MB, Suzuki RK, Sand TT. Percutaneous injection of autologous bone marrow concentrate cells significantly reduces lumbar discogenic pain through 12 months. Stem Cells 2015; 33(1): 146-56.
[http://dx.doi.org/10.1002/stem.1845] [PMID: 25187512]

CHAPTER 4

Current Bioengineering Strategies for Injured or Degenerative Intervertebral Discs

Alvaro Dowling[1,*] and **Marcelo Molina**[2]

[1] *Orthopaedic Spine Surgeon, Director of Endoscopic Spine Clinic, Santiago, Chile*

[2] *Department of Orthopaedic Surgery, Faculdade de Medicina de Ribeirão Preto - USP (School of Medicine of Ribeirão Preto - University of São Paulo), Ribeirão Preto, SP, Brazil*

Abstract: The functionality of the intervertebral disc can be compromised due to aging and injuries. Synthetic and composite materials are investigated for disc repair to reduce pain. Synthetic materials or composite implants lack interaction with the disc's biological components and have yet to gain widespread usage or achieve desirable outcomes in treating intervertebral disc disorders. This chapter examines bioengineering approaches to disc repair, including cell-enhanced materials or biologically derived acellular materials that allow for cellular interactions and remodeling within the intervertebral disc. While still in its early stages, bioengineering techniques utilizing innovative biomaterials are showing promise as potential alternatives for the clinical treatment of intervertebral disc disorders.

Keywords: Annulus fibrosus, Disc degeneration, Degenerative disc disease, Fusion, Herniation, Intervertebral disc, Nucleus pulposus, Spine.

INTRODUCTION

The intervertebral disc (IVD) has historically been implicated in dorsalgia and has consequently undergone rigorous scientific scrutiny for the innovation of novel therapeutic modalities. The degenerative cascade within the IVD encompasses proteoglycan diminution, aberrations in extracellular matrix topography, annular fissures, formation of extruded discal fragments, and decrement in discal elevation [1 - 4]. Such morphological perturbations can culminate in radicular nerve encroachment, spinal canal stenosis, and facet joint infringement, thereby manifesting as nociceptive experiences and neurological insufficiencies [5, 6]. Additionally, the inflammatory microenvironment and neoinnervation observed within compromised discs have been postulated as etiological agents of discogenic dorsalgia [7]. Consequently, the multifaceted genesis of discogenic

---
***** **Corresponding author: Álvaro Dowling:** Orthopaedic Spine Surgeon, Director of Endoscopic Spine Clinic, Santiago, Chile; E-mail: adowling@dws.cl

Kai-Uwe Lewandrowski & William Omar Contreras López (Eds.)

back pain involves intricate interplay amongst biomechanical attributes of the IVD, systemic inflammation, and neurophysiological systems (both peripheral and central) [8].

In light of their prospective efficacy in symptom alleviation and functional restitution, tissue engineering and regenerative medicine approaches have elicited considerable scholarly attention as pre-surgical interventions aimed at decelerating or even reversing the ongoing trajectory of IVD degradation and its concomitant nociceptive and dysfunctional symptomatology. These paradigms possess the unique merit of concurrently targeting the biomechanical, immunological, and neurophysiological dimensions implicated in IVD pathophysiology.

Contrary to the prevailing perception that the intervertebral disc (IVD) possesses a restricted regenerative aptitude following trauma (as illustrated in Fig. **1**), emergent insights into IVD ontogenesis, cellular biology, and mechanisms of degeneration portend the feasibility of cellularly-mediated rejuvenation [4]. Research has elucidated that the intrinsic cellular constituencies of the IVD exhibit a responsiveness to biomechanical provocations, such as substrate rigidity, and to an array of chemotactic and pro-inflammatory molecules, including but not limited to, chemokines and cytokines that modulate metabolic pathways and extracellular matrix assembly [9, 10]. Furthermore, aging-associated infiltration of macrophages and monocytes within the IVD has been demonstrated to modulate disc cell phenotypic expression, biosynthetic activity, and longevity. Bioengineering modalities represent a propitious avenue for directing cellular assimilation into implantable materials, representing a notable enhancement over erstwhile "inert" prosthetic devices that culminated in suboptimal clinical outcomes. There exists an escalating academic focus geared toward the refinement of both biological and bioengineering methodologies that capitalize on the endogenous cellular components resident within the IVD.

In this chapter, the authors proffer a succinct survey of clinical investigations that employ biomaterials as vectors for either cellular or pharmacological delivery. These investigations elucidate approaches for either the complete or partial restitution of the intervertebral disc (IVD) using cellularly-augmented as well as acellular, biologically-derived substrates that facilitate cellular-material interaction and architectural reorganization. Various preclinical and clinical inquiries have scrutinized the ramifications of infusing both allogeneic and autologous progenitor and stem cell lineages into the IVD milieu [11, 12]. Although the objectives aligned with cellular or drug deployment may intersect those of engineered biomaterials, such as restoring discal elevation, mitigating neural encroachments, or reversing radiological manifestations of pathology, the complex landscape of regulatory approval coupled with the intense requirement for precise cellular introduction into the IVD has engendered work that transcends a consensus-oriented conceptualization of best practices.

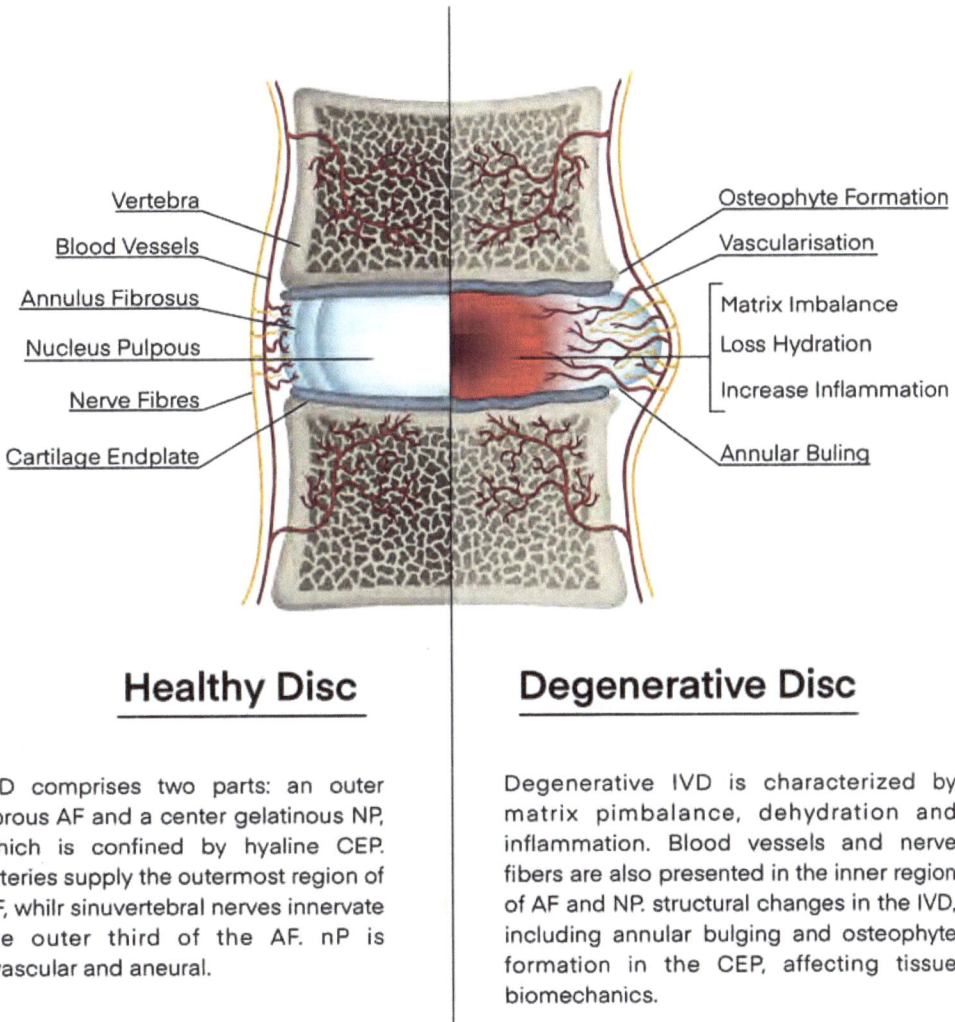

Healthy Disc

Degenerative Disc

IVD comprises two parts: an outer fibrous AF and a center gelatinous NP, which is confined by hyaline CEP. Arteries supply the outermost region of AF, whilr sinuvertebral nerves innervate the outer third of the AF. nP is avascular and aneural.

Degenerative IVD is characterized by matrix pimbalance, dehydration and inflammation. Blood vessels and nerve fibers are also presented in the inner region of AF and NP. structural changes in the IVD, including annular bulging and osteophyte formation in the CEP, affecting tissue biomechanics.

Fig. (1). In a healthy disc (left panel), the annulus fibrosus (outer layer) and nucleus pulposus (inner gel-like core) maintain their structural integrity and provide cushioning, flexibility, and shock absorption. In a degenerative lumbar intervertebral disc (right panel), the annulus fibrosus develops fissures leading to disc bulging or herniation. The nucleus pulposus may lose hydration and elasticity, becoming less capable of absorbing mechanical stresses resulting in reduced disc height and impaired disc function. Degenerative discs often are associated with osteophytes, spinal instability, nerve compression, and chronic low back pain.

In this context, the authors will delineate evolving methodologies and innovative breakthroughs involving biomaterials that are either in contemporary utilization or under development for the therapeutic intervention of IVD disorders, inclusive of annulus fibrosus restoration, nucleus pulposus substitution or intradiscal substance administration, and hybrid techniques. Although these innovative approaches remain in an incipient stage of maturation, the authors discern recurrent paradigms and dissect procedural efficacies to lay the groundwork for future biomaterial-centric initiatives with conceivable translational benefits for human clinical application.

Annulus Fibrosus Repair

An aberrant annulus fibrosus is architecturally composed of an inner and outer stratification (as depicted in Fig. **2**). The intrinsic regenerative proclivity of annulus fibrosus (AF) tissue post-traumatic disruption or laceration remains markedly constrained. In the context of intervertebral disc (IVD) deterioration, decrement in discal elevation can potentiate augmented biomechanical stress upon the AF, manifesting both in terms of compressive and tensile forces. Such alterations in mechanical solicitation engender microtraumatic defects, typified by minuscule fissurations or diminutive lacerations, which are susceptible to progressive exacerbation and may ultimately become discernible through radiological modalities like magnetic resonance imaging (MRI) or computed tomography (CT) scans. If such AF lacerations remain unaddressed, there exists the potential for dislocation of AF particulates accompanied by the extrusion of nucleus pulposus (NP) constituents. While microdiscectomy serves as a viable surgical intervention for the excision of these dislocated fragments that may impinge upon neural architecture, a neglected AF rupture could serve as a catalyst for recurrent disc herniation or aberrant kinematics of the IVD [13].

Methodologies for the repair of the annulus fibrosus (AF) disruptions have been proffered, targeting the locus of herniation with the objective of re-establishing intervertebral disc (IVD) functionality while attenuating the probability of recurrent herniation. A salient advantage of AF repair resides in its potential for facilitating the integration of the implanted repair construct with the contiguous osseous structures. This is facilitated by the direct insertion of AF fibrous elements into the endplates of adjacent vertebral entities, thereby permitting robust fixation. Evaluative protocols for engineered solutions tailored to AF repair predominantly focus on ascertaining the robustness of the integration interface between the reparative and the native tissue matrices, exemplified by metrics like suture pull-out tensile strength. The tensile load-bearing characteristics of the entire vertebral motion segment in an *In vitro* environment have been quantified in the context of AF repair implementations. However, the correlative association between these biomechanical indices and *In vivo* functional outcomes—such as the incidence rates of IVD re-herniation, kinematics of individual motion segments, and the subjective experience of nociception—remains an area of nebulous understanding.

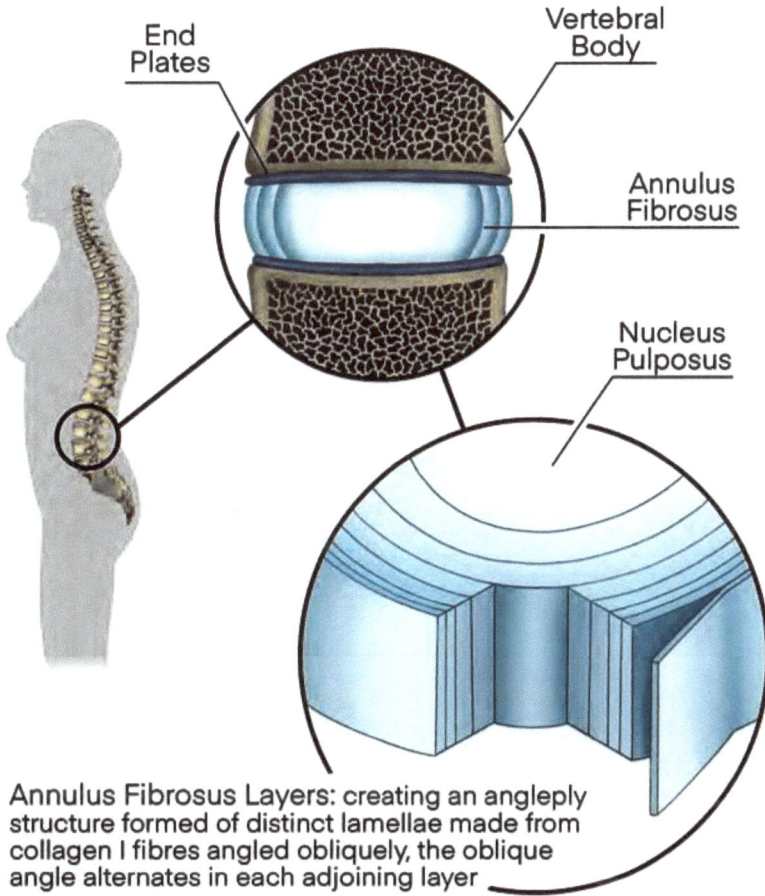

Fig. (2). The annulus fibrosus consists of two distinct layers: the outer annulus fibrosus and the inner annulus fibrosus. The outer annulus fibrosus forms the disc's outermost layer and is composed of several concentric rings of fibrous tissue. These rings, known as lamellae, are arranged in a crisscross pattern, providing strength and stability to the disc. The collagen fibers within the lamellae are predominantly oriented in a parallel fashion, enhancing the disc's resistance to tensile forces. The inner annulus fibrosus exhibits a more disorganized arrangement of collagen fibers. This region contains a higher concentration of proteoglycans, contributing to the disc's ability to retain water and maintain hydration. The inner annulus fibrosus also serves as a transition zone between the annulus fibrosus and the central nucleus pulposus [14].

Preliminary interventions aimed at the amelioration of lacerated annulus fibrosus (AF) tissues predominantly employ sophisticated suturing apparatuses, as delineated in Table **1**. Such devices, which may bear the European Conformity (CE) insignia or possess circumscribed approval from the United States Food and Drug Administration (FDA), necessitate the surgical deposition of bespoke sutures or polymeric meshwork precisely over the loci of annular defects. Subsequent to their placement, these devices are conventionally anchored to osseous structures to ensure stabilization, as exemplified by technologies such as XClose® Surgical Repair, Inclose™ Surgical Mesh, and Barricaid™. Efficacious outcomes have been demonstrated in terms of precluding nucleus pulposus (NP) extrusion [15] and reinstating tensile resilience to compromised AF tissue, primarily as corroborated by *In vitro* investigations. Clinical evaluations have revealed a paucity of adverse incidents and a diminution in the rates of recurrent herniation. However, the widespread adoption of these devices remains impeded by factors such as surgical intricacy, protracted procedure duration, and fiscal constraints [13]. Nevertheless, a converging opinion posits that less convoluted methodologies, capable of more comprehensively targeting the compromised AF than the acellular suturing techniques presently discussed, harbor the potential for mitigating the risk of re-herniation.

Table 1. Annular Repair Methods & Products (Adopted from Bowles *et al.*) [16].

Method	Description	Results
Suture Repair Methods		
XClose™ tissue repair	Polymeric suture with soft tissue anchors.	Reduced recurrent disc herniation rate up to 2 years; no adverse events [17].
Barricaid™	Polymer mesh with titanium anchor to vertebral body rim.	At 2-year follow-up, tear closure was associated with no recurrent disc herniation and maintenance of disc height [18].
Patch- or Void-filling Methods		
PTMC scaffold covered with a sutured PU membrane	Human MSCs	Restored disc height in IVD degeneration model and prevented recurrent NP herniation; MSCs seeded onto PTMC had elevated markers of AF phenotype [19].
Porous silk fibroin	Bovine AF cells	Cells attached and produced matrix; conjugation with RGD peptide had no effect on cell attachment or morphology [20].
Electrospun PCL	Bovine AF cells	Reproduced the anisotropic, angle-ply laminate structure of AF; cells aligned along predominant fiber direction; integration was shown with engineered NP *In vivo* [21 - 23].
BMG with PPCLM	Murine AF cells	Supported AF cell survival, alignment, and matrix accumulation; stiffness and degradation were adjusted by post polymerization time; gelatin component assisted integration and tensile strength [24].
POM	Murine AF cells	Supported cell infiltration, elongation, and matrix accumulation; tensile strength and degradation time increased with polymerization time [24].

(Table 1) cont.....

Method	Description	Results
PDLLA/Bioglass	Human AF cells	Foam supported cell cultures and supported cell proliferation and sGAG, collagen type I and collagen type II production [25].
Electrospun PU and PCL	Bovine AF cells	Electrospinning increased "yield strain," promoted AF cell phenotype with the retention of collagen and glycosaminoglycan compared with films [26].
Fibrin cross-linked with genipin	Human AF cells	Demonstrated suitable mechanical properties that restored compressive properties to IVD; promoted adhesion and elongation; maintained viability of cell population; had a slower *In vitro* degradation rate [27].
Photochemically crosslinked collagen in shape of needle	Placed following intradiscal delivery of MSCs in microsphere carriers	Restored compressive properties to IVD, reduced cell leakage, withstood torsional push-out test. In rabbit model, needle shape revealed placement of the device [28].
Collagen cross-linked with riboflavin	No cells	Retained in defect under loading and contributed to restored compressive moduli of IVD [29].

Abbreviations: AF, annulus fibrosus; BMG composite bone gelatin; IVD, intervertebral disc; MSC, mesenchymal stem cell; NA, not applicable; NP, nucleus pulposus PCL, poly(ε-caprolactone); PDLLA: poly-D,L-lactic acid; POM, poly(1,8-octanediol malate); PPCLM, poly(poly-caprolactone triol malate); PTMC; poly(trimethylene carbonate); PU; poly(ester-urethane); RGD, arginylglycylaspartic acid; sGAG: sulfated glycosaminoglycans.

Techniques for filling voids in the annulus fibrosus (AF) have been devised, employing a panoply of materials, either cell-free or cellularly augmented. Such methodologies predominantly utilize hydrogel formulations encompassing diverse substances like alginate, agarose, gelatin, and collagen, in addition to porous matrices synthesized from polyglycolic acid (PGA), polylactic acid (PLA), poly(ε-caprolactone), silk, hyaluronic acid, and glycosaminoglycans, as cataloged in Table 1. These injectable hydrogels exhibit malleability to conform to variegated defect dimensions and geometries, and may be further customized through cross-linking with biocompatible agents like genipin or riboflavin, targeting fibrin and collagen matrices, respectively [30, 31]. Complementary strategies, such as shape-memory alginate constructs [32], have been postulated, which undergo volumetric expansion into the defect upon rehydration. Preclinical investigations have substantiated the efficacy of genipin-crosslinked fibrin hydrogels in recapitulating compressive biomechanical attributes of the IVD in an *In vitro* milieu. A needle-like plug comprised of crosslinked collagen has been engineered for defect occlusion [28], demonstrating sufficient mechanical stability and efficacious containment of cellular efflux in *Ex vivo* push-out assays. Subsequent *In vivo* studies employing this collagen plug within a rabbit AF defect model have corroborated its therapeutic promise [28].

Injectable hydrogels intended for AF repair cultivate an ambient milieu conducive to AF cellular viability and the biosynthesis of extracellular matrix (ECM), thereby implicating cellularly mediated bio-remodeling of the implanted construct as an adjunctive factor in ensuring extended implant longevity and enhanced clinical outcomes. Notably, these materials predominantly sustain cells in a spheroidal morphology, a state that predisposes towards the secretion of a hyaline cartilage-like ECM, as opposed to a more structured fibrocartilaginous arrangement, save for contracted and aligned collagen gels [33]. The long-term clinical ramifications of this feature, particularly in relation to implant survival periods exceeding one year, remain indeterminate. Although mechanical assays have authenticated the capability of these hydrogels to rehabilitate IVD kinematics, the lack of an inherently aligned collagenous matrix might circumscribe their aptitude for efficient tensile stress transference across defect sites during biomechanical loading and motility. The characterization of imperative performance indicators for these hydrogels, extending beyond preclinical *In vitro* assessments, remains an active area of investigation. Nonetheless, their relative ease of application and generally favorable safety profile in disparate anatomical contexts render them attractive candidates.

Tissue Engineering for Annular Repair

The engineering of annulus fibrosus (AF) repair methodologies capable of mimicking the innate collagenous fiber architecture constitutes a pivotal objective in regenerative medicine. One paradigm entails the utilization of a decellularized extracellular matrix featuring highly organized fibers—exemplified by small intestinal submucosa—serving as a bone-anchored patch *via* titanium osseous fasteners [34]. This modality has manifested robust integration at the site of AF defect, enabling augmented intervertebral disc (IVD) pressurization in preclinical investigations and ensuring sustained tissue hydration in *In vivo* models for durations exceeding 24 weeks. Efforts to replicate this oriented fibrous architecture employing synthetic substrates or alternative bioactive materials have been pursued *via* techniques such as electrospinning [35 - 38], collagen-induced contraction [33, 39], sericin-reinforced fiber winding [40, 41], and the architectural incorporation of anisotropic honeycomb configurations into scaffold constructs [42]. Electrospinning, in particular, has demonstrated efficacy in recapitulating the AF's multilamellar architecture, achieving fibrous alignment, and imparting anisotropic mechanical attributes [22]. Nonetheless, the deployment of specific polymers, like poly(ε-caprolactone), in the electrospinning process has been challenged by questions concerning mechanical robustness and optimal integration with native tissue matrices. Current investigative thrusts are trained on devising composite, tissue-engineered paradigms proficient in mimicking the mechanical resilience, structural orientation, and bio-integrative capabilities of native AF tissues, bearing semblance to injectable void-repair modalities [23, 43]. Ongoing scholarly inquiries in this field are venturing into the exploration of synergistic strategies that amalgamate attributes of both the annulus fibrosus and nucleus pulposus to surmount the extant challenges in AF repair.

Nucleus Augmentation and Injectables

For more than four decades, the investigative scrutiny has been cast upon injectable biomaterials as adjunctive modalities to discectomy procedures. Pioneering inquiries by Nachemson (1962) [44] and Schneider and Oyen (1974) [45, 46] evaluated the applicability of room-temperature vulcanizing silicone and silicone elastomers as infusions into compromised intervertebral discs. Subsequent advancements have ushered in an array of injectable scaffolding substitutes tailored for nucleus pulposus restoration, inclusive of hyaluronic acid matrices, fibrin adhesives, alginate constructs, elastin-mimetic polypeptides, and collagen Type I hydrogels, among others. A litany of patents has been conferred for formulations like cross-linkable silk-elastin copolymers, polyurethane-encapsulated balloon systems, aldehyde-stabilized bovine serum albumin matrices, collagen-poly(ethylene glycol) conjugates, chitosan-derived structures, and an assortment of recombinant and light-curable polymeric configurations [47].

The underlying imperatives for nucleus pulposus augmentation post-discectomy encompass the deterrence of disc height diminution and the resultant biomechanical and biochemical aberrations engendered by volumetric compromise. The optative infusion of a flowable biomaterial serves not only to reestablish the void ensuing from surgical disc excision but also to conserve structural disc height. Depending on the compositional attributes, such infusible substances are capable of facile integration with surgical lacunae and adhesion to adjoining tissues. Optimal injectable scaffolds should facilitate the uniform incorporation of cellular constituents and therapeutic bioactives. Complementary strategies may leverage an array of growth factors like BMP, TGF, and IGF, in addition to anti-inflammatory cytokine and protease inhibitors, to counterbalance matrix degradation and attenuate its repercussions on the contiguous tissue and neural milieu, specifically nociceptive structures. The structural robustness, biodegradability, and biocompatibility of the injectable material are indispensable attributes. Additionally, the material should offer convenient handling characteristics, such as minimal setting time, negligible thermal fluctuations, and low-viscosity formulation conducive to facile injection and disc space accessibility. The scaffold ought to proffer the requisite mechanical attributes to furnish physical support, facilitate matrix genesis, and undergo timely degradation. Biocompatibility remains paramount, necessitating that neither the primordial scaffold nor its degradation byproducts evoke protracted immune responses, elicit immunotoxic phenomena, or manifest cytotoxicity. Customarily, candidate biomaterials are instilled as highly viscous fluids and subsequently solidified *via* strategies like thermoresponsive or pH-responsive cross-linking, photopolymerization, or solidifying agent addition, culminating in a gelatinous matrix. The setting kinetics should accommodate precise implantation without unduly extending procedural duration, and any thermogenic alterations during material solidification must be constrained to ensure the well-being of adjacent tissues.

Nucleus Replacement and Regeneration

Substances employed for the replacement of the nucleus pulposus (NP) predominantly concentrate on either injectable synthetic or biologically-sourced materials that are designed to reinstate the structural elevation and biomechanical equanimity of the intervertebral disc (IVD) while preserving the architectural integrity of the annulus fibrosus (AF) [12, 48, 49]. Synthetic variants, conceived explicitly for this application, aspire to emulate the material characteristics inherent to the native anatomical constituents. Such compatibility is indispensable for ensuring seamless integration with juxtaposed structures, retention of implant positioning devoid of migration or slippage phenomena, and the recapitulation of the native motion dynamics and mechanical attributes of the functional spinal unit. The prerequisites for efficacious clinical transition include resilience, withstanding multitudinous load cycles devoid of any morphological degradation, and minimal generation of wear particulates to avert the induction of immune responses. Conversely, biomaterials of biological provenance are susceptible to cellularly mediated degradation, culminating in the temporal remodeling of the NP implant. Evaluative criteria for implant efficacy employed in the former category may retain relevance here, albeit with diminished emphasis on long-term durability owing to the intrinsic remodeling capabilities. Moreover, selected biomaterials may serve dual functions as vehicles for cellular delivery to the NP, thereby establishing an environment amenable to cellularly orchestrated NP tissue regeneration. The methodologies, empirically substantiated findings, and therapeutic outcomes pertaining to each of these paradigms are elaborated upon in the ensuing sections (Tables **2** & **3**).

Table 2. Nucleus pulposus repair or replacement devices (Adopted from Bowles *et al.*) [16].

Polymer	Trade Name/ Clinical Trials?	Measurement Outcomes/Comments
Injectable Synthetic Polymers		
Copolymeric hydrogel (PAN and polyacrylamide) encased in a polyethylene fiber jacket	PDN, Yes	No longer in use
Semihydrated poly(vinyl) alcohol	Aquarelle, Yes	No longer in use
Copolymer of poly(vinyl alcohol) [and poly(vinyl pyrrolidone) or modified PAN] reinforced by a Dacron mesh	NeuDisc™, Yes	Restored compressive stiffness
Hydrating PAN	NucleoFix™, Yes	Marketed under CE mark
Consists of inflatable silicone membrane and a tubular fiber graft with one-way valve to prevent flowable, curable silicon from leaking out [50, 51]	PerQdisc™, Yes	Marketed under CE mark, used for surgical replacement of a single NP between spinal lumbar discs L1-S1 using an anterior or lateral transpsoas approach.
***In situ* Forming (or Cross-linked) Synthetic and Biologically Based Polymers**		
In situ curing polymer using inflatable polyurethane "balloon"	DASCOR™, Yes	Restored multidirectional segment flexibility
In situ curing polymerized water-in-oil emulsion composite	DiscCell™, Yes	From *In vitro* work: restored motion segment stability[a]
Glutaraldehyde cross-linked albumin	Biodisc™, Yes	Uncertain status
Hydrogel of a chemically cross-linked elastin and silk polypeptide	NuCore™, Yes	Maintenance of disc height; significantly reduced leg and back pain; improved function scores in discectomy patients
Oxidized hyaluronic acid gelatin implant [52]	Preclinical	Restored motion segment stability; no changes in stiffness
Thiol-modified hyaluronan and elastin-like polypeptide [53]	Preclinical	Restored stiffness
Sulfonate-containing glycosaminoglycan surrogates [54]	NA	Restored stiffness; maintained disc height under compression
Silk fibroin/polyurethane composite [55]	Preclinical	Mechanical properties stable over time; higher stiffness than native NP but conducive for cell support
PNIPAAm-PEG hydrogels [56]	NA	Enhanced recovery from compressive strain, was thermoresponsive, sustained drug release
Chitosan gels [57]	NA	Supported matrix accumulation for native cells and retention of proteoglycan
Hyaluronic acid/collagen hydrogel [58]	Preclinical	Implant did not improve disc height; increased scarring and inflammation in AF

(Table 2) cont.....

Polymer	Trade Name/ Clinical Trials?	Measurement Outcomes/Comments
Hyaluronan polymers [59]	Preclinical	Prevented fibrotic changes; supported cell growth; no mechanical outcomes
Hyaluroan / PEG crosslinked copolymer [60]	NA	Engineered design that could be targeted to maintain NP or AF cell phenotype in vitro
Collagen type II / hyaluronan-PEG crosslinked hydrogel [61]	NA	Supported maintenance of cell phenotype and biosynthesis for native NP cells

Abbreviations: AF, anulus fibrosus; CE, European Conformity; NP, nucleus pulposus; PAN, polyacrylonitrile; PEG, polyethylene glycol; PNIPPAm, poly(N-isopropyl acrylamide).

Table 3. Bioengineering strategies for AF / NP repair or replacement. (Adopted from Bowles *et al.*) [16].

Anulus Fibrosus	Nucleus Pulposus	Bone	Outcome
PGA/PLA, ovine AF cells (isotropic)	Alginate, ovine NP cells	NA	First research to demonstrate tissue-engineered composite IVD, ECM production, and compressive mechanical properties on the order of native ovine IVD [79].
PLLA/HA, MSCs (isotropic)	HA, MSCs	NA	First paper to demonstrate a composite IVD structure using electrospun fibers; *In vitro* study demonstrated histological evidence of an AF and NP region with collagen I, II, and aggrecan production [80].
Demineralized bone matrix rabbit AF cells (isotropic)	Collagen (II)/hyaluronate/chondroitin-6-sulfate rabbit NP cells	NA	Composite IVD subcutaneously implanted into aythmic mice demonstrated NP and AF region with collagen and proteoglycan deposition [81].
Contracted collagen gel, ovine AF cells (anisotropic)	Alginate, ovine NP cells	NA	Composite IVD implanted in a rat-tail and lumbar model showed integration, disc height maintenance, and mechanical properties on the order of the native controls in all implants in the tail model, and disc height maintenance in 50% of the implants in the lumbar model [30, 33, 39, 82].

(Table 3) cont.....

Anulus Fibrosus	Nucleus Pulposus	Bone	Outcome
Toroidal scaffolds of porous silk	Fibrin/hyaluron crosslinked hydrogel	NA	In vitro study demonstrated histological evidence of an AF from implanted AF cells, and NP from implanted chondrocytes, with phenotypically appropriate gene expression [40, 83].
Multiple lamellae of photocrosslinked collagen membranes	Collagen-glycosaminoglycan co-precipitate	NA	Composite IVD tested mechanically in compression for comparison with native IVD; results showed a role for collagen lamellae in preserving height recovery following loading, and transient behaviors in creep and recovery [40, 83].
Electrospun PCL, MSCs (anisotropic)	Agarose, MSCs	NA	Composite IVD with AF and NP regions showed aligned PCL fiber and lamella AF organization that mimicked those of the native IVD; *In vitro* study demonstrated organization and appropriate ECM deposition in the composite IVD constructs [80].
Electrospun PCL, acellular (anisotropic)	No material acellular	NA	Construct with organized AF architecture was implanted in a rat-tail model showing maintenance of disc height in 50% of samples without fixation and 100% with fixation [21, 23].
Contracted collagen gel, MSCs (anisotropic)	Collagen–GAG gel coprecipitate MSC	Osteogenic MSCs	Created an engineered IVD with AF/NP/osteochondral subunits with appropriate histological features of each region [84].

Abbreviations: AF, anulus fibrosus; ECM, extracellular matrix; GAG, glycosaminoglycan; HA, hyaluronic acid; IVD, intervertebral disc; MSC, mesenchymal stem cell; NA, not applicable; NP, nucleus pulposus; PCL, poly(ε-caprolactone); PGA, polyglycolic acid; PLA, polylactic acid.

Initially, endeavors in nucleus pulposus (NP) augmentation or substitution were largely predicated on the deployment of biomaterials with the principal objective of reinstating intervertebral disc height and biomechanical function of the motion segment, whilst largely eschewing considerations pertaining to cellular outcomes or biological ramifications. Archetypal methodologies aimed to recapitulate the hydration levels, intra-discal pressure, and disc elevation through the utilization of in situ-hydrating synthetic polymers, formulated to emulate the physicochemical attributes of endogenous glycosaminoglycans present within the NP. A salient exemplar in this regard is a copolymeric hydrogel enveloped within a polyethylene fibrous sheath (PDN™), boasting a protracted history of clinical deployment and serving as a referential paradigm for NP prosthesis. Subsequent implantable devices, composed of semi-hydrated poly(vinyl) alcohol (PVA) or co-polymers thereof with poly(vinyl pyrrolidone) (PVP), have been conceived along analogous conceptual lines [62]. Notwithstanding, the regulatory control over polymer swelling has posed formidable challenges, with unrestrained expansion precipitating adverse outcomes such as increased rigidity, end-plate overloading, fractures, subsidence of the device, and ultimate mechanical failure [63, 64].

Concurrently, the PerQdisc Nucleus Replacement Device, developed by SST, is undergoing evaluation in clinical settings specifically targeting patients afflicted by degenerative disc disease (DDD) of the lumbar spine, manifesting as debilitating back pain and devoid of stenotic or unstable complications [50, 51]. The clinical investigation aims to furnish this patient cohort with hitherto elusive surgical interventions, ameliorating discogenic lumbar discomfort whilst conserving disc elevation and kinematic range. Encompassing an enrollment of 72 subjects distributed across seven South American research trials, the data harvested from these LOPAIN2 trials will serve as the foundation for subsequent CE Mark accreditation under the European Medical Device Regulation (MDR).

Simultaneously, an emergent subclass of biomaterials, coined as 'in situ-forming synthetic polymers,' has gained traction in NP prosthesis research. Upon intradiscal injection, these substances undergo a phase transition, morphing from a liquidous to either gelatinous or solid state, thereby minimizing potential harm to the surrounding annulus fibrosus (AF) during the implantation procedure [62, 65, 66]. Various cross-linking methodologies have been explored, encompassing chemical, thermal, and pH-responsive mechanisms. For example, chemically cross-linked polymers deployed for NP implants include silk and elastin copolymeric sequences amalgamated with cross-linking agents (NuCore™) [65] and albumin-derived proteins subjected to glutaraldehyde cross-linking (BioDisc™).

While a multitude of these investigative strategies have been subjected to human clinical evaluation, a paucity have successfully navigated the labyrinthine pathways to market authorization. These materials are predominantly formulated to meet mechanical design metrics, including the restitution of disc rigidity, kinematic range, neutral axial alignment, or elevation. However, the interplay between these implanted materials and the native cellular milieu, as well as their assimilation into the adjoining structural anatomy, remains conspicuously understudied. With the advancement of these biomaterials, novel interrogatives concerning integration fidelity, biological reciprocity, and mechanical load distribution are likely to surface.

Biomaterials

Explorations in the realm of biomaterials as vectors for NP regeneration have garnered considerable attention, principally attributed to the diminution in NP cellular density and phenotypic alterations, factors that culminate in NP degradation and compromised biomechanical integrity of the motion segment [67, 68]. While cellular supplementation within the NP milieu has been exhaustively investigated across both preclinical and clinical landscapes, an accord regarding the optimal cellular composition to achieve long-term therapeutic efficacy remains elusive [11, 12]. Moreover, despite the nascent promise exhibited by cellular augmentation devoid of a biomaterial scaffold, the preponderance of investigative focus has been dedicated to cellular delivery mediated through biomaterial substrates. The operative mechanisms by which these transplanted cells enhance functional outcomes post-NP replacement remain inadequately delineated.

When contemplating the design of biomaterials, pivotal considerations must encompass the procedural intricacies and resultant functional outcomes of cellular transplantation for NP remediation. Preliminary comparative analyses have been conducted, contrasting methodologies such as the encapsulation of mesenchymal stem cells (MSCs) within atelocollagen gels against their direct intra-discal injection within animal models symptomatic of intervertebral disc (IVD) degeneration. Such studies substantiate that cellular deployment in tandem with a collagenous carrier preserves disc elevation, magnetic resonance signal integrity, and histomorphological resemblance to native tissues over extended durations [69]. Furthermore, preserving the structural integrity of the extracellular matrix (ECM) emerges as a sine qua non for the implanted cells' viability.

The utilization of bioactive indigenous materials like intestinal submucosa evinces that the incorporation of native ECM constituents can offer a conducive milieu for the sustenance of endogenous cellular populations [70 - 72]. These seminal discoveries have heralded the conceptualization and actualization of biomaterial platforms amalgamating biologically-derived substances and explicit ECM elements [73]. Conversely, when adjudicating the selection criteria for such biomaterials, considerations traditionally skew toward operational handling characteristics and safety profiles, often at the expense of biological, degradative, or bio-inductive attributes essential for NP regeneration.

Numerous commercially available substrates, encompassing fibrin gels, Gelfoam™, crosslinked or high-molecular-weight hyaluronan solutions, and hyaluronic acid sponges, have been deployed in preclinical evaluations [11]. Particularly, hyaluronan, in its liquid or gel states, has procured wider clinical validation as a vehicle for intra-discal delivery of allogeneic mesenchymal precursor cells or autologous bone marrow-derived stem cells [74, 75]. Derivatives of hyaluronan, achieved *via* cross-linking, are also undergoing scrutiny for the risk-mitigated transplantation of ex vivo-amplified autologous IVD cells [75].

Transitioning from *In vitro* to preclinical research paradigms, heightened scrutiny has been directed toward identifying the quintessential characteristics of biomaterials conducive for efficacious cellular delivery within the NP domain. Certain investigative consortia have engineered biocompatible scaffold systems incorporating native ECM constituents, such as hyaluronan, proteoglycans, or collagens, aimed at nurturing the NP cellular phenotype [60, 61, 76]. For instance, scaffolds laden with polymerizing fibrin and the growth factor transforming growth factor β (TGF-β) in conjunction with allogeneic MSCs have exhibited superior abilities in preserving disc height and mitigating apoptosis when compared to either entity utilized in isolation [77]. Given the ubiquity of TGF-β within healthy intervertebral discs, its incorporation within biomaterial substrates might be contributory to the documented efficacies. Likewise, injectable matrices constituted of pentosan polysulfate, a glycosaminoglycan analog, have shown promise in supporting progenitor cells [78].

Annulus Fibrosus/nucleus Pulposus Bioengineering Strategies

Total disc arthroplasty serves as an avant-garde modality for the comprehensive replacement of the intricately structured annulus fibrosus-nucleus pulposus-endplate units [67, 68]. Comprising well-vetted materials traditionally employed in arthroplastic procedures, such as biocompatible metals optimized for osseointegration and polyethylenes conducive for articular functionality, these prosthetic constructs aspire to reestablish natural biomechanical motion and uphold the physiological well-being of adjacent intervertebral discs. Nevertheless, the wide-scale adoption of these devices remains stymied, owing primarily to their surgical intricacy, propensity for implant migration, and the associated challenges that beset their eventual explantation.

There is a discernible pivot in research activities toward the conceptualization and realization of holistic disc replacements employing biodegradable substrates and biomimetic strategies that engender cellular viability and facilitate neo-tissue formation. It should be noted, however, that these nascent approaches predominantly reside within the confines of preclinical experimentation and *In vitro* investigational paradigms.

The amalgamation of diverse bioengineering paradigms aimed at nucleus pulposus (NP) substitution and annulus fibrosus (AF) remediation presents an intriguing avenue for the development of composite intervertebral disc (IVD) replacements. Despite its theoretical appeal, the scientific landscape has offered only limited empirical investigations into this multi-disciplinary concept. Illustratively, one exploratory study employed a polyglycolic acid/polylactic acid (PGA/PLA) matrix seeded with cells for the AF conjoined with an alginate-based NP, resulting in favorable outcomes with respect to matrix biosynthesis and compressive mechanical attributes. Notwithstanding, this construct failed to recapitulate the intricate collagenous organization inherently present within the native AF. Additional forays into generating holistic disc constructs, while eschewing the characteristic AF architecture, employed a demineralized bone matrix gelatin matrix for the AF component and a complex of collagen II, hyaluronate, and chondroitin-6-sulfate for the NP, both seeded with respective cellular types [81]. The ramifications of omitting an organized, fibrous AF on the functional longevity and biomechanical efficacy of such composite discs remain enigmatic, albeit it would undoubtedly compromise the AF's intrinsic ability to bear tensile stresses during NP pressurization and mechanical loading.

Recent scientific endeavors have increasingly gravitated toward constructing composite IVDs that incorporate the variable fibrous organization emblematic of the AF [33, 39, 21, 80, 86]. Initial undertakings utilized a hyaluronic acid gel core replete with cellular constituents, enveloped by an electrospun nanofibrous scaffold to simulate an integrated NP-AF construct [80]. Subsequent designs featured silk scaffolds with engineered pores and oriented lamellar structures seeded with AF cells, juxtaposed against a fibrin-hyaluronan gel serving as the NP component [40, 83, 87]. Though these configurations have demonstrated a commendable facsimile of both morphological and key biological functionalities, only structures with explicitly oriented AF were proficient in replicating pivotal biomechanical parameters such as integration robustness and compressive resilience. Advancements have included composite IVDs employing an organized AF architecture utilizing materials like contracted collagen gel, silk, and electrospun poly-ε-caprolactone (PCL). A more recent study deployed crosslinked collagen membranes as AF lamellae, amalgamated with a collagen-glycosaminoglycan coprecipitate for emulating the native NP milieu [88]. This extensive evaluation elucidated that an optimal configuration of ten AF-like lamellae was instrumental in maintaining specific biomechanical properties during compressive loading, thereby substantiating the indispensable role of an organized AF in tissue-engineered composite constructs.

The transplantation of an entirely tissue-engineered intervertebral disc (IVD) into the caudal vertebral column of rodent subjects revealed a primary integration predominantly *via* interactions with the annulus fibrosus (AF). This yielded a matrix biosynthesis and biomechanical compressive properties closely resembling those of the indigenous IVD [76]. Nonetheless, when subjected to evaluation within the lumbar vertebral region, a mere 50% of the implanted constructs succeeded in preserving disc space, whereas the remaining half exhibited disc space atrophy followed by spondylodesis [82]. This differential outcome insinuates that the biomechanical complexities inherent to the lumbar spinal environment could potentially attenuate the procedure's overall efficacy as opposed to caudal implementations. A subsequent study entailing the implantation of an electrospun poly-ε-caprolactone (PCL) disc into the caudal disc space revealed maintained disc height when accompanied by spinal stabilization; however, suboptimal integration with the native matrix was observed, leading to implant displacement in approximately half of the instances [23]. Subsequent investigative efforts ought to prioritize the incorporation of electrospun fibrous materials with autochthonous tissues to ensure proficient tensile load transference. Additional studies employing more anthropomimetic models are imperative for for the discovery of implant integration dynamics and establishing design parameters that preclude post-implantation disc migration. Furthermore, the utilization of diminutive disc dimensions in rodent models could obfuscate nutritional inadequacies and impede functional matrix ontogenesis, particularly when extrapolating these observations for human clinical applications [89].

The congruency between the artificial IVD and the endogenous osseous endplates stands as a pivotal determinant in the operational success of composite IVD constructs. The feasibility of achieving rigid osteointegration supersedes that of AF or NP fixation. Preliminary inquiries into multi-component IVD tissue engineering have scrutinized the interface between fabricated NP tissue and a calcium polyphosphate substrate, serving as a surrogate for vertebral endplate integration, yielding auspicious outcomes in proteoglycan content and compressive mechanical attributes [122]. Nevertheless, the critical variable of integration strength was not specifically assessed. Innovative strategies have evolved to encompass the regeneration of comprehensive motion segments, inclusive of a bony endplate region, concomitant with AF and NP components [90]. Such complexly engineered segments could ostensibly integrate directly with the vertebral corpus, thereby obviating the nociceptive neural ingress commonly associated with native IVDs. Despite incremental advancements in the sophistication of regenerative disc replacement methodologies, further research remains essential for evaluating the functional durability of these constructs within the pathological IVD spaces commonly encountered in the human clinical context.

DISCUSSION

Diverse biomaterial-centric methodologies for the restoration and substitution of intervertebral disc (IVD) tissues have been posited. Evidently, engineering paradigms that singularly depend on synthetic constituents or composite prostheses, whilst disregarding the intricate biological facets of the IVD, encounter restricted acceptance owing to operational intricacies and suboptimal clinical outcomes. This underscores the imperative of concurrently evaluating biological processes and clinical practicability along with conceptual design in the formulation of IVD disorder interventions. Innovative strategies that facilitate cellular symbiosis and permit temporal remodeling of introduced biomaterials, thereby adapting to biomechanical and biological stimuli, are emerging as propitious therapeutic alternatives. Procedural simplifications *via* injectable, defect-occlusive, in situ fixation techniques, and minimally invasive implantation modalities are anticipated to manifest superior success rates. The exigent mechanical burden prerequisites and labyrinthine amalgamation with chondral and annulus fibrosus architectures present formidable challenges to efficacious IVD remediation. Additionally, the milieu featuring inflammation, acidic pH, hypoxic tension, and restricted nutrient accessibility further compromise cell-centric approaches. Surmounting these obstacles necessitates innovative insights and methodologies for interfacing and modulating IVD physiology, concomitant with advancements in biomaterial sciences.

Contemporary scholarly discourses suggest a predilection for bioengineering tactics that employ polymers, extracellular matrix derivatives, and proteinaceous substances for annulus fibrosus reconstruction, nucleus pulposus substitution, or amalgamated modalities. Nevertheless, without meticulously delineated success metrics, deducing definitive conclusions remains premature. Despite this, several unifying principles emerge from this research epoch: a) Emulating the lamellar configuration of the orientation-specific collagenous annulus fibrosis augments the biomechanical integrity of composite annulus fibrosis/nucleus pulposus regenerative strategies, particularly since the lamellar annulus fibrosis is adept at counteracting deformation under nucleus pulposus pressurization; b) Maintaining the aforementioned lamellar structure in annulus fibrosis repair may be non-essential, as defect-sealing and integrated "plug" strategies have demonstrated efficacy; c) For nucleus pulposus substitution as an isolated procedure, recapitulating the hydrational attributes of glycosaminoglycans may be dispensable for disc height preservation—alternative materials have showcased utility, although recovery capabilities from mechanical stresses *via* re-hydration or analogous mechanisms could enhance implant longevity; d) Osteointegration with vertebral bodies and endplates could offer a preferred paradigm for annulus fibrosis and composite annulus fibrosis/nucleus pulposus regenerative tactics, benefiting from the well-vascularized environment absent in healthy IVDs—although the induction of vascularity or neural integration within regenerating IVDs may not be requisite for analgesia and matrix preservation during healing; e) Biomaterial approaches that incorporate a precisely regulated display of bioactive moieties—such as sequestered growth factors, pharmacogenomics, peptide sequences, or extracellular matrix proteins—complement strategies directly manipulating incorporated progenitor or primary cells, for instance, through gene transference.

CONCLUSION

Clearly defined outcomes and design goals should guide future research in IVD treatment. The preponderance of IVD regenerative and restorative methodologies has been principally preoccupied with the reconstitution of vital anatomical landmarks characteristic of a healthy IVD and functional motion segment. Such pivotal markers include optimal disc height, magnetic resonance imaging signal intensity, the decompression of spinal cord and nerve roots, and the re-establishment of kinematic freedom without prosthesis malpositioning or translocation. These benchmarks, amenable to assessment *via* radiological imaging modalities, are anticipated to persist as indispensable primary endpoints for the clinical actualization of any prospective regenerative paradigm. Tactics that solely emulate IVD matrix synthesis, cellular viability, or histological alignment without reinvigorating quintessential aspects of salubrious IVD architecture are unlikely to effectuate a substantive impact on the clinical management of IVD maladies. Finally, the extant paucity of exhaustive comprehension vis-à-vis the etiopathogenesis of IVD disorders and their nociceptive correlates considerably obfuscates the enterprise of IVD regeneration and remediation. Bioengineering stratagems must evolve in concert with foundational research endeavors to more adeptly delineate design imperatives and synthesized resolutions pertinent to the treatment of IVD afflictions and concomitant pathologies.

REFERENCES

[1]   Boos N, Weissbach S, Rohrbach H, Weiler C, Spratt KF, Nerlich AG. Classification of age-related changes in lumbar intervertebral discs: 2002 Volvo Award in basic science. Spine 2002; 27(23): 2631-44.
[http://dx.doi.org/10.1097/00007632-200212010-00002] [PMID: 12461389]

[2]   Yasuma T, Koh S, Okamura T, Yamauchi Y. Histological changes in aging lumbar intervertebral discs. Their role in protrusions and prolapses. J Bone Joint Surg Am 1990; 72(2): 220-9.
[http://dx.doi.org/10.2106/00004623-199072020-00009] [PMID: 2303508]

[3]   Andersson G. Low Back Pain: A Scientific and Clinical Overview 1996.

[4]   Urban JPG, Roberts S. Degeneration of the intervertebral disc. Arthritis Res 2003; 5(3): 120-30.
[http://dx.doi.org/10.1186/ar629] [PMID: 12723977]

[5]   Hurri H, Karppinen J. Discogenic pain. Pain 2004; 112(3): 225-8.
        [http://dx.doi.org/10.1016/j.pain.2004.08.016] [PMID: 15561376]

[6]   Woolf AD, Pfleger B. Burden of major musculoskeletal conditions. Bull World Health Organ 2003;
        81(9): 646-56.
        [PMID: 14710506]

[7]   Risbud MV, Shapiro IM. Role of cytokines in intervertebral disc degeneration: pain and disc content.
        Nat Rev Rheumatol 2014; 10(1): 44-56.
        [http://dx.doi.org/10.1038/nrrheum.2013.160] [PMID: 24166242]

[8]   Lotz JC, Ulrich JA. Innervation, inflammation, and hypermobility may characterize pathologic disc
        degeneration: review of animal model data. J Bone Joint Surg Am 2006; 88 (Suppl. 2): 76-82.
        [http://dx.doi.org/10.2106/00004623-200604002-00016] [PMID: 16595449]

[9]   Setton LA, Chen J. Mechanobiology of the intervertebral disc and relevance to disc degeneration. J
        Bone Joint Surg Am 2006; 88 (Suppl. 2): 52-7.
        [PMID: 16595444]

[10]   Hwang PY, Chen J, Jing L, Hoffman BD, Setton LA. The role of extracellular matrix elasticity and
        composition in regulating the nucleus pulposus cell phenotype in the intervertebral disc: a narrative
        review. J Biomech Eng 2014; 136(2)021010
        [http://dx.doi.org/10.1115/1.4026360] [PMID: 24390195]

[11]   Sakai D, Andersson GBJ. Stem cell therapy for intervertebral disc regeneration: obstacles and
        solutions. Nat Rev Rheumatol 2015; 11(4): 243-56.
        [http://dx.doi.org/10.1038/nrrheum.2015.13] [PMID: 25708497]

[12]   Benneker LM, Andersson G, Iatridis JC, *et al.* Cell therapy for intervertebral disc repair: advancing
        cell therapy from bench to clinics. Eur Cell Mater 2014; 27s: 5-11.
        [http://dx.doi.org/10.22203/eCM.v027sa02] [PMID: 24802611]

[13]   Guterl CC, See EY, Blanquer SBG, *et al.* Challenges and strategies in the repair of ruptured annulus
        fibrosus. Eur Cell Mater 2013; 25: 1-21.
        [http://dx.doi.org/10.22203/eCM.v025a01] [PMID: 23283636]

[14]   Schollmeier G, Lahr-Eigen R, Lewandrowski KU. Observations on fiber-forming collagens in the
        anulus fibrosus. Spine 2000; 25(21): 2736-41.
        [http://dx.doi.org/10.1097/00007632-200011010-00004] [PMID: 11064517]

[15]   Bron JL, Helder MN, Meisel HJ, Van Royen BJ, Smit TH. Repair, regenerative and supportive
        therapies of the annulus fibrosus: achievements and challenges. Eur Spine J 2009; 18(3): 301-13.
        [http://dx.doi.org/10.1007/s00586-008-0856-x] [PMID: 19104850]

[16]   Bowles RD, Setton LA. Biomaterials for intervertebral disc regeneration and repair. Biomaterials
        2017; 129: 54-67.
        [http://dx.doi.org/10.1016/j.biomaterials.2017.03.013] [PMID: 28324865]

[17]   Bailey A, Araghi A, Blumenthal S, Huffmon GV. Prospective, multicenter, randomized, controlled
        study of anular repair in lumbar discectomy: two-year follow-up. Spine 2013; 38(14): 1161-9.
        [http://dx.doi.org/10.1097/BRS.0b013e31828b2e2f] [PMID: 23392414]

[18]   Vukas D, Grahovac G, Barth M, Bouma G, Vilendecic M, Ledic D. Effect of anular closure on disk
        height maintenance and reoperated recurrent herniation following lumbar diskectomy: two-year data. J
        Neurol Surg A Cent Eur Neurosurg 2015; 76(3): 211-8.
        [http://dx.doi.org/10.1055/s-0034-1393930] [PMID: 25587701]

[19]   Pirvu T, Blanquer SBG, Benneker LM, *et al.* A combined biomaterial and cellular approach for
        annulus fibrosus rupture repair. Biomaterials 2015; 42: 11-9.
        [http://dx.doi.org/10.1016/j.biomaterials.2014.11.049] [PMID: 25542789]

[20]   Chang G, Kim HJ, Kaplan D, Vunjak-Novakovic G, Kandel RA. Porous silk scaffolds can be used for

tissue engineering annulus fibrosus. Eur Spine J 2007; 16(11): 1848-57.
[http://dx.doi.org/10.1007/s00586-007-0364-4] [PMID: 17447088]

[21]   Nerurkar NL, Sen S, Huang AH, Elliott DM, Mauck RL. Engineered disc-like angle-ply structures for intervertebral disc replacement. Spine 2010; 35(8): 867-73.
[http://dx.doi.org/10.1097/BRS.0b013e3181d74414] [PMID: 20354467]

[22]   Nerurkar NL, Baker BM, Sen S, Wible EE, Elliott DM, Mauck RL. Nanofibrous biologic laminates replicate the form and function of the annulus fibrosus. Nat Mater 2009; 8(12): 986-92.
[http://dx.doi.org/10.1038/nmat2558] [PMID: 19855383]

[23]   Martin JT, Milby AH, Chiaro JA, *et al.* Translation of an engineered nanofibrous disc-like angle-ply structure for intervertebral disc replacement in a small animal model. Acta Biomater 2014; 10(6): 2473-81.
[http://dx.doi.org/10.1016/j.actbio.2014.02.024] [PMID: 24560621]

[24]   Wan Y, Feng G, Shen FH, Laurencin CT, Li X. Biphasic scaffold for annulus fibrosus tissue regeneration. Biomaterials 2008; 29(6): 643-52.
[http://dx.doi.org/10.1016/j.biomaterials.2007.10.031] [PMID: 17997480]

[25]   Helen W, Merry CLR, Blaker JJ, Gough JE. Three-dimensional culture of annulus fibrosus cells within PDLLA/Bioglass® composite foam scaffolds: Assessment of cell attachment, proliferation and extracellular matrix production. Biomaterials 2007; 28(11): 2010-20.
[http://dx.doi.org/10.1016/j.biomaterials.2007.01.011] [PMID: 17250887]

[26]   Wismer N, Grad S, Fortunato G, Ferguson SJ, Alini M, Eglin D. Biodegradable electrospun scaffolds for annulus fibrosus tissue engineering: effect of scaffold structure and composition on annulus fibrosus cells in vitro. Tissue Eng Part A 2014; 20(3-4)
[http://dx.doi.org/10.1089/ten.tea.2012.0679] [PMID: 24131280]

[27]   Guterl CC, Torre OM, Purmessur D, *et al.* Characterization of mechanics and cytocompatibility of fibrin-genipin annulus fibrosus sealant with the addition of cell adhesion molecules. Tissue Eng Part A 2014; 20(17-18): 2536-45.
[http://dx.doi.org/10.1089/ten.tea.2012.0714] [PMID: 24684314]

[28]   Chik TK, Ma XY, Choy TH, *et al.* Photochemically crosslinked collagen annulus plug: A potential solution solving the leakage problem of cell-based therapies for disc degeneration. Acta Biomater 2013; 9(9): 8128-39.
[http://dx.doi.org/10.1016/j.actbio.2013.05.034] [PMID: 23751592]

[29]   Borde B, Grunert P, Härtl R, Bonassar LJ. Injectable, high□density collagen gels for annulus fibrosus repair: An *in vitro* rat tail model. J Biomed Mater Res A 2015; 103(8): 2571-81.
[http://dx.doi.org/10.1002/jbm.a.35388] [PMID: 25504661]

[30]   Grunert P, Borde BH, Hudson KD, Macielak MR, Bonassar LJ, Härtl R. Annular repair using high-density collagen gel: a rat-tail *in vivo* model. Spine 2014; 39(3): 198-206.
[http://dx.doi.org/10.1097/BRS.0000000000000103] [PMID: 24253790]

[31]   Schek RM, Michalek AJ, Iatridis JC. Genipin-crosslinked fibrin hydrogels as a potential adhesive to augment intervertebral disc annulus repair. Eur Cell Mater 2011; 21: 373-83.
[http://dx.doi.org/10.22203/eCM.v021a28] [PMID: 21503869]

[32]   Guillaume O, Daly A, Lennon K, Gansau J, Buckley SF, Buckley CT. Shape-memory porous alginate scaffolds for regeneration of the annulus fibrosus: Effect of TGF-β3 supplementation and oxygen culture conditions. Acta Biomater 2014; 10(5): 1985-95.
[http://dx.doi.org/10.1016/j.actbio.2013.12.037] [PMID: 24380722]

[33]   Bowles RD, Williams RM, Zipfel WR, Bonassar LJ. Self-assembly of aligned tissue-engineered annulus fibrosus and intervertebral disc composite *via* collagen gel contraction. Tissue Eng Part A 2010; 16(4): 1339-48.
[http://dx.doi.org/10.1089/ten.tea.2009.0442] [PMID: 19905878]

[34]   Ledet EH, Jeshuran W, Glennon JC, *et al.* Small intestinal submucosa for anular defect closure: long-term response in an *in vivo* sheep model. Spine 2009; 34(14): 1457-63.
        [http://dx.doi.org/10.1097/BRS.0b013e3181a48554] [PMID: 19525836]

[35]   Nerurkar NL, Elliott DM, Mauck RL. Mechanics of oriented electrospun nanofibrous scaffolds for annulus fibrosus tissue engineering. J Orthop Res 2007; 25(8): 1018-28.
        [http://dx.doi.org/10.1002/jor.20384] [PMID: 17457824]

[36]   Li WJ, Mauck RL, Cooper JA, Yuan X, Tuan RS. Engineering controllable anisotropy in electrospun biodegradable nanofibrous scaffolds for musculoskeletal tissue engineering. J Biomech 2007; 40(8): 1686-93.
        [http://dx.doi.org/10.1016/j.jbiomech.2006.09.004] [PMID: 17056048]

[37]   Koepsell L, Zhang L, Neufeld D, Fong H, Deng Y. Electrospun nanofibrous polycaprolactone scaffolds for tissue engineering of annulus fibrosus. Macromol Biosci 2011; 11(3): 391-9.
        [http://dx.doi.org/10.1002/mabi.201000352] [PMID: 21080441]

[38]   Attia M, Santerre JP, Kandel RA. The response of annulus fibrosus cell to fibronectin-coated nanofibrous polyurethane-anionic dihydroxyoligomer scaffolds. Biomaterials 2011; 32(2): 450-60.
        [http://dx.doi.org/10.1016/j.biomaterials.2010.09.010] [PMID: 20880584]

[39]   Bowles RD, Gebhard HH, Härtl R, Bonassar LJ. Tissue-engineered intervertebral discs produce new matrix, maintain disc height, and restore biomechanical function to the rodent spine. Proc Natl Acad Sci USA 2011; 108(32): 13106-11.
        [http://dx.doi.org/10.1073/pnas.1107094108] [PMID: 21808048]

[40]   Park SH, Gil ES, Mandal BB, Cho H, Kluge JA, Min BH, *et al.* Annulus fibrosus tissue engineering using lamellar silk scaffolds. J Tissue Eng Regen Med 2012; 6(Suppl 3): s24-33.

[41]   Bhattacharjee M, Miot S, Gorecka A, *et al.* Oriented lamellar silk fibrous scaffolds to drive cartilage matrix orientation: Towards annulus fibrosus tissue engineering. Acta Biomater 2012; 8(9): 3313-25.
        [http://dx.doi.org/10.1016/j.actbio.2012.05.023] [PMID: 22641105]

[42]   Sato M, Kikuchi M, Ishihara M, *et al.* Tissue engineering of the intervertebral disc with cultured annulus fibrosus cells using atelocollagen honeycombshaped scaffold with a membrane seal (ACHMS scaffold). Med Biol Eng Comput 2003; 41(3): 365-71.
        [http://dx.doi.org/10.1007/BF02348444] [PMID: 12803304]

[43]   Ionescu LC, Mauck RL. Porosity and cell preseeding influence electrospun scaffold maturation and meniscus integration in vitro. Tissue Eng Part A 2013; 19(3-4): 538-47.
        [http://dx.doi.org/10.1089/ten.tea.2012.0052] [PMID: 22994398]

[44]   Nachemson A. Some mechanical properties of the lumbar intervertebral discs. Bull Hosp Jt Dis 1962; 23: 130-43.
        [PMID: 13937019]

[45]   Schneider PG, Oyen R. [Proceedings: Disk displacement. Experimental studies--clinical consequences]. Z Orthop Ihre Grenzgeb 1974; 112(4): 791-2. [Proceedings: Disk displacement. Experimental studies--clinical consequences].
        [PMID: 4280754]

[46]   Schneider PG, Oyen R. [Surgical replacement of the intervertebral disc. First communication: replacement of lumbar discs with silicon-rubber. Theoretical and experimental investigations (author's transl)]. Z Orthop Ihre Grenzgeb 1974; 112(5): 1078-86. [Surgical replacement of the intervertebral disc. First communication: replacement of lumbar discs with silicon-rubber. Theoretical and experimental investigations (author's transl)].
        [PMID: 4280830]

[47]   Cappello JE SR. inventorSynthetic proteins for In vivo drug delivery and tissue augmentation 2002.

[48]   Mehrkens A, Müller AM, Valderrabano V, Schären S, Vavken P. Tissue engineering approaches to degenerative disc disease – A meta-analysis of controlled animal trials. Osteoarthritis Cartilage 2012;

20(11): 1316-25.
[http://dx.doi.org/10.1016/j.joca.2012.06.001] [PMID: 22789805]

[49] Iatridis JC, Nicoll SB, Michalek AJ, Walter BA, Gupta MS. Role of biomechanics in intervertebral disc degeneration and regenerative therapies: what needs repairing in the disc and what are promising biomaterials for its repair? Spine J 2013; 13(3): 243-62.
[http://dx.doi.org/10.1016/j.spinee.2012.12.002] [PMID: 23369494]

[50] Golan JD, Martens F, Griebel J, LoPresti DC, Hess MG, Ahrens M. Long-term outcomes following lumbar nucleus replacement. Int J Spine Surg 2021; 15(6): 1096-102.
[http://dx.doi.org/10.14444/8196] [PMID: 35078882]

[51] Hess G, Golan J, Mozsko S, Duarte J, Jarzem P, Martens F, Eds. EARLY CLINICAL RESULTS OF A NOVEL NUCLEUS REPLACEMENT DEVICE Orthopaedic Proceedings. The British Editorial Society of Bone & Joint Surgery 2021.

[52] Malhotra NR, Han WM, Beckstein J, Cloyd J, Chen W, Elliott DM. An injectable nucleus pulposus implant restores compressive range of motion in the ovine disc. Spine 2012; 37(18): E1099-105.
[http://dx.doi.org/10.1097/BRS.0b013e31825cdfb7] [PMID: 22588378]

[53] Leckie AE, Akens MK, Woodhouse KA, Yee AJM, Whyne CM. Evaluation of thiol-modified hyaluronan and elastin-like polypeptide composite augmentation in early-stage disc degeneration: comparing 2 minimally invasive techniques. Spine 2012; 37(20): E1296-303.
[http://dx.doi.org/10.1097/BRS.0b013e318266ecea] [PMID: 22772576]

[54] Sivan SS, Roberts S, Urban JPG, *et al.* Injectable hydrogels with high fixed charge density and swelling pressure for nucleus pulposus repair: Biomimetic glycosaminoglycan analogues. Acta Biomater 2014; 10(3): 1124-33.
[http://dx.doi.org/10.1016/j.actbio.2013.11.010] [PMID: 24270091]

[55] Hu J, Chen B, Guo F, *et al.* Injectable silk fibroin/polyurethane composite hydrogel for nucleus pulposus replacement. J Mater Sci Mater Med 2012; 23(3): 711-22.
[http://dx.doi.org/10.1007/s10856-011-4533-y] [PMID: 22231270]

[56] Thomas JD, Fussell G, Sarkar S, Lowman AM, Marcolongo M. Synthesis and recovery characteristics of branched and grafted PNIPAAm–PEG hydrogels for the development of an injectable load-bearing nucleus pulposus replacement. Acta Biomater 2010; 6(4): 1319-28.
[http://dx.doi.org/10.1016/j.actbio.2009.10.024] [PMID: 19837195]

[57] Roughley P, Hoemann C, DesRosiers E, Mwale F, Antoniou J, Alini M. The potential of chitosan-based gels containing intervertebral disc cells for nucleus pulposus supplementation. Biomaterials 2006; 27(3): 388-96.
[http://dx.doi.org/10.1016/j.biomaterials.2005.06.037] [PMID: 16125220]

[58] Omlor GW, Nerlich AG, Lorenz H, *et al.* Injection of a polymerized hyaluronic acid/collagen hydrogel matrix in an *in vivo* porcine disc degeneration model. Eur Spine J 2012; 21(9): 1700-8.
[http://dx.doi.org/10.1007/s00586-012-2291-2] [PMID: 22531895]

[59] Revell PA, Damien E, Di Silvio L, Gurav N, Longinotti C, Ambrosio L. Tissue engineered intervertebral disc repair in the pig using injectable polymers. J Mater Sci Mater Med 2007; 18(2): 303-8.
[http://dx.doi.org/10.1007/s10856-006-0693-6] [PMID: 17323162]

[60] Jeong CG, Francisco AT, Niu Z, Mancino RL, Craig SL, Setton LA. Screening of hyaluronic acid–poly(ethylene glycol) composite hydrogels to support intervertebral disc cell biosynthesis using artificial neural network analysis. Acta Biomater 2014; 10(8): 3421-30.
[http://dx.doi.org/10.1016/j.actbio.2014.05.012] [PMID: 24859415]

[61] Halloran DO, Grad S, Stoddart M, Dockery P, Alini M, Pandit AS. An injectable cross-linked scaffold for nucleus pulposus regeneration. Biomaterials 2008; 29(4): 438-47.
[http://dx.doi.org/10.1016/j.biomaterials.2007.10.009] [PMID: 17959242]

[62]　Thomas J, Lowman A, Marcolongo M. Novel associated hydrogels for nucleus pulposus replacement. J Biomed Mater Res A 2003; 67A(4): 1329-37.
[http://dx.doi.org/10.1002/jbm.a.10119] [PMID: 14624520]

[63]　Bertagnoli R, Sabatino CT, Edwards JT, Gontarz GA, Prewett A, Parsons JR. Mechanical testing of a novel hydrogel nucleus replacement implant. Spine J 2005; 5(6): 672-81.
[http://dx.doi.org/10.1016/j.spinee.2004.12.004] [PMID: 16363077]

[64]　Bao QB, Yuan HA. New technologies in spine: nucleus replacement. Spine 2002; 27(11): 1245-7.
[http://dx.doi.org/10.1097/00007632-200206010-00020] [PMID: 12045526]

[65]　Boyd LM, Carter AJ. Injectable biomaterials and vertebral endplate treatment for repair and regeneration of the intervertebral disc. Eur Spine J 2006; 15(Suppl 3): S414-21.
[http://dx.doi.org/10.1007/s00586-006-0172-2]

[66]　Pereira DR, Silva-Correia J, Oliveira JM, Reis RL. Hydrogels in acellular and cellular strategies for intervertebral disc regeneration. J Tissue Eng Regen Med 2013; 7(2): 85-98.
[http://dx.doi.org/10.1002/term.500] [PMID: 22072398]

[67]　Cunningham BW, Dmitriev AE, Hu N, McAfee PC. General principles of total disc replacement arthroplasty: seventeen cases in a nonhuman primate model. Spine 2003; 28(20) (Suppl.): S118-24.
[http://dx.doi.org/10.1097/00007632-200310151-00005] [PMID: 14560183]

[68]　Geisler FH, McAfee PC, Banco RJ, *et al.* Prospective, Randomized, Multicenter FDA IDE Study of CHARITÉ Artificial Disc versus Lumbar Fusion: Effect at 5-year Follow-up of Prior Surgery and Prior Discectomy on Clinical Outcomes Following Lumbar Arthroplasty. SAS J 2009; 3(1): 17-25.
[http://dx.doi.org/10.1016/S1935-9810(09)70003-9] [PMID: 25802625]

[69]　Meisel HJ, Ganey T, Hutton WC, Libera J, Minkus Y, Alasevic O. Clinical experience in cell-based therapeutics: intervention and outcome. Eur Spine J 2006; 15(Suppl 3): S397-405.
[http://dx.doi.org/10.1007/s00586-006-0169-x]

[70]　Sakai D, Mochida J, Yamamoto Y, *et al.* Transplantation of mesenchymal stem cells embedded in Atelocollagen® gel to the intervertebral disc: a potential therapeutic model for disc degeneration. Biomaterials 2003; 24(20): 3531-41.
[http://dx.doi.org/10.1016/S0142-9612(03)00222-9] [PMID: 12809782]

[71]　Sakai D, Mochida J, Iwashina T, *et al.* Differentiation of mesenchymal stem cells transplanted to a rabbit degenerative disc model: potential and limitations for stem cell therapy in disc regeneration. Spine 2005; 30(21): 2379-87.
[http://dx.doi.org/10.1097/01.brs.0000184365.28481.e3] [PMID: 16261113]

[72]　Crevensten G, Walsh AJL, Ananthakrishnan D, *et al.* Intervertebral disc cell therapy for regeneration: mesenchymal stem cell implantation in rat intervertebral discs. Ann Biomed Eng 2004; 32(3): 430-4.
[http://dx.doi.org/10.1023/B:ABME.0000017545.84833.7c] [PMID: 15095817]

[73]　Le Visage C, Yang SH, Kadakia L, Sieber AN, Kostuik JP, Leong KW. Small intestinal submucosa as a potential bioscaffold for intervertebral disc regeneration. Spine 2006; 31(21): 2423-30.
[http://dx.doi.org/10.1097/01.brs.0000238684.04792.eb] [PMID: 17023850]

[74]　NCT01290367 Safety and Preliminary Efficacy Study of Mesenchymal Precursor Cells (MPCs) in Subjects With Lumbar Back Pain [06042023] Available from: wwwclinicaltrialsgov

[75]　NCT02338271 Autologous Adipose Derived Stem Cell Therapy for Intervertebral Disc Degeneration [Available from: wwwclinicaltrialsgov

[76]　Collin EC, Grad S, Zeugolis DI, *et al.* An injectable vehicle for nucleus pulposus cell-based therapy. Biomaterials 2011; 32(11): 2862-70.
[http://dx.doi.org/10.1016/j.biomaterials.2011.01.018] [PMID: 21276612]

[77]　Yang H, Wu J, Liu J, *et al.* Transplanted mesenchymal stem cells with pure fibrinous gelatin-transforming growth factor-β1 decrease rabbit intervertebral disc degeneration. Spine J 2010; 10(9):

802-10.
[http://dx.doi.org/10.1016/j.spinee.2010.06.019] [PMID: 20655810]

[78]   Frith JE, Cameron AR, Menzies DJ, *et al.* An injectable hydrogel incorporating mesenchymal precursor cells and pentosan polysulphate for intervertebral disc regeneration. Biomaterials 2013; 34(37): 9430-40.
[http://dx.doi.org/10.1016/j.biomaterials.2013.08.072] [PMID: 24050877]

[79]   Mizuno H, Roy AK, Vacanti CA, Kojima K, Ueda M, Bonassar LJ. Tissue-engineered composites of anulus fibrosus and nucleus pulposus for intervertebral disc replacement. Spine 2004; 29(12): 1290-7.
[http://dx.doi.org/10.1097/01.BRS.0000128264.46510.27] [PMID: 15187626]

[80]   Nesti LJ, Li WJ, Shanti RM, *et al.* Intervertebral disc tissue engineering using a novel hyaluronic acid-nanofibrous scaffold (HANFS) amalgam. Tissue Eng Part A 2008; 14(9): 1527-37.
[http://dx.doi.org/10.1089/ten.tea.2008.0215] [PMID: 18707229]

[81]   Zhuang Y, Huang B, Li CQ, *et al.* Construction of tissue-engineered composite intervertebral disc and preliminary morphological and biochemical evaluation. Biochem Biophys Res Commun 2011; 407(2): 327-32.
[http://dx.doi.org/10.1016/j.bbrc.2011.03.015] [PMID: 21382343]

[82]   Bowles RD, Gebhard HH, Dyke JP, *et al.* Image□based tissue engineering of a total intervertebral disc implant for restoration of function to the rat lumbar spine. NMR Biomed 2012; 25(3): 443-51.
[http://dx.doi.org/10.1002/nbm.1651] [PMID: 21387440]

[83]   Park SH, Gil ES, Cho H, *et al.* Intervertebral disk tissue engineering using biphasic silk composite scaffolds. Tissue Eng Part A 2012; 18(5-6): 447-58.
[http://dx.doi.org/10.1089/ten.tea.2011.0195] [PMID: 21919790]

[84]   Chik TK, Chooi WH, Li YY, *et al.* Bioengineering a multicomponent spinal motion segment construct--a 3D model for complex tissue engineering. Adv Healthc Mater 2015; 4(1): 99-112.
[http://dx.doi.org/10.1002/adhm.201400192] [PMID: 24846571]

[85]   Mizuno H, Roy AK, Zaporojan V, Vacanti CA, Ueda M, Bonassar LJ. Biomechanical and biochemical characterization of composite tissue-engineered intervertebral discs. Biomaterials 2006; 27(3): 362-70.
[http://dx.doi.org/10.1016/j.biomaterials.2005.06.042] [PMID: 16165204]

[86]   Lazebnik M, Singh M, Glatt P, Friis LA, Berkland CJ, Detamore MS. Biomimetic method for combining the nucleus pulposus and annulus fibrosus for intervertebral disc tissue engineering. J Tissue Eng Regen Med 2011; 5(8): e179-87.
[http://dx.doi.org/10.1002/term.412] [PMID: 21774081]

[87]   Chang G, Kim HJ, Vunjak-Novakovic G, Kaplan DL, Kandel R. Enhancing annulus fibrosus tissue formation in porous silk scaffolds. J Biomed Mater Res A 2010; 92A(1): 43-51.
[http://dx.doi.org/10.1002/jbm.a.32326] [PMID: 19165797]

[88]   Choy ATH, Chan BP. A Structurally and Functionally Biomimetic Biphasic Scaffold for Intervertebral Disc Tissue Engineering. PLoS One 2015; 10(6)e0131827
[http://dx.doi.org/10.1371/journal.pone.0131827] [PMID: 26115332]

[89]   Huang YC, Urban JPG, Luk KDK. Intervertebral disc regeneration: do nutrients lead the way? Nat Rev Rheumatol 2014; 10(9): 561-6.
[http://dx.doi.org/10.1038/nrrheum.2014.91] [PMID: 24914695]

[90]   Séguin CA, Grynpas MD, Pilliar RM, Waldman SD, Kandel RA. Tissue engineered nucleus pulposus tissue formed on a porous calcium polyphosphate substrate. Spine 2004; 29(12): 1299-306.
[http://dx.doi.org/10.1097/01.BRS.0000127183.43765.AF] [PMID: 15187628]

CHAPTER 5

Current Therapy Strategies for Vertebral Endplates

Alvaro Dowling[1,*] and **Marcelo Molina**[2]

[1] *Orthopaedic Spine Surgeon, Director of Endoscopic Spine Clinic, Santiago, Chile*

[2] *Department of Orthopaedic Surgery, Faculdade de Medicina de Ribeirão Preto - USP (School of Medicine of Ribeirão Preto - University of São Paulo), Ribeirão Preto, SP, Brazil*

Abstract: The vertebral endplate is a critical component of the intervertebral disc, and its dysfunction can lead to various spinal disorders and chronic back pain. The structure and function of the vertebral endplate play an important role in disc nutrition, biomechanical support, and waste removal. Endplate-related conditions and their respective pathophysiologies may play a role in painful degeneration, fractures, and Modic changes. This chapter summarizes current concepts of therapeutic strategies with an emphasis on regenerative medicine application. It discusses using mesenchymal stem cells, platelet-rich plasma, growth factors, and tissue engineering approaches for endplate regeneration and repair. Diagnostic strategies for assessing vertebral endplate disorders and palliative as well as regenerative treatment strategies are discussed. The current evidence, ongoing research, and prospects in endplate-based therapies are highlighted.

Keywords: Annulus fibrosus, Disc degeneration, Degenerative disc disease, Fusion, Herniation, Intervertebral disc, Nucleus pulposus, Spine.

INTRODUCTION

Insufficient nutrient influx coupled with catabolic waste accrual are salient factors in the pathogenesis of intervertebral disc degeneration [1-6]. Given the disc's avascular constitution, it predominantly relies on vertebral endplates as essential conduits for nutrient facilitation [7, 8]. This solute transfer is orchestrated *via* an intricate network involving capillary beds and vascular interconnections between the osseous marrow recesses and the hyaline cartilaginous structure of the endplates [6, 9-12]. These vascular interfaces are imperative for cellular metabolic functions and the biofabrication of extracellular matrix components. Moreover, the effective expulsion of metabolic byproducts, notably lactic acid, is quintes-

* **Corresponding author: Álvaro Dowling:** Orthopaedic Spine Surgeon, Director of Endoscopic Spine Clinic, Santiago, Chile; E-mail: adowling@dws.cl

Kai-Uwe Lewandrowski & William Omar Contreras López (Eds.)

sential for averting their intradiscal accumulation [13]. Further, osmotic regulation *via* endplate-mediated water diffusion maintains intradiscal pressure equilibrium, which in turn contributes to disc height and mechanical functionality [14, 15].

Substantial empirical substantiation posits a robust correlative link between disc degenerative phenomena and concomitant alterations in adjoining endplates. Studies, exemplified by those conducted by Nachemson *et al.*, unveil a significant association between reduced endplate permeability and degenerative disc maladies [16]. Histological annotations indicate that disc degeneration is often presaged by lesions and microfractures within the endplates [17-19]. Additionally, age-associated calcification of endplate cartilage and the ensuing occlusion of nutrient conduits have been empirically observed. Radiological diagnostics, encapsulated by variations in MRI signal intensities in the vertebral marrow and morphological endplate alterations, manifest a strong linkage to degenerative disc conditions [22, 23]. Further, the aperture density within endplates has been ascertained to have a significant correlation with the degree of observed morphological deterioration [24].

Common interventional paradigms for mitigating disc degeneration encompass discectomy followed by scaffold implantation within the intradiscal environment. However, the efficacious implementation of these regenerative scaffolds is inexorably contingent upon the structural and functional integrity of the endplates. In instances where endplates exhibit sclerotic or hypertrophic characteristics, the anticipated restorative efficacy of the scaffold becomes critically compromised, owing predominantly to impeded fluidic and nutrient permeation. Thus, a compromised foundational architecture in the form of defective endplates ultimately undermines the holistic objectives oriented towards disc remediation.

Physiology

Endplates are composite structures characterized by both osseous and hyaline cartilaginous elements, discernible from embryonic developmental phases [25]. The osseous segment undergoes co-ossification with adjoining vertebral entities, while the cartilaginous component persists throughout standard ontogeny, eliciting noteworthy scientific attention. This cartilage portion is constituted by a hydrogel-like matrix replete with proteoglycan macromolecules, buttressed by a reticulum of collagen fibrils. Contrary to articular cartilage in diarthrodial joints, these collagenous fibrils refrain from direct osseous anchoring to the vertebral corpus [26]. Nevertheless, the endplate retains its proximal interface with the intervertebral disc *via* the inner annulus fibrosus lamellae [27]. During axial skeletal maturation, capillary networks transiently invade the endplates, furnishing requisite nutrients to the disc [25]. These vasculatures regress upon the attainment ofskeletal maturity, rendering mature discs largely dependent on solute diffusion across the endplates for sustenance and metabolic reciprocity [28].

Expansive scientific exploration has interrogated the endplate's biochemical constitution under physiological homeostasis and diverse degenerative paradigms [29, 30]. Of the various collagen subtypes identified within the disc, Type X collagen accrues particular significance in endplate pathophysiology, serving as a surrogate marker for hypertrophic chondrocytes and participating in calcification cascades [31]. Intriguingly, targeted abrogation of one Collagen II gene allele in murine models precipitates diminished glycosaminoglycan content within endplates, engendering abnormally thickened and precociously calcified structures [32]. These proteoglycan moieties play pivotal roles in modulating osmotic dynamics and maintaining hydric equilibrium within endplate cartilaginous matrices [33]. Their diminution correlates with concomitant proteoglycan deficits within the nucleus pulposus, implicating proteoglycan attrition as a likely precursor to disc degenerative processes [34].

Additional biochemical alterations in the endplates during skeletogenesis may impart a contributory role in the etiopathogenesis of conditions like scoliosis [35-37]. Comprehensive metabolic and nutritional studies of the disc have employed diverse *In vitro* models, substantiating the endplate's cardinal role in metabolic orchestration [16]. Notably, lateral peripheries of the endplate adjacent to vertebral rims exhibit reduced permeability *vis-a-vis* its central or annular counterparts [9, 28]. Morphometric analyses employing post-mortem human specimens have revealed a differential distribution of microvascular networks, with central endplate regions possessing augmented capillary densities relative to peripheral disc areas [3, 38]. This circulatory infrastructure, visualized through specialized injection techniques, corroborates that primary nutrient influx into the disc is mediated by diffusional transfer of minute solutes from these microvessels [7, 39]. However, this permeability is selective, governed by molecular dimensions and ionic polarity. The nucleus pulposus' high proteoglycan content endows it with a net negative electrostatic charge, thereby facilitating the ingress of cations like sodium and calcium, in addition to neutral entities like glucose and oxygen, whilst obstructing the transit of anions such as sulfate and chloride, as well as larger macromolecules like immunoglobulins and enzymatic compounds.

Endplate and Skeletal Maturity

Upon the attainment of skeletal maturity, the cartilaginous architecture of the endplate undergoes pronounced metamorphosis, culminating in substantive mineralization—a process subsequently reversed through osteoclastic resorption and osseous substitution [20, 40]. This emergent tissue composition impinges detrimentally on the indispensable solute diffusion and nutritive exchange between vertebral marrow and intervertebral disc architecture [41]. Such calcification phenomena precipitate the effacement of intraluminal capillaries within the endplate, further constricting vital metabolic interchange.

With chronological aging, endplate morphologies typically manifest adaptive and pathological alterations, which may correlate with perturbations in the nucleus pulposus and annulus fibrosus, particularly during late-stage disc degenerative [42]. Early-stage microscopic features commonly include the advent of horizontal lacerations and cavitations traversing the endplate, sporadically accompanied by chondrocyte necrosis. In certain instances, neovascularization is discernible in the proximity of osseous endplate demarcations. As a terminal event, cartilaginous elements capitulate to ossification processes.

In scenarios where cartilage maintains a vestige of its physiological integrity, vascular infiltrations into the endplate result in nuclear compensation within these resultant vacuities; notably, these vascular anomalies seldom compromise the osseous surface. By the fifth decade, extrusions of nuclear material into vertebral marrow become observable, concomitant with the emergence of focal osseous sclerosis owing to active tissue remodeling. The ultimate trajectory often culminates in complete cartilaginous attrition. In an animal paradigm designed to emulate spondylolysis, evidence of disc degeneration—inclusive of endplate erosion—was observed, accompanied by an upsurge in apoptotic activity among endplate chondrocytes. This portends the plausible involvement of programmed cellular demise in the pathogenesis of age-affiliated disc degenerative phenomena [43].

Vascularity

Vascular dynamics within the endplate region are not merely subject to passive mechanisms; the presence of muscarinic receptors has been corroborated, serving to modulate nutrient influx into the disc under variegated physiological conditions [5]. Ancillary investigations have also discerned the existence of neural fibrils and vascular networks within the endplates and subjacent osseous strata of degenerative discs, implying a plausible nexus between tissue reparative processes and dorsalgia [44, 45]. Intriguingly, post-maturation revascularization capabilities of the endplate have been substantiated in specific species, both under basal conditions [12] and under pathological exigencies [46]. In the context of the latter, despite the revascularization ostensibly representing a reparative effort, it failed to ameliorate the inexorable degenerative trajectory incited by disruptions in the annulus fibrosus.

Notably, the neoangiogenesis within the endplate is potentiated by the activation of matrix metalloproteinases (MMPs), enzymes intrinsically involved in extracellular matrix degradation. These enzymes are customarily sequestered in an inactive state by endogenous tissue inhibitors, underscoring the intricate balance of enzymatic activity and restraint crucial to tissue homeostasis [47-51].

Neuroanatomy of the Vertebral Endplate

Microscopic exploration has elucidated the existence of dually organized neurovascular assemblages, as well as insular intraosseous neural configurations within vertebral anatomical units [52-54]. These nerve plexuses, referred to as basivertebral nerves (BVNs), emanate as offshoots from the sinuvertebral nerves and ingress the vertebral structure *via* the posterior basivertebral foramina. Within the osteological unit, approximately at one-third the distance from the posterior to the anterior diameter, these BVNs ramify to furnish neural enervation to the entirety of the vertebral corpus, including the vertebral endplate (VEP) [52, 53]. These BVNs and their tributaries manifest nociceptive neuropeptides such as Substance P and calcitonin gene-related peptides, thereby intimating their presumptive role in the conduction of dolorific stimuli [44, 52, 53]. Empirical assessments have identified that specific VEP irregularities, predominantly of types 1 and 2, manifest an elevated neural density [55] and augmented prevalence of nociceptive neuropeptides in contrast to normative VEP specimens [44, 52, 53, 55], thereby suggesting a role for BVNs in the pathogenesis of chronic lower back pain (CLBP).

Supplementary inquiries have scrutinized potential alternative or adjunctive neural sources for VEP innervation [56]. Various studies have proposed extra-BVN neural structures within the posterior region of the VEP as emanating branches from the sinuvertebral nerve, and alternative neural inroads penetrating the anterior osseous cortex as another potential enervating source [52, 54]. Furthermore, the gray rami communicans, which typically provide innervation to the peripheral anterolateral annulus fibrosus, may also participate in the enervation of the contiguous periphery of theVEP [57]. These avenues for alternative neural sources bear potential clinical import.

The postulated role of the VEP in the pathophysiology of CLBP has engendered the advancement of minimally invasive therapeutic modalities aimed at mitigating nociceptive transmission within the VEP. Among these is the radiofrequency ablation (RFA) of the BVN, performed under fluoroscopic control through a unilateral transpedicular approach. A strategically positioned curved stylet delineates the path towards the BVN, enabling the insertion of a bipolar RFA electrode. Subsequent thermal escalation of the electrode to 85°C over a 15-

minute interval facilitates the ablation of the BVN, culminating in the generation of a spherical lesion within the osteological unit, with an approximate volume of one cubic centimeter. Preclinical models [58] and subsequent human trials have corroborated the procedure's efficacy *via* post-procedural magnetic resonance imaging assessments [58-61].

Endplate Failure Modes

Post-mortem examinations have corroborated the notion that discrete sectors of the endplate may disassociate from the vertebral corpus and undergo herniation in conjunction with affiliated annular fibers [62, 63]. The vicinity in proximity to the epiphyseal ring—serving as the anchoring point for annular fibers into the vertebral entity—emerges as a structurally vulnerable locus, substantiating its frequent designation as a fracture epicenter in the adolescent population [64]. Both finite element analysis [65] and meticulous microscopic scrutiny [42] have validated these findings. Mechanical insufficiency of the endplate is predominantly observed at the juncture of its attachment to the subjacent subchondral osseous structure. This susceptibility is attributable to the suboptimal interfacing of collagen fibrils with the bone matrix [26]. Empirical endeavours employing adolescent porcine spinal models have recapitulated analogous outcomes following mechanical compression [66-68].

Among the frequently discerned endplate irregularities is Schmorl's node (Fig. **1**), typified by a vertical intrusion of nuclear material into the adjoining vertebral construct [21]. These nodes have been identified in an excess of 70% of vertebral autopsies, with prevalence unaffected by age stratification, implying their genesis early in life [69]. Notably, the male predominance of these nodes reverses post-sixty year, aligning with the timeframe during which vertebral discs are increasingly susceptible to structural compromise, such as osteoporotic alterations [54]. Despite the general absence of natural perforations in most endplates, Schmorl postulated that these lesions emerge from localized regions of fragility engendered by cartilaginous degeneration [21]. In instances devoid of direct traumatic insult or neoplastic degradation, the endplates remain integral, and the prevailing opinion attributes this integrity to residual scar tissue subsequent to the occlusion of diminutive vascular pathways during spinal development. Significantly, endplates harboring Schmorl's nodes exhibit a heightened frequency of marrow edema, insinuating their potential contributory role in ancillary pathologies, such as Scheuermann's disease.

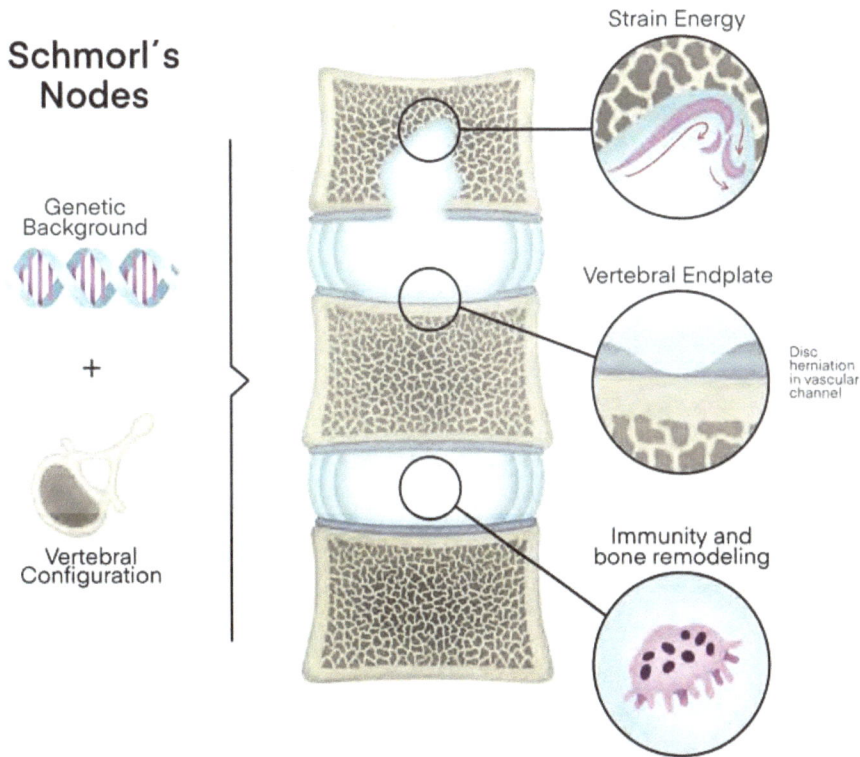

Fig. (1). A Schmorl's node is a vertical protrusion of nucleus contents into the adjacent vertebral body. Schmorl's nodes are found in over 70% of spines during the autopsy, with an equal frequency above and below the age of 50, suggesting their occurrence early in life. They are twice as common in adult men implying an association with occupational trauma. After age 60, Schmorl's nodes become twice as common in women suggesting a correlation with age-related changes, such as osteoporosis. Schmorl's nodes arise from focal weak spots caused by degenerate cartilage. Vascular channels within the nodes have been observed, indicating a potential role of angiogenesis in their formation and progression. Inflammatory immune responses, including the activation of immune cells and the release of proinflammatory cytokines, have been implicated in the pathogenesis of Schmorl's nodes. Remodeling of the extracellular matrix, mediated by enzymes such as matrix metalloproteinases, may contribute to the degenerative changes associated with the nodes.

Termed Modic changes, represent a specific category of anomalies affecting the vertebral endplate as well as the osseous marrow, initially delineated by Dr. Michael Modic in the late 20th century [23]. These alterations have been systematically compartmentalized into three distinct typologies. Type I Modic alterations are distinguished by an amplification of signal intensity in T2-weighted magnetic resonance imaging (MRI), indicative of marrow edema and vascular proliferation. Conversely, Type II alterations manifest as a diminution of signal intensity in both T1- and T2-weighted MRI, a hallmark of fatty infiltration supplanting the bone marrow. Type III alterations are characterized by augmented signal intensity in T1-weighted MRI scans, serving as a proxy for subchondral osseous sclerosis [70-72]. Notably, these changes are frequently concomitant with symptomatology of lumbar discomfort and have been implicated in both the genesis and progression of spondylotic disc maladies. However, a comprehensive elucidation of the underlying pathophysiological mechanisms and clinical relevance of Modic alterations necessitates further scholarly investigation [72] (Fig. **2**).

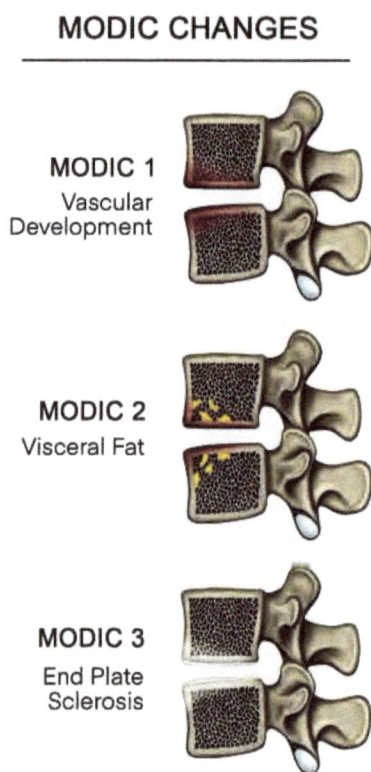

Fig. (2). Modic type I changes are characterized by increased signal intensity on T2-weighted magnetic resonance imaging (MRI), representing edema and vascularization within the bone marrow. Modic type II changes exhibit decreased signal intensity on both T1- and T2-weighted MRI, indicating fatty replacement of the bone marrow. Modic type III changes show increased signal intensity on T1-weighted MRI and represent subchondral bone sclerosis.

Rationale for Endplate Treatment

Interventions aimed at disc augmentation, repair, and regenerative therapy may necessitate targeted remediation of vertebral endplates to approximate their pre-injury or pre-degenerative physiological states as closely as feasible. The therapeutic modalities applied to the endplate are contingent upon the specific form of endplate deterioration, as well as the nature of the biomaterial matrix designated for the intradiscal intervention. One conceivable therapeutic avenue involves the chemical decalcification of sclerotic, hypertrophied, and impermeable vertebral endplates. An alternative modality could encompass basivertebral nerve (BVN) ablation.

Articular cartilaginous calcification in endplates imposes constraints on fluidic transference, a hindrance potentially ameliorated by the injection of chelating agents with high calcium affinity. Subsequent to an optimal incubation period, these decalcifying agents, along with their metabolic derivatives, may be evacuated from the intervertebral space. Furthermore, macro-proteoglycans such as aggrecan can occlude the trans-endplate diffusion of specific solutes. This permeability impediment can be counteracted by enzymatic degradation using trypsin or similar catalytic proteins, often in concomitance with calcification treatment.

Tissue engineering approaches, which amalgamate cellular systems, biocompatible scaffolding, and an array of growth factors or cytokines, hold promise for the reconstructive regeneration of tissues and organs. Hence, preliminary treatment of vertebral endplates could potentiate cellular infiltration into the introduced scaffolds. Such pretreatment measures may also facilitate the osteointegration of specific disc prosthetics, which can be pre-seeded with autologous disc cells prior to implantation.

Increasing Endplate Vascularity

The presence of a robust vasculature within the endplate domain is imperative for the efficacious conveyance of essential nutrients and the subsequent biological performance of the intervertebral disc. Pharmacological interventions may be employed to potentiate vascular proliferation within the tissue matrices, incorporating bioactive substances such as vascular endothelial growth factors (VEGF) and other pro-angiogenic cytokines. These bioactive molecules are readily assimilated by the cellular and extracellular components of the endplate, necessitating only minimal incubation periods and obviating the need for subsequent removal. Concurrently, genetic therapeutic strategies may be invoked to enact transient transfection of native cellular entities, notably endothelial cells, for the targeted secretion of angiogenic cytokines [73, 74]. Given its protracted bioactive duration, this vascular-augmenting approach is optimally reserved for the concluding phase of a comprehensive endplate remediation regimen.

Enhanced Biointegration

Optimal Interfacing of Biomaterials in Disc Prosthetics: Ensuring efficacious integration between scaffold biomaterials and surrounding anatomical structures—including the pivotal endplate contact zones—is quintessential for the stable anchorage and long-term viability of intradiscal prosthetic implants. Both solid and in situ-curable, injectable scaffold constructs fundamentally rely on osteointegration at the graft-host juncture. This osteointegrative interaction is particularly salient at the interface conjoining the prosthetic device and vertebral endplate [75-77].

However, the endogenous cartilaginous matrices of both the endplate and annulus fibrosus are replete with an array of macro- and micro-proteoglycans that can obfuscate optimal bio-integration. Within the milieu of articular cartilage regeneration, enzymatic disintegration of peripherally adjacent cartilaginous matrices has been posited to facilitate interdigitation with neosynthesized matrix elements. Empirical investigations indicate that enzymatically-mediated matrix degradation—specifically *via* protease application—paves the way for facile infiltration of reconstituted repair tissues by reducing structured aqueous and matrix components [78].

For the establishment of a well-integrated graft-tissue interphase, enzymatic preconditioning of afflicted endplates, utilizing enzymatic agents such as trypsin or hyaluronidase, may prove beneficial. These enzymes encourage the outgrowth of cartilaginous tissue buds from adjacent, untreated tissues into the enzymatically modified graft area. Protocols involving sequential enzymatic degradation—initially with hyaluronidase, followed by trypsin—have demonstrated the effective extraction of proteoglycans without consequential compromise of the foundational collagen fiber network.

Subsequent to an appropriate enzymatic incubation interval, residual solutions, and enzymatic byproducts are evacuated from the discal chamber, succeeded by thorough irrigation with an isotonic saline medium. Alternative targeting of extracellular matrix constituents may also be executed *via* the utilization of specific proteolytic enzymes. Furthermore, implant integration can be augmented through secondary cellular infiltration from ectopic sources such as non-articulating knee cartilage. This involves cellular migration into the scaffold from surrounding native tissues, rather than direct cellular implantation onto or within the scaffold. Preconditioning of cartilaginous explants with trypsin has been empirically demonstrated to foster accelerated chondrocyte proliferation and rapid reconstitution of matrix components denatured during enzymatic treatment [14].

Clinical Studies

At the time of the writing of this chapter in June 2023, a paucity of peer-reviewed literature exists regarding controlled clinical trials explicitly targeting endplate regeneration. An exception can be cited in a technical note accompanied by a case report proffered by Kirchner *et al.* in 2017 [79]. The research group employed a synergistic therapeutic modality encompassing vertebral intraosseous (VIO) and intradiscal (ID) administrations of Plasma Rich in Growth Factors (PRGF-Endoret), a subclass of leukocyte-depleted platelet-rich plasma, as an interventional strategy for the amelioration of discogenic pain syndromes [79] (Fig. **3**).

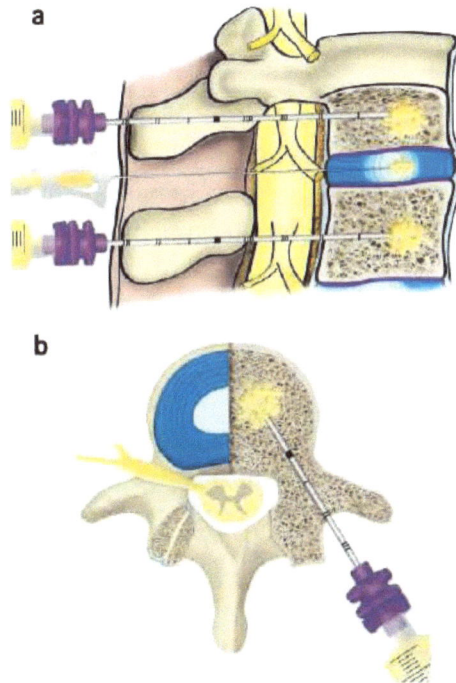

Fig. (3). Explanation of the technique employed for the intraosseous infiltration of PRGF: a) Sagittal view: In cases where the disc lesion is located near two damaged endplates with Modic type I or II lesions, Schmörl hernias, or fracture sequelae [27], the regeneration of the disc lesion can be more effective, faster, and safer by performing an intraosseous infiltration in the two adjacent vertebral bodies along with the disc. Only 4-5 ml of PRGF (F2) is infiltrated, and the needle tip does not need to be near the endplate since this volume is sufficient to fill the entire vertebral body. b) Axial view: This view demonstrates the transpedicular approach of the needle (15 G, 1.8 mm × 90 mm), which reaches the intraosseous level of the vertebral body, just slightly more than 1 cm from the back wall. The trocar-biopsy needle system is positioned using a low-speed power driver. Reproduced under Creative Commons Attribution 4.0 International License from Kirchner *et al.* [79], which permits unrestricted use, distribution, and reproduction in any medium, provided appropriate credit to the original author(s) and the source. No changes were made to the image or legend. Creative Commons license (http://creativecommons.org/licenses/by/4.0/).

Kirchner *et al.* delineate the vertebral endplate as a bipartite structural entity, composed of a cartilaginous endplate (CEP) and a vertebral subchondral bone (VSB). This composite edifice serves as a partitioning barrier, functionally segregating the vertebral osseous structure from the intervertebral disc (IVD), thereby mitigating the potential for nuclear pulposus herniation into adjacent neural elements. Distinct from the IVD, the endplate's central region within the VSB possesses abundant innervation, concomitant with the neighboring vertebral marrow. The VSB is instrumental in conserving spinal biomechanical integrity and ensuring the metabolic sustenance of the IVD [80].

Operating on the hypothesis that alterations in the biomechanical and bio-chemical attributes of both the IVD and VSB are inextricably linked with the pathogenesis of spinal pain syndromes and degenerative disc disease (DDD), the authors embarked on an investigation aimed at elucidating the therapeutic potential of an innovative regenerative approach targeting lumbar disc degenerative pathology.

The therapeutic protocol deployed by Kirchner *et al.* was predicated on dual cardinal tenets: a) the physiological and architectural relevance of the intervertebral disc (IVD) and vertebral subchondral bone (VSB) in spinal biomechanics and degenerative pathology, and b) the methodological congruence with established intraosseous PRGF infusions previously elucidated in the context of osteoarthritic afflictions of the knee [81] and hip [82] for analgesic interventions [20]. Accordingly, a combinatorial approach was instituted involving intradiscal [83] and vertebral intraosseous platelet-rich plasma (PRP) injections to galvanize the reparative processes of compromised spinal architecture [84]. The underlying hypothesis posited that targeted amelioration of endplate (EP) abnormalities would expedite the regenerative trajectory of symptomatic IVDs, owing to the nutrient influx primarily mediated by the EP itself [80].

Structural and functional spinal evolution was scrupulously monitored *via* magnetic resonance imaging (MRI). For instance, in a singular patient case, vertebral intraosseous PRGF administrations were undertaken at L3 and L4 loci under localized anesthesia. Serial dosages were subsequently extended to encompass the L4/L5 and L5/S1 intervertebral domains, with consequential alleviation in pain and functional impairment indices.

Six-month follow-up MRI analysis revealed unchanged global disc desiccation and degenerative severity at the L3/4 juncture, albeit with marginal attenuation in discal protrusion dimensions along the craniocaudal (CC) axis. No indicators of thecal sac or radicular encroachment were noted. Although the data remain anecdotal, the results substantiate extant literature on the spontaneous involution of herniated lumbar disc material subsequent to PRP administration. Nonetheless, the exact mechanistic underpinnings necessitate further elucidation.

Scant evidence exists concerning intravertebral herniations, such as Schmorl's nodes (SNs) [85], with sporadic reports substantiating MRI-mediated visual improvements in disc degeneration and herniation following PRP interventions [86, 87]. The documented clinical vignette offers an illustration of discernible MRI ameliorations in SN regression post-PRGF treatment. As a biologically inspired regimen targeting both spinal regenerative processes and symptomatic relief, PRGF modalities could potentially illuminate the physiological mechanisms governing discal and intravertebral herniation resolution [87]. Kirchner's avant-garde methodology underscores the imperative of employing standardized, high-resolution imaging and quantification strategies for the objective assessment of lumbar spinal pathoanatomy, thereby facilitating the correlation between analgesic efficacy, functional recuperation, and the regenerative potential of adjacent spinal architectures [88].

Pertaining to the therapeutic intervention of basivertebral nerve (BVN) ablation, an array of clinical investigations, encompassing evidence from randomized controlled trials, have been promulgated in the extant literature [58-61, 89-91]. These scientific inquiries uniformly necessitated primary inclusion criteria including, but not limited to, chronic lumbosacral pain (CLBP) of a minimum duration of six months refractory to non-surgical management, the negation of alternative etiologies for pain as ascertained by the presiding clinician, an Oswestry Disability Index (ODI) baseline score exceeding 30, a Numerical Rating Scale (NRS) nociceptive assessment of four or beyond on a decadic scale, as well as the verification of Modic alterations (MC) of either type one or two within the vertebral endplates (VEPs) across the L3 to S1 spinal segments (Fig. **4**).

Typical primary exclusion stipulations commonly precluded individuals manifesting radicular nociception, symptomatic spinal canal narrowing, prolapsed nucleus pulposus exceeding 5 millimeters, or spondylolisthetic shift greater than 2 millimeters. Select studies further delineated exclusionary criteria to omit individuals with prior lumbar surgical interventions, while alternate studies incorporated patients with historical discectomies or laminectomies provided the radicular symptoms had been satisfactorily ameliorated (Table **1**).

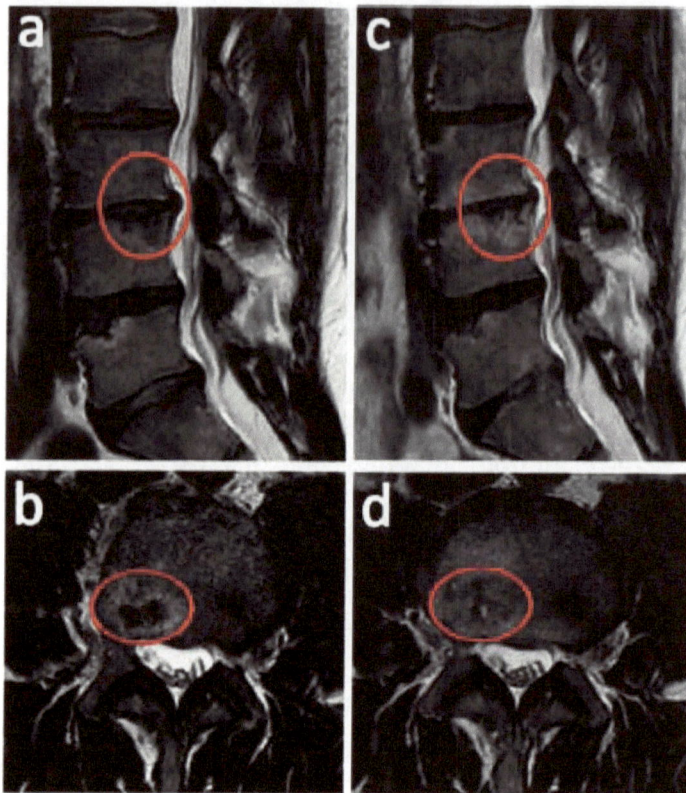

Fig. (4). MRI scan before and after platelet-rich plasma treatment. Initial MRI a sagittal and b axial T2-weighted images (T2WI) (in yellow letters). Six months later, a substantial reduction of Schmörl's node diameter (SND) was shown on c sagittal and d axial T2WI at the lumbar spinal level L3/L4. Red circles delineate SN size. Reproduced under Creative Commons Attribution 4.0 International License from Kirchner *et al.* [79], which permits unrestricted use, distribution, and reproduction in any medium, provided appropriate credit to the original author(s) and the source. No changes were made to image or legend. Creative Commons license (http://creativecommons.org/licenses/by/4.0/).

The paramount metric of therapeutic efficacy across these studies was predicated on alterations in ODI scores at the three-month postoperative mark, with nociceptive indices and other functional measures relegated to secondary outcome categorization. Response rates, both in terms of ODI amelioration and nociceptive diminution, constituted the focal endpoints subjected to analytic scrutiny in the current review. While the operational definition of clinically meaningful differences in ODI and pain indices exhibited minor heterogeneity across trials, a universal benchmark was instituted, mandating a nadir of a ten-point decrement in ODI and a 1.5-point diminution in either the Visual Analog Scale (VAS) or NRS as the minimal clinically significant variation. The present chapter collates and interprets response rates predicated upon extant data as synthesized by Michalik *et al.* [56].

Table 1. Outcomes in currently published BVN clinical trials; adopted from Michalik *et al.* [56].

Trials	N	Follow-Up [months]	Responder Rate (95% CI)	
			Pain Relief	Functional Improvement
Khalil *et al.* (2019) pragmatic randomized controlled trial) [61]	51	3	≥2-point NRS reduction: 73% (60–85%) ≥50% NRS reduction: 63% (49–76%)	≥20-point ODI reduction: 63% (49–76%)
Fischgrund *et al.* (2018)*,† (explanatory randomized controlled trial) [60]	128	3	≥50% VAS reduction: BVN RFA group: 45% (37–54%) Sham group: 37% (26–48%)	≥20-point ODI reduction: BVN RFA group: 48% (39–56%) Sham group: not reported
Fischgrund *et al.* (2019) [89]	128	24	≥1.5-point VAS reduction: 57% (49–66%)	≥20-point ODI reduction: 58% (48–67%)
Fischgrund *et al.* (2020) [90]	117	60	≥50% VAS reduction: 66% (57–75%)	≥15-point ODI reduction: 77% (69–85%)
Becker *et al.* (2017) [58]	16	12	Not reported	≥10-point reduction ODI: 81% (62–100%)
Truumees *et al.* (2019) [59]	28	3	≥2-point NRS reduction: 75.0% (59–91%)	≥20-point ODI reduction: 75.0% (59–91%)
		6	Not reported	≥20-point ODI reduction: 84% (68–100%)
Macadaeg *et al.* (2020) [91]	45	12	≥2-point NRS reduction: 80% (63–89%) ≥50% NRS reduction: 69% (95% CI not reported)	≥20 point reduction ODI: 84% (71–94%)

In a meticulously designed, multicenter, prospective, randomized, double-blind, sham-controlled investigation, denominated as the SMART Trial, Fischgrund *et al.* engaged 225 subjects [60]. Initial per-protocol statistical scrutiny revealed that the cohort receiving basivertebral nerve radiofrequency ablation (BVN RFA) demonstrated a statistically significant enhancement in Oswestry Disability Index (ODI) scores at the three-month evaluative juncture when contrasted with the sham control group (P=0.019). Notably, 48% of individuals in the BVN RFA arm achieved a decrement of 20 points or greater in ODI during this time frame. However, this differential impact waned, failing to achieve statistical significance, at subsequent six-month and one-year intervals.

With regard to analgesic outcomes, nearly half of the participants subjected to BVN RFA manifested a pain reduction of 50% or more at the aforementioned three-month mark, juxtaposed against 37% in the sham control. Although Visual

Analog Scale (VAS) scores did not reveal a statistically significant difference at three months (P=0.083), they did so at both six (P=0.008) and twelve-month (P=0.038) time points in favor of BVN RFA.

The intent-to-treat analysis did not corroborate these per-protocol findings at the three-month juncture (P=0.107). Several etiological factors accounted for this analytical discrepancy, primarily encompassing procedural inaccuracies, targeting failures during BVN RFA implementation, and instances of non-adherence to study protocols. It should be noted that the efficacy of placebo or sham treatments can be influenced by neurobiological factors and patient expectations. However, sham interventions are generally not endorsed as therapeutic modalities for chronic low back pain (CLBP), and a robust sham response is generally unforeseen in open-label investigations.

Moreover, after reaching the one-year milestone, subjects in the sham arm were presented with the option for treatment crossover; 73% opted for BVN RFA. Subsequent analyses beyond the one-year mark reverted to intra-group comparisons, contrasting BVN RFA outcomes with baseline metrics. At the 24-month evaluation, response rates stood at 58% and 57% for improvements in ODI and VAS, respectively. Furthermore, longitudinal data culled from an average follow-up duration of 6.4 years affirms the sustained therapeutic efficacy and durability of BVN RFA treatment, with 77% and 66% of subjects demonstrating substantial enhancements in ODI and analgesic relief, respectively [89, 90].

In a rigorously orchestrated, multicenter, randomized study known as INTRACEPT, Khalil *et al.* juxtaposed the efficaciousness of basivertebral nerve radiofrequency ablation (BVN RFA) with conventional therapeutic modalities [61]. The study deployed a 1:1 randomization protocol across 140 recruited participants. Conservative management encompassed a plethora of interventions including pharmacotherapy, physiotherapy, chiropractic manipulation, acupuncture, and epidural injections. An interim appraisal, executed upon 60% of participants reaching the primary endpoint of a three-month follow-up, was subjected to evaluation by an autonomous data management committee. Given the statistically significant clinical superiority of BVN RFA, the committee proffered an early cessation of recruitment and suggested treatment crossover for the standard care arm. Data harvested at the three-month juncture encompassed 104 participants—51 allocated to BVN RFA and 53 to conventional care. Remarkably, the BVN RFA cohort exhibited a 63% responder rate, defined by an enhancement of 20 points or more in ODI metrics, in stark contrast to a 14% response rate in the conventional care group (P < 0.001). Additionally, notable proportions (63% and 73%, respectively) reported pain amelioration of at least

50% and a minimum two-point improvement in the Numeric Rating Scale (NRS), as opposed to 34% in the conventional care arm (P < 0.001).

Simultaneously, Becker *et al.* conducted a prospective, observational, single-cohort inquiry comprising 16 subjects, all of whom underwent BVN RFA [58]. Mean ODI scores plummeted significantly from an initial baseline of 52 to 23 at the three-month review (P < 0.001) and displayed temporal stability up to the 12-month observational milestone. Concurrently, average Visual Analog Scale (VAS) scores underwent a salient decrement, declining from an initial 61 to 45 at the same three-month point (P < 0.05). Furthermore, at the one-year follow-up, a staggering 81% of subjects reported a decrement of 10 points or more in ODI scores.

Truumees *et al.*, in another investigative endeavor, undertook a prospective, open-label, single-arm clinical trial involving 28 participants subjected to BVN RFA treatment [59]. At the three-month evaluation, an overwhelming 75% of participants achieved both a 20-point or greater improvement in ODI and a minimum two-point increment in NRS. Extending this observation to a six-month follow-up, 84% registered a 20-point or greater amelioration in ODI metrics. Furthermore, data disseminated for the 12-month assessment revealed that 84% sustained this level of improvement in ODI scores, while 80% maintained at least a two-point advancement in NRS. An additional 69% reported pain reduction by at least 50%, substantiating the therapeutic longevity of BVN RFA.

The safety panorama of Bipolar Radiofrequency Ablation (BVN RFA) appears overwhelmingly benign, with scant incidence of severe adverse sequelae [60]. A singular case of vertebral body compression fracture has been cited, occurring in a patient undergoing hormone therapy and diagnosed with osteopenia; this fracture proceeded to uneventful convalescence. For individuals manifesting a heightened risk for compromised bone mineral density, preemptive assessment *via* dual-energy X-ray absorptiometry is judiciously advised [60]. Moreover, isolated iatrogenic incidents such as radicular trauma induced by trocar malposition and a solitary instance of retroperitoneal hemorrhage, ascribed to errant trocar localization, have been documented [60]. Ephemeral and mild phenomena, including motor or sensory deficits, paresthesias, and limb discomfort, have been sporadically noted across multiple studies [58, 59, 61]. Yet, there are no reported severe device- or technique-associated complications or substantial neurological impairments [58, 59, 61].

While theoretical apprehensions might be posited regarding the inadvertent propagation of the ablative lesion into the spinal canal, such concerns remain unsubstantiated. Extant clinical trials have not revealed any symptomatic corroborations, and post-procedure magnetic resonance imaging consistently affirms a discrete demarcation between the lesion and the posterior vertebral body wall [60]. Preexisting literature has substantiated the safety parameters of analogous bipolar RFA interventions within the spinal axis [92]. Therefore, it stands to reasoned extrapolation that BVN RFA would likely demonstrate comparable, if not superior, safety indices. This is further supported by the anatomical disposition of the targeted lesion in propinquity to the epidural venous plexus and cerebrospinal fluid, which function as thermal dissipators, thereby mitigating the potential for thermal insult to the cauda equina.

While data on protracted clinical outcomes are extant, a comprehensive explication of the long-term ramifications of Bipolar Radiofrequency Ablation (BVN RFA) remains pending [60]. There exists apprehension vis-à-vis Charcot spinal arthropathy, a pathology characterized by impaired deep pain and proprioceptive sensations within the vertebral architecture, consequent to attenuated afferent neural traffic [93]. Yet, the empirical record is devoid of cases of Charcot spinal arthropathy subsequent to BVN RFA procedures, ostensibly implicating the preservation of neural pathways in anatomical structures such as the intervertebral disc (IVD), facet joints, and perhaps segments of the vertebral endplate (VEP) in mitigating this risk [52].

For patients manifesting spondylolisthesis, theoretical speculation posits a heightened propensity for detrimental reductions in afferent neuronal input. However, this correlation has not achieved empirical substantiation to date. Prudence is, therefore, urged for this patient subset, given the idiosyncratic segmental instability that is categorically excluded from extant clinical investigations. Of particular note, magnetic resonance imaging conducted at a 6-month postoperative juncture failed to identify accelerated IVD degeneration, avascular necrosis, or spinal cord insults [60]. Nonetheless, an imperative for longitudinal imaging surveillance persists, to elucidate these variables with greater granularity [60].

DISCUSSION

There are many emerging therapeutic modalities for both the palliation and regeneration of vertebral endplates. These range from the deployment of recombinant proteins, cytokines, and growth factors to intricate molecular interventions, gene transfer techniques, cellular therapies, and basivertebral nerve ablation. To explain the scope of these therapeutic approaches is beyond the scope of this chapter. Nevertheless, it is worth stressing that most of these therapies are presently conceptualized within the broader anatomical and pathological context of the entire intervertebral disc, acknowledging the intricate biomechanical interplay within the spinal motion segment.

Except for the application of plasma rich in growth factors (PRGF-Endoret) for transpedicular infiltrations into the vertebral body, as suggested by Kirchner *et al.* [79], most regenerative strategies remain preclinical, poised for clinical application pending the outcome of rigorous empirical evaluation. Even upon validation, these treatments may not engender complete reversal of the degenerative processes; rather, they may aim to mitigate or forestall their inexorable clinical manifestations.

The crux lies in the judicious identification of intervention targets, which may span genes, bioactive molecules, or specific cellular entities, and most pertinently, individual pain generators. In this regard, the mitigative impact of basivertebral nerve ablation on pain scores corroborates the potential relevance of endplate-based pain generators [56, 58 - 61, 89 - 91]. Delineating between discogenic and vertebral endplate pain, however, presents an analytic challenge. While anesthetic discography offers a less invasive diagnostic option, the utility of intradiscal anesthetics under various pathophysiological conditions merits further investigation [95-98], particularly given the altered solute transport observed in the presence of Modic changes (MCs).

Several clinical trials have deployed a transpedicular approach with varying degrees of targeting success, the nuances of which may influence therapeutic outcomes [59 - 61]. Concomitant variations in procedural technique, as well as potential alternative innervation mechanisms [52, 54, 57], could contribute to incomplete denervation and subsequent persistent pain following basivertebral nerve ablation.

Conclusively, the clinical efficacies observed in basivertebral nerve ablation trials lend credence to the hypothesis that intervertebral discs may not constitute the singular etiological agents of back pain. As regenerative medicine burgeons, so too do expectations for biologically grounded solutions to degenerative diseases, obviating the need for more invasive surgical interventions. In light of this, patient selection criteria, informed by a myriad of variables ranging from genetic predispositions to occupational exposures, assume paramount importance for optimized therapeutic outcomes. Further studies elucidating the intricate relationships between endplate diffusion and cell nutrition are indispensable for the refinement of these emerging therapies.

CONCLUSION

Future research endeavors in the domain of intervertebral disc (IVD) therapeutics ought to be rigorously guided by well-articulated outcome metrics and design objectives. To date, the principal focus of regenerative and replacement strategies for IVD has been the restitution of salient anatomical hallmarks inherent to a eubiotic IVD and spinal motion segment. These encompass the preservation of normative disc height, magnetic resonance imaging signal intensity, unobstructed spinal cord, and nerve root pathways, and the maintenance of a physiological range of motion devoid of prosthesis malposition or dislocation. Such criteria, amenable to quantification through radiographic modalities, will undoubtedly persist as indispensable primary endpoints in the clinical actualization of prospective regenerative methodologies.

Tactics solely aimed at emulating matrix production, cellular viability, or tissue alignment within the IVD, while failing to re-establish these critical anatomical features, are unlikely to wield significant therapeutic efficacy in the treatment of IVD maladies. Complicating these endeavors is an extant deficit in our comprehensive understanding of IVD pathological ontogenesis and its symptomatic contributions, underscoring the need for a concomitant advance in bioengineering techniques. This synergistic development in bioengineering and foundational research is crucial for the informed establishment of design imperatives and engineered solutions aimed at ameliorating IVD disorders and their attendant pathologies.

REFERENCES

[1]   Adams MA, Bogduk N, Burton K, Dolan P. The Biomechanics of Back Pain-E-Book: Elsevier health sciences 2012.

[2]   Brodin H. Paths of nutrition in articular cartilage and intervertebral discs. Acta Orthop Scand 1955; 24(3): 177-83.
[PMID: 14387660]

[3]   Maroudas A, Stockwell RA, Nachemson A, Urban J. Factors involved in the nutrition of the human lumbar intervertebral disc: cellularity and diffusion of glucose in vitro. J Anat 1975; 120(Pt 1): 113-30.
[PMID: 1184452]

[4]   Urban JPG, Smith S, Fairbank JCT. Nutrition of the intervertebral disc. Spine 2004; 29(23): 2700-9.
[http://dx.doi.org/10.1097/01.brs.0000146499.97948.52] [PMID: 15564919]

[5]   Wallace AL, Wyatt BC, McCarthy ID, Hughes SPF. Humoral regulation of blood flow in the vertebral endplate. Spine 1994; 19(12): 1324-8.
[http://dx.doi.org/10.1097/00007632-199406000-00004] [PMID: 8066511]

[6]   Whalen JL, Parke WW, Mazur JM, Stauffer ES. The intrinsic vasculature of developing vertebral end plates and its nutritive significance to the intervertebral discs. J Pediatr Orthop 1985; 5(4): 403-10.
[http://dx.doi.org/10.1097/01241398-198507000-00003] [PMID: 4019751]

[7]   Urban JPG, Holm S, Maroudas A. Diffusion of small solutes into the intervertebral disc: as in vitro study. Biorheology 1978; 15(3-4): 203-23.

[http://dx.doi.org/10.3233/BIR-1978-153-409] [PMID: 737323]

[8]   Urban JPG, Maroudas A. The measurement of fixed charged density in the intervertebral disc. Biochim Biophys Acta, Gen Subj 1979; 586(1): 166-78.
[http://dx.doi.org/10.1016/0304-4165(79)90415-X]

[9]   Crock HV, Goldwasser M. Anatomic studies of the circulation in the region of the vertebral end-plate in adult Greyhound dogs. Spine 1984; 9(7): 702-6.
[http://dx.doi.org/10.1097/00007632-198410000-00009] [PMID: 6505840]

[10]   Donisch EW, Trapp W. The cartilage endplates of the human vertebral column (some considerations of postnatal development). Anat Rec 1971; 169(4): 705-15.
[http://dx.doi.org/10.1002/ar.1091690409] [PMID: 4102248]

[11]   Hassler O. The human intervertebral disc. A micro-angiographical study on its vascular supply at various ages. Acta Orthop Scand 1969; 40(6): 765-72.
[http://dx.doi.org/10.3109/17453676908989540] [PMID: 5394000]

[12]   Oki S, Matsuda Y, Shibata T, Okumura H, Desaki J. Morphologic differences of the vascular buds in the vertebral endplate: scanning electron microscopic study. Spine 1996; 21(2): 174-7.
[http://dx.doi.org/10.1097/00007632-199601150-00003] [PMID: 8720400]

[13]   Bibby SRS, Jones DA, Ripley RM, Urban JPG. Metabolism of the intervertebral disc: effects of low levels of oxygen, glucose, and pH on rates of energy metabolism of bovine nucleus pulposus cells. Spine 2005; 30(5): 487-96.
[http://dx.doi.org/10.1097/01.brs.0000154619.38122.47] [PMID: 15738779]

[14]   Adams MA, Hutton WC. The effect of posture on the fluid content of lumbar intervertebral discs. Spine 1983; 8(6): 665-71.
[http://dx.doi.org/10.1097/00007632-198309000-00013] [PMID: 6685921]

[15]   Paajanen H, Lehto I, Alanen A, Erkintalo M, Komu M. Diurnal fluid changes of lumbar discs measured indirectly by magnetic resonance imaging. J Orthop Res 1994; 12(4): 509-14.
[http://dx.doi.org/10.1002/jor.1100120407] [PMID: 8064481]

[16]   Nachemson A, Lewin T, Maroudas A, Freeman MAR. *In vitro* diffusion of dye through the end-plates and the annulus fibrosus of human lumbar inter-vertebral discs. Acta Orthop Scand 1970; 41(6): 589-607.
[http://dx.doi.org/10.3109/17453677008991550] [PMID: 5516549]

[17]   Boos N, Weissbach S, Rohrbach H, Weiler C, Spratt KF, Nerlich AG. Classification of age-related changes in lumbar intervertebral discs: 2002 Volvo Award in basic science. Spine 2002; 27(23): 2631-44.
[http://dx.doi.org/10.1097/00007632-200212010-00002] [PMID: 12461389]

[18]   Pritzker KPH. Aging and degeneration in the lumbar intervertebral disc. Orthop Clin North Am 1977; 8(1): 65-77.
[http://dx.doi.org/10.1016/S0030-5898(20)30936-6] [PMID: 857227]

[19]   Vernon-Roberts B, Pirie CJ. Healing trabecular microfractures in the bodies of lumbar vertebrae. Ann Rheum Dis 1973; 32(5): 406-12.
[http://dx.doi.org/10.1136/ard.32.5.406] [PMID: 4270883]

[20]   Bernick S, Cailliet R. Vertebral end-plate changes with aging of human vertebrae. Spine 1982; 7(2): 97-102.
[http://dx.doi.org/10.1097/00007632-198203000-00002] [PMID: 7089697]

[21]   Chandraraj S, Briggs CA, Opeskin K. Disc herniations in the young and end-plate vascularity. Clin Anat 1998; 11(3): 171-6.
[http://dx.doi.org/10.1002/(SICI)1098-2353(1998)11:3<171::AID-CA4>3.0.CO;2-W]   [PMID: 9579589]

[22]   Kokkonen SM, Kurunlahti M, Tervonen O, Ilkko E, Vanharanta H. Endplate degeneration observed on

magnetic resonance imaging of the lumbar spine: correlation with pain provocation and disc changes observed on computed tomography diskography. Spine 2002; 27(20): 2274-8.
[http://dx.doi.org/10.1097/00007632-200210150-00017] [PMID: 12394906]

[23]   Modic MT, Steinberg PM, Ross JS, Masaryk TJ, Carter JR. Degenerative disk disease: assessment of changes in vertebral body marrow with MR imaging. Radiology 1988; 166(1): 193-9.
[http://dx.doi.org/10.1148/radiology.166.1.3336678] [PMID: 3336678]

[24]   Benneker LM, Heini PF, Alini M, Anderson SE, Ito K. 2004 Young Investigator Award Winner: vertebral endplate marrow contact channel occlusions and intervertebral disc degeneration. Spine 2005; 30(2): 167-73.
[http://dx.doi.org/10.1097/01.brs.0000150833.93248.09] [PMID: 15644751]

[25]   Taylor JR. Growth of human intervertebral discs and vertebral bodies. J Anat 1975; 120(Pt 1): 49-68.
[PMID: 1184458]

[26]   Inoue H. Three-dimensional architecture of lumbar intervertebral discs. Spine 1981; 6(2): 139-46.
[http://dx.doi.org/10.1097/00007632-198103000-00006] [PMID: 7280814]

[27]   Hukins D. Biology of the Intervertebral Disc. Boca Raton, FL: CRC Press 1988; Vol. 1. In the press

[28]   Holm S, Maroudas A, Urban JPG, Selstam G, Nachemson A. Nutrition of the intervertebral disc: solute transport and metabolism. Connect Tissue Res 1981; 8(2): 101-19.
[http://dx.doi.org/10.3109/03008208109152130] [PMID: 6453689]

[29]   Antoniou J, Goudsouzian NM, Heathfield TF, *et al.* The human lumbar endplate. Evidence of changes in biosynthesis and denaturation of the extracellular matrix with growth, maturation, aging, and degeneration. Spine 1996; 21(10): 1153-61.
[http://dx.doi.org/10.1097/00007632-199605150-00006] [PMID: 8727189]

[30]   Bayliss M, Johnstone B, Jayson M. The lumbar spine and back pain Biochemistry of the intervertebral disc. 4th ed., Churchill Livingstone 1992.

[31]   Aigner T, Greskötter KR, Fairbank JCT, von der Mark K, Urban JPG. Variation with age in the pattern of type X collagen expression in normal and scoliotic human intervertebral discs. Calcif Tissue Int 1998; 63(3): 263-8.
[http://dx.doi.org/10.1007/s002239900524] [PMID: 9701632]

[32]   Sahlman J, Inkinen R, Hirvonen T, *et al.* Premature vertebral endplate ossification and mild disc degeneration in mice after inactivation of one allele belonging to the Col2a1 gene for Type II collagen. Spine 2001; 26(23): 2558-65.
[http://dx.doi.org/10.1097/00007632-200112010-00008] [PMID: 11725236]

[33]   Pearce RH, Grimmer BJ, Adams ME. Degeneration and the chemical composition of the human lumbar intervertebral disc. J Orthop Res 1987; 5(2): 198-205.
[http://dx.doi.org/10.1002/jor.1100050206] [PMID: 3572589]

[34]   Roberts S, Urban JPG, Evans H, Eisenstein SM. Transport properties of the human cartilage endplate in relation to its composition and calcification. Spine 1996; 21(4): 415-20.
[http://dx.doi.org/10.1097/00007632-199602150-00003] [PMID: 8658243]

[35]   Antoniou J, Arlet V, Goswami T, Aebi M, Alini M. Elevated synthetic activity in the convex side of scoliotic intervertebral discs and endplates compared with normal tissues. Spine 2001; 26(10): E198-206.
[http://dx.doi.org/10.1097/00007632-200105150-00002] [PMID: 11413439]

[36]   Pedrini-Mille A, Pedrini VA, Tudisco C, Ponseti IV, Weinstein SL, Maynard JA. Proteoglycans of human scoliotic intervertebral disc. J Bone Joint Surg Am 1983; 65(6): 815-23.
[http://dx.doi.org/10.2106/00004623-198365060-00014] [PMID: 6863364]

[37]   Roberts S, Menage J, Eisenstein SM. The cartilage end□plate and intervertebral disc in scoliosis: Calcification and other sequelae. J Orthop Res 1993; 11(5): 747-57.
[http://dx.doi.org/10.1002/jor.1100110517] [PMID: 8410475]

[38]   Crock HV, Yoshizawa H. The blood supply of the lumbar vertebral column. Clin Orthop Relat Res 1976; &NA;(115): 6-21.
[http://dx.doi.org/10.1097/00003086-197603000-00003] [PMID: 1253499]

[39]   Urban JPG, Holm S, Maroudas A, Nachemson A. Nutrition of the intervertebral disk. An *in vivo* study of solute transport. Clin Orthop Relat Res 1977; 129(129): 101-14.
[http://dx.doi.org/10.1097/00003086-197711000-00012] [PMID: 608268]

[40]   Oda J, Tanaka H, Tsuzuki N. Intervertebral disc changes with aging of human cervical vertebra. From the neonate to the eighties. Spine 1988; 13(11): 1205-11.
[http://dx.doi.org/10.1097/00007632-198811000-00001] [PMID: 3206279]

[41]   Roberts S, McCall IW, Menage J, Haddaway MJ, Eisenstein SM. Does the thickness of the vertebral subchondral bone reflect the composition of the intervertebral disc? Eur Spine J 1997; 6(6): 385-9.
[http://dx.doi.org/10.1007/BF01834064] [PMID: 9455665]

[42]   Vernon-Roberts B, Jayson M. The lumbar spine and back pain Pathology of Intervertebral Discs and Apophyseal Joints New York. Churchill Livingstone 1987.

[43]   Ariga K, Miyamoto S, Nakase T, *et al.* The relationship between apoptosis of endplate chondrocytes and aging and degeneration of the intervertebral disc. Spine 2001; 26(22): 2414-20.
[http://dx.doi.org/10.1097/00007632-200111150-00004] [PMID: 11707702]

[44]   Brown MF, Hukkanen MVJ, McCarthy ID, *et al.* Sensory and sympathetic innervation of the vertebral endplate in patients with degenerative disc disease. J Bone Joint Surg Br 1997; 79-B(1): 147-53.
[http://dx.doi.org/10.1302/0301-620X.79B1.0790147] [PMID: 9020464]

[45]   Fagan A, Moore R, Vernon Roberts B, Blumbergs P, Fraser R. ISSLS prize winner: The innervation of the intervertebral disc: a quantitative analysis. Spine 2003; 28(23): 2570-6.
[http://dx.doi.org/10.1097/01.BRS.0000096942.29660.B1] [PMID: 14652473]

[46]   Moore RJ, Osti OL, Vemon-Roberts B, Fraser RD. Changes in endplate vascularity after an outer anulus tear in the sheep. Spine 1992; 17(8): 874-8.
[http://dx.doi.org/10.1097/00007632-199208000-00003] [PMID: 1523489]

[47]   Crean JKG, Roberts S, Jaffray DC, Eisenstein SM, Duance VC. Matrix metalloproteinases in the human intervertebral disc: role in disc degeneration and scoliosis. Spine 1997; 22(24): 2877-84.
[http://dx.doi.org/10.1097/00007632-199712150-00010] [PMID: 9431623]

[48]   Goupille P, Jayson MIV, Valat JP, Freemont AJ. Matrix metalloproteinases: the clue to intervertebral disc degeneration? Spine 1998; 23(14): 1612-26.
[http://dx.doi.org/10.1097/00007632-199807150-00021] [PMID: 9682320]

[49]   Kang JD, Stefanovic-Racic M, McIntyre LA, Georgescu HI, Evans CH. Toward a biochemical understanding of human intervertebral disc degeneration and herniation. Contributions of nitric oxide, interleukins, prostaglandin E2, and matrix metalloproteinases. Spine 1997; 22(10): 1065-73.
[http://dx.doi.org/10.1097/00007632-199705150-00003] [PMID: 9160463]

[50]   Roberts S, Caterson B, Menage J, Evans EH, Jaffray DC, Eisenstein SM. Matrix metalloproteinases and aggrecanase: their role in disorders of the human intervertebral disc. Spine 2000; 25(23): 3005-13.
[http://dx.doi.org/10.1097/00007632-200012010-00007] [PMID: 11145811]

[51]   Weiler C, Nerlich A, Zipperer J, Bachmeier B, Boos N. 2002 SSE Award Competition in Basic Science: Expression of major matrix metalloproteinases is associated with intervertebral disc degradation and resorption. Eur Spine J 2002; 11(4): 308-20.
[http://dx.doi.org/10.1007/s00586-002-0472-0] [PMID: 12193991]

[52]   Bailey JF, Liebenberg E, Degmetich S, Lotz JC. Innervation patterns of PGP 9.5-positive nerve fibers within the human lumbar vertebra. J Anat 2011; 218(3): 263-70.
[http://dx.doi.org/10.1111/j.1469-7580.2010.01332.x] [PMID: 21223256]

[53]   Fras C, Kravetz P, Mody DR, Heggeness MH. Substance P–containing nerves within the human

vertebral body. Spine J 2003; 3(1): 63-7.
[http://dx.doi.org/10.1016/S1529-9430(02)00455-2] [PMID: 14589248]

[54] Antonacci MD, Mody DR, Heggeness MH. Innervation of the human vertebral body: a histologic study. J Spinal Disord 1998; 11(6): 526-31.
[http://dx.doi.org/10.1097/00002517-199812000-00013] [PMID: 9884299]

[55] Fields AJ, Liebenberg EC, Lotz JC. Innervation of pathologies in the lumbar vertebral end plate and intervertebral disc. Spine J 2014; 14(3): 513-21.
[http://dx.doi.org/10.1016/j.spinee.2013.06.075] [PMID: 24139753]

[56] Michalik A, Conger A, Smuck M, Maus TP, McCormick ZL. Intraosseous Basivertebral Nerve Radiofrequency Ablation for the Treatment of Vertebral Body Endplate Low Back Pain: Current Evidence and Future Directions. Pain Med 2021; 22 (Suppl. 1): S24-30.
[http://dx.doi.org/10.1093/pm/pnab117] [PMID: 34308955]

[57] Bogduk N. The innervation of the lumbar spine. Spine 1983; 8(3): 286-93.
[http://dx.doi.org/10.1097/00007632-198304000-00009] [PMID: 6226119]

[58] Becker S, Hadjipavlou A, Heggeness MH. Ablation of the basivertebral nerve for treatment of back pain: a clinical study. Spine J 2017; 17(2): 218-23.
[http://dx.doi.org/10.1016/j.spinee.2016.08.032] [PMID: 27592808]

[59] Truumees E, Macadaeg K, Pena E, *et al.* A prospective, open-label, single-arm, multi-center study of intraosseous basivertebral nerve ablation for the treatment of chronic low back pain. Eur Spine J 2019; 28(7): 1594-602.
[http://dx.doi.org/10.1007/s00586-019-05995-2] [PMID: 31115683]

[60] Fischgrund JS, Rhyne A, Franke J, *et al.* Intraosseous basivertebral nerve ablation for the treatment of chronic low back pain: a prospective randomized double-blind sham-controlled multi-center study. Eur Spine J 2018; 27(5): 1146-56.
[http://dx.doi.org/10.1007/s00586-018-5496-1] [PMID: 29423885]

[61] Khalil JG, Smuck M, Koreckij T, *et al.* A prospective, randomized, multicenter study of intraosseous basivertebral nerve ablation for the treatment of chronic low back pain. Spine J 2019; 19(10): 1620-32.
[http://dx.doi.org/10.1016/j.spinee.2019.05.598] [PMID: 31229663]

[62] Moore RJ, Vernon-Roberts B, Fraser RD, Osti OL, Schembri M. The origin and fate of herniated lumbar intervertebral disc tissue. Spine 1996; 21(18): 2149-55.
[http://dx.doi.org/10.1097/00007632-199609150-00018] [PMID: 8893441]

[63] Tanaka M, Nakahara S, Inoue H. A pathologic study of discs in the elderly. Separation between the cartilaginous endplate and the vertebral body. Spine 1993; 18(11): 1456-62.
[http://dx.doi.org/10.1097/00007632-199318110-00009] [PMID: 8235816]

[64] Beggs I, Addison J. Posterior vertebral rim fractures. Br J Radiol 1998; 71(845): 567-72.
[http://dx.doi.org/10.1259/bjr.71.845.9691906] [PMID: 9691906]

[65] Natarajan RN, Ke JH, Andersson GBJ. A model to study the disc degeneration process. Spine 1994; 19(3): 259-64.
[http://dx.doi.org/10.1097/00007632-199402000-00001] [PMID: 8171355]

[66] Lundin O, Ekström L, Hellström M, Holm S, Swärd L. Injuries in the adolescent porcine spine exposed to mechanical compression. Spine 1998; 23(23): 2574-9.
[http://dx.doi.org/10.1097/00007632-199812010-00012] [PMID: 9854756]

[67] Lundin O, Ekström L, Hellström M, Holm S, Swärd L. Exposure of the porcine spine to mechanical compression: differences in injury pattern between adolescents and adults. Eur Spine J 2000; 9(6): 466-71.
[http://dx.doi.org/10.1007/s005860000164] [PMID: 11189914]

[68] Rolander SD, Blair WE. Deformation and fracture of the lumbar vertebral end plate. Orthop Clin North Am 1975; 6(1): 75-81.

[http://dx.doi.org/10.1016/S0030-5898(20)31202-5] [PMID: 1113982]

[69]   Hilton RC, Ball J, Benn RT. Vertebral end-plate lesions (Schmorl's nodes) in the dorsolumbar spine. Ann Rheum Dis 1976; 35(2): 127-32.
[http://dx.doi.org/10.1136/ard.35.2.127] [PMID: 942268]

[70]   Jensen OK, Nielsen CV, Sørensen JS, Stengaard-Pedersen K. Type 1 Modic changes was a significant risk factor for 1-year outcome in sick-listed low back pain patients: a nested cohort study using magnetic resonance imaging of the lumbar spine. Spine J 2014; 14(11): 2568-81.
[http://dx.doi.org/10.1016/j.spinee.2014.02.018] [PMID: 24534386]

[71]   Jensen RK, Jensen TS, Grøn S, *et al.* Prevalence of MRI findings in the cervical spine in patients with persistent neck pain based on quantification of narrative MRI reports. Chiropr Man Therap 2019; 27(1): 13.
[http://dx.doi.org/10.1186/s12998-019-0233-3] [PMID: 30873276]

[72]   Jensen RK, Leboeuf-Yde C. Is the presence of Modic changes associated with the outcomes of different treatments? A systematic critical review. BMC Musculoskelet Disord 2011; 12(1): 183.
[http://dx.doi.org/10.1186/1471-2474-12-183] [PMID: 21831312]

[73]   Nishida K, Gilbertson LG, Evans CH, Kang JD. Spine Update. Spine 2000; 25(10): 1308-14.
[http://dx.doi.org/10.1097/00007632-200005150-00021] [PMID: 10806514]

[74]   Yoon ST. The potential of gene therapy for the treatment of disc degeneration. Orthop Clin North Am 2004; 35(1): 95-100.
[http://dx.doi.org/10.1016/S0030-5898(03)00097-X] [PMID: 15062722]

[75]   Bos PK, DeGroot J, Budde M, Verhaar JAN, van Osch GJVM. Specific enzymatic treatment of bovine and human articular cartilage: Implications for integrative cartilage repair. Arthritis Rheum 2002; 46(4): 976-85.
[http://dx.doi.org/10.1002/art.10208] [PMID: 11953975]

[76]   van de Breevaart Bravenboer J, In der Maur CD, Bos PK, *et al.* Improved cartilage integration and interfacial strength after enzymatic treatment in a cartilage transplantation model. Arthritis Res Ther 2004; 6(5): R469-76.
[http://dx.doi.org/10.1186/ar1216] [PMID: 15380046]

[77]   Quinn TM, Hunziker EB. Controlled enzymatic matrix degradation for integrative cartilage repair: effects on viable cell density and proteoglycan deposition. Tissue Eng 2002; 8(5): 799-806.
[http://dx.doi.org/10.1089/10763270260424150] [PMID: 12459058]

[78]   Caplan AI, Elyaderani M, Mochizuki Y, Wakitani S, Goldberg VM. Principles of cartilage repair and regeneration. Clin Orthop Relat Res 1997; (342): 254-69.
[http://dx.doi.org/10.1097/00003086-199709000-00033] [PMID: 9308548]

[79]   Kirchner F, Pinar A, Milani I, Prado R, Padilla S, Anitua E. Vertebral intraosseous plasma rich in growth factor (PRGF-Endoret) infiltrations as a novel strategy for the treatment of degenerative lesions of endplate in lumbar pathology: description of technique and case presentation. J Orthop Surg Res 2020; 15(1): 72.
[http://dx.doi.org/10.1186/s13018-020-01605-w] [PMID: 32093768]

[80]   Huang YC, Urban JPG, Luk KDK. Intervertebral disc regeneration: do nutrients lead the way? Nat Rev Rheumatol 2014; 10(9): 561-6.
[http://dx.doi.org/10.1038/nrrheum.2014.91] [PMID: 24914695]

[81]   Sánchez M, Anitua E, Delgado D, *et al.* A new strategy to tackle severe knee osteoarthritis: Combination of intra-articular and intraosseous injections of Platelet Rich Plasma. Expert Opin Biol Ther 2016; 16(5): 627-43.
[http://dx.doi.org/10.1517/14712598.2016.1157162] [PMID: 26930117]

[82]   Fiz N, Pérez JC, Guadilla J, *et al.* Intraosseous Infiltration of Platelet-Rich Plasma for Severe Hip Osteoarthritis. Arthrosc Tech 2017; 6(3): e821-5.

[http://dx.doi.org/10.1016/j.eats.2017.02.014] [PMID: 28706837]

[83]   Anitua E, Kirchner F. Intradiscal and intra articular facet infiltrations with plasma rich in growth factors reduce pain in patients with chronic low back pain. J Craniovertebr Junction Spine 2016; 7(4): 250-6.
[http://dx.doi.org/10.4103/0974-8237.193260] [PMID: 27891035]

[84]   Anitua E, Padilla S. Biologic therapies to enhance intervertebral disc repair. Regen Med 2018; 13(1): 55-72.
[http://dx.doi.org/10.2217/rme-2017-0111] [PMID: 29355455]

[85]   Mattei TA, Rehman AA. Schmorl's nodes: current pathophysiological, diagnostic, and therapeutic paradigms. Neurosurg Rev 2014; 37(1): 39-46.
[http://dx.doi.org/10.1007/s10143-013-0488-4] [PMID: 23955279]

[86]   Lutz GE. Increased Nuclear T2 Signal Intensity and Improved Function and Pain in a Patient One Year After an Intradiscal Platelet–Rich Plasma Injection. Pain Med 2017; 18(6): 1197-9.
[http://dx.doi.org/10.1093/pm/pnw299] [PMID: 28339718]

[87]   Akeda K, Ohishi K, Masuda K, et al. Intradiscal Injection of Autologous Platelet-Rich Plasma Releasate to Treat Discogenic Low Back Pain: A Preliminary Clinical Trial. Asian Spine J 2017; 11(3): 380-9.
[http://dx.doi.org/10.4184/asj.2017.11.3.380] [PMID: 28670405]

[88]   Fields AJ, Battié MC, Herzog RJ, et al. Measuring and reporting of vertebral endplate bone marrow lesions as seen on MRI (Modic changes): recommendations from the ISSLS Degenerative Spinal Phenotypes Group. Eur Spine J 2019; 28(10): 2266-74.
[http://dx.doi.org/10.1007/s00586-019-06119-6] [PMID: 31446492]

[89]   Fischgrund JS, Rhyne A, Franke J, et al. Intraosseous Basivertebral Nerve Ablation for the Treatment of Chronic Low Back Pain: 2-Year Results From a Prospective Randomized Double-Blind Sham-Controlled Multicenter Study. Int J Spine Surg 2019; 13(2): 110-9.
[http://dx.doi.org/10.14444/6015] [PMID: 31131209]

[90]   Fischgrund JS, Rhyne A, Macadaeg K, et al. Long-term outcomes following intraosseous basivertebral nerve ablation for the treatment of chronic low back pain: 5-year treatment arm results from a prospective randomized double-blind sham-controlled multi-center study. Eur Spine J 2020; 29(8): 1925-34.
[http://dx.doi.org/10.1007/s00586-020-06448-x] [PMID: 32451777]

[91]   Macadaeg K, Truumees E, Boody B, et al. A prospective, single arm study of intraosseous basivertebral nerve ablation for the treatment of chronic low back pain: 12-month results. N Am Spine Soc J 2020; 3100030
[http://dx.doi.org/10.1016/j.xnsj.2020.100030] [PMID: 35141598]

[92]   Gazis AN, Beuing O, Franke J, Jöllenbeck B, Skalej M. Bipolar radiofrequency ablation of spinal tumors: predictability, safety and outcome. Spine J 2014; 14(4): 604-8.
[http://dx.doi.org/10.1016/j.spinee.2013.06.081] [PMID: 24139752]

[93]   Dahdaleh NS, Lee D. Charcot spinal arthropathy. J Craniovertebr Junction Spine 2018; 9(1): 9-19.
[http://dx.doi.org/10.4103/jcvjs.JCVJS_130_17] [PMID: 29755231]

[94]   Heggeness MH, Doherty BJ. Discography causes end plate deflection. Spine 1993; 18(8): 1050-3.
[http://dx.doi.org/10.1097/00007632-199306150-00015] [PMID: 8367772]

[95]   Boswell MV, Shah RV, Everett CR, et al. Interventional techniques in the management of chronic spinal pain: evidence-based practice guidelines. Pain Physician 2005; 1(8): 1-47.
[http://dx.doi.org/10.36076/ppj.2006/9/1] [PMID: 16850041]

[96]   Fukui S, Iwashita N, Nitta K, Tomie H, Nosaka S. The results of percutaneous intradiscal high-pressure injection of saline in patients with extruded lumbar herniated disc: comparison with microendoscopic discectomy. Pain Med 2012; 13(6): 762-8.

[http://dx.doi.org/10.1111/j.1526-4637.2012.01400.x] [PMID: 22621436]

[97] Gallucci M, Limbucci N, Zugaro L, *et al.* Sciatica: treatment with intradiscal and intraforaminal injections of steroid and oxygen-ozone versus steroid only. Radiology 2007; 242(3): 907-13.
[http://dx.doi.org/10.1148/radiol.2423051934] [PMID: 17209164]

[98] Noriega DC, Ardura F, Hernández-Ramajo R, *et al.* Intervertebral Disc Repair by Allogeneic Mesenchymal Bone Marrow Cells. Transplantation 2017; 101(8): 1945-51.
[http://dx.doi.org/10.1097/TP.0000000000001484] [PMID: 27661661]

CHAPTER 6

The Current Concept for Stem Cell Therapy in Spinal Cord Injury

Alvaro Dowling[1,*] and **Marcelo Molina**[2]

[1] *Orthopaedic Spine Surgeon, Director of Endoscopic Spine Clinic, Santiago, Chile*

[2] *Department of Orthopaedic Surgery, Faculdade de Medicina de Ribeirão Preto - USP (School of Medicine of Ribeirão Preto - University of São Paulo), Ribeirão Preto, SP, Brazil*

Abstract: Spinal cord injury with neurological deficits is devastating to patients and their families. After the immediate treatment that may involve spinal decompression and stabilization surgeries, patients are typically left with long-term disability. Intense research has focused on spinal cord regeneration, tissue repair, and reinnervation to improve function. Stem cell-based therapies are at the center of this effort. This chapter summarizes common spinal cord injury (SCI) patterns, including complete and incomplete SCIs, and their classification-based prognosis and treatments. They review the types of stem cells used in preclinical and clinical trials in the treatment of SCI and the associated ethical concerns and summarize the current state of the art of stem cell-based SCI treatments.

Keywords: Classification, Prognosis, Spinal cord injury, Stem cells, Treatment.

INTRODUCTION

Spinal cord injuries (SCIs) represent a formidable public health problem, manifesting an incidence range of 40 to 80 cases per million individuals annually, according to existing epidemiological data [1]. Predominantly afflicting a younger demographic, these injuries occasion irremediable neurological deficits that exert an onerous toll on patients, healthcare providers, and medical infrastructures alike. While prophylactic measures targeting vehicular mishaps, unlawful conduct, and secondary etiological factors such as neoplastic or degenerative pathologies are indisputably vital, the true challenge confronting the scientific community lies in the domain of therapeutic intervention, especially in the absence of a universally recognized, efficacious treatment modality.

---

* **Corresponding author Álvaro Dowling:** Orthopaedic Spine Surgeon, Director of Endoscopic Spine Clinic, Santiago, Chile; E-mail: adowling@dws.cl

Recent years have witnessed salient advancements in specialized, multidisciplinary methodologies for addressing SCI. Noteworthy among emerging organizational entities committed to this specialized sector of neurological injury is the International Association of Neurorestoratology (IANR). Such professional assemblies underscore the efforts to surmount a yet unresolved clinical impasse.

Within the scope of contemporary neurological practice, the re-establishment of functional capabilities post-SCI remains a daunting enterprise. This necessitates the employment of a spectrum of neurorestorative tactics throughout the acute, subacute, and chronic temporal stages of SCI, aimed at the reversing functional losses.

Primary Injury

The spinal cord of mammals is organized into ten laminae of neurons, named dorsoventrally, according to the Rexed description [2]. The neurons are mostly multipolar and vary in size. In the dorsal laminae, sensory neurons receive inputs from the dorsal root ganglion cells and project them to other spinal levels or the upper centers of the sensory pathways.

Within the dorsal laminae, sensory neurons act as afferent conduits for dorsal root ganglion cells, directing somatosensory information to alternate spinal echelons or more rostral sensorimotor processing centers. Conversely, the ventral laminae house substantial populations of cholinergic motor neurons, which orchestrate myogenic contractions *via* efferent axonal pathways. An intermediary locus is occupied by morphologically diverse interneurons, recipients of both descending corticospinal projections and recurrent axonal fibers from spinal motoneurons, thereby modulating motoneuronal discharge patterns [3, 4]. Neuronal constituents within the spinal cord forge intricate intraspinal circuitries under the governance of descending neural pathways, with the reflex arc representing the most rudimentary of such closed-loop systems.

During the acute temporal phase of SCI, the underlying traumatic etiology may encompass a variety of mechanical insults, such as contusions, lacerations, tensile forces, compressional impacts, or outright cellular obliteration. These initial traumatic events culminate in the primary injury phase, characterized by disintegration of neural circuitries [5]. In the immediate post-injury interval, typically within the first two hours [6], cellular constituents, including both neurons and glial entities at the lesion nexus, succumb to either necrotic or apoptotic fates [7]. Ergo, therapeutic objectives in post-SCI management should prioritize the restitution of native intraspinal circuitry, followed by the facilitation of regenerative growth in descending pathways, to re-establish volitional governance over these circuits. It is unequivocally acknowledged that the most pivotal juncture in the pathophysiological trajectory of SCI pertains to the secondary injury phase. This latter phase is typified by an unchecked, maladaptive cascade involving aberrant molecular signaling pathways, inflammatory cascades, vascular aberrations, and consequent cellular dysregulations, further exacerbating the initial insult [8-11].

Secondary Injury

Within the context of an injured spinal cord, a spectrum of destructive mechanisms disturbs the local microenvironment, the severity of which is contingent upon the characteristics of the primary injury. In terms of vascular pathology, there occurs a widespread attenuation of blood perfusion attributable to phenomena such as vasospasms, focal microhemorrhagic events, and thrombotic incidents, collectively leading to a comprehensive compromise of the blood-spinal cord barrier integrity [8, 12]. Concurrently, a dysregulation in ionic equilibrium manifests around cellular membranes and associated ion transport machinery. Specifically, an efflux of potassium ions (K+) is observed in the extracellular milieu, concomitant with an intracellular accrual of sodium (Na+) and calcium ions (Ca2+) [8, 13]. These perturbations result in the attenuation of neuronal signal transduction capabilities.

An acidotic milieu further exacerbates this dysfunctional state by facilitating the ingress of water molecules into the cellular compartment, culminating in cytotoxic edema and subsequent cellular demise [14-16]. The injurious cascade also precipitates the release of multiple biochemical entities, including reactive oxygen species and various neurotransmitters. Immunologically, the breach in the blood-brain barrier inaugurates the recruitment and infiltration of immune cells—such as T lymphocytes, macrophages, microglia, and neutrophils—into the neuronal matrix, thereby adopting a proinflammatory phenotype. The ensuing milieu is further enriched by the secretion of a cadre of proinflammatory cytokines, including but not limited to, Interleukin-1 beta (IL-1β), Interleukin-1 alpha (IL-1α), Tumor Necrosis Factor-alpha (TNF-α), and Interleukin-6 (IL-6). These factors collectively contribute to a localized cellular assembly that fosters neurodegenerative processes [17-19].

Chronic Phase and Neurodegeneration

In the chronic phase of spinal cord injury (SCI), a hallmark feature is the fibrotic encapsulation engendered by gliotic processes and the accretion of extracellular matrix components, thereby attenuating functional capacity. Bioactive molecules harboring anti-proliferative properties are liberated, targeting specific neuronal receptor complexes. The demise of oligodendrocytes during the primary injury event is of particular importance, given that the resulting myelin detritus harbors axonal growth-inhibitory molecules such as Nogo-A protein and myelin-associated glycoprotein (MAG) [20-23].

Additional constituents, including proteoglycans, exhibit specific roles in the chronic phase; while the majority act as impediments to axonal regenerative efforts, a subset serves to demarcate and circumscribe the scar tissue, thus mitigating the potential for exacerbating tissue damage [24, 25].

Within this inflammatory environment, the phagocytic clearance of cellular debris emerges as a pivotal determinant of neuroregenerative success. The phenotypic modulation of macrophages— ranging from pro-inflammatory M1 subtypes elicited by IFN-γ and TNF-α to the Th1 phenotype, as well as the more nuanced anti-inflammatory M2 subtypes (encompassing M2a, b, and c phenotypes)— constitutes a multifactorial and decisive element in shaping the trajectory of neurologic recovery [17-19, 26].

Remarkably, while mammalian systems exhibit limited neuronal regenerative capabilities within the context of SCI, certain lower vertebrates such as the axolotl (a species of salamander) manifest intrinsic regenerative capacities. These are mediated through specific molecular regulators that modulate glial responses post-injury and facilitate glial cell migration and proliferation to reconstitute neural tissue and stimulate axonal elongation [27]. The identification of cellular mechanisms governing neural regeneration thus becomes imperative for enhancing SCI repair. Strategies aimed at modulating intraneuronal signaling cascades and extracellular conditions are essential for augmenting axonal regrowth and facilitating the reestablishment of intraspinal as well as ascending and descending neural pathways [25]. Attaining mastery over glial scar formation, modifying perineuronal networks, and the judicious regulation of post-SCI neuroinflammatory responses remain indispensable yet elusive goals in the comprehensive strategy for spinal cord restoration [29]. Lastly, factors such as axonal sprouting, synaptic plasticity, and neural remodeling—each subject to autonomous and non-autonomous regulatory influences—can be differentially modulated by a myriad of cellular and molecular entities within the disparate compartments of the injured spinal cord [30].

American Spinal Cord Injury Association Scale

The American Spinal Cord Injury Association (ASIA) is the international standard for neurological classification, and it is based on sensory and motor assessment [31-33]. The Asia Impairment Scale (ASIA) involves sensory and motor examination level for both sides of the body, and whether the injury is incomplete or complete.

Determination of Neurological Level of Injury

Determined by the most caudal segment of the cord with intact sensation and antigravity muscle function strength (Grade 3/5 or more) on both sides, with normal motor and sensory status rostrally (Grade 5/5). Motor Level is determined by the most caudal normal myotome with at least Grade 3/5 on motor examination [34]. The sensory level is the most caudal intact dermatome for pin-prick and light touch sensation. In the case of a discrepancy in sides, the neurological level of injury is considered the most cephalad segment of the four groups.

ASIA Impairment Scale

The American Spinal Injury Association Impairment Scale (AIS), an analytical schema promulgated by the American Spinal Injury Association (ASIA), serves as a canonical metric for the quantification and delineation of spinal cord injury (SCI) severity. The AIS divides SCI into 5 subcategories, each representative of a unique confluence of sensory and motoric impairments, thereby furnishing clinicians, academicians, and afflicted individuals with an invaluable lexicon for the precise articulation of SCI prognostication and gradation [32]. The scale traverses a continuum from AIS Grade A, indicative of a comprehensive absence of both sensory and motor functions distal to the injury locus, to AIS Grade E, which connotes a neurologically unremarkable profile devoid of deficits [31].

SCI can further be classified into "Complete" or "Incomplete", contingent upon the presence or absence of "sacral sparing," delineated by residual sensory or motor function within the most caudal sacral segment. Such assessments may encompass evaluations of deep anal pressure or volitional contraction of the anal sphincter. The AIS nomenclature is delineated as follows (Fig. 1):

1. AIS A (Complete): Embodies a comprehensive SCI, typified by the total loss of sensory and motor faculties distal to the injured spinal segment.

2. AIS B (Sensory Incomplete): Denotes preservation of limited sensory functions below the lesion site, but with a lack of any conserved motor capabilities. The individual may retain tactile or pressure perception in specified zones, albeit without volitional control over these regions.

3. AIS C (Motor Incomplete): Signifies a partial conservation of motor faculties below the level of injury. Here, voluntary movement is evident in a majority of key muscle groups below the neurological level, albeit the musculature is insufficiently robust to counter gravitational forces.

Fig. (1). The ASIA Impairment scale was developed by the American Spinal Injury Association (ASIA). It categorizes spinal cord injuries (SCIs) into five levels based on the degree of sensory and motor function impairment, and provides a standardized method for assessing and describing the severity of SCIs.

4. AIS D (Motor Incomplete): This grade exhibits enhanced motor function compared to AIS C, characterized by the presence of volitional movement in a majority of key muscles below the neurological level, being sufficiently robust to overcome gravitational forces.

5. AIS E (Normal): Designates an unremarkable neurological evaluation, devoid of any sensory or motor deficits, implying complete sensory and motor functionality below the level of injury.

The AIS serves as a seminal tool for the stratification of SCI, offering precise gauges for both clinical and research milieus.

The stratification of spinal cord injury (SCI) is carried out through an algorithmic assessment paradigm, outlined in Fig. (2), incorporating a multi-step evaluative process:

Steps in classification

The following order is recommended for determining the classification of individuals with SCL.

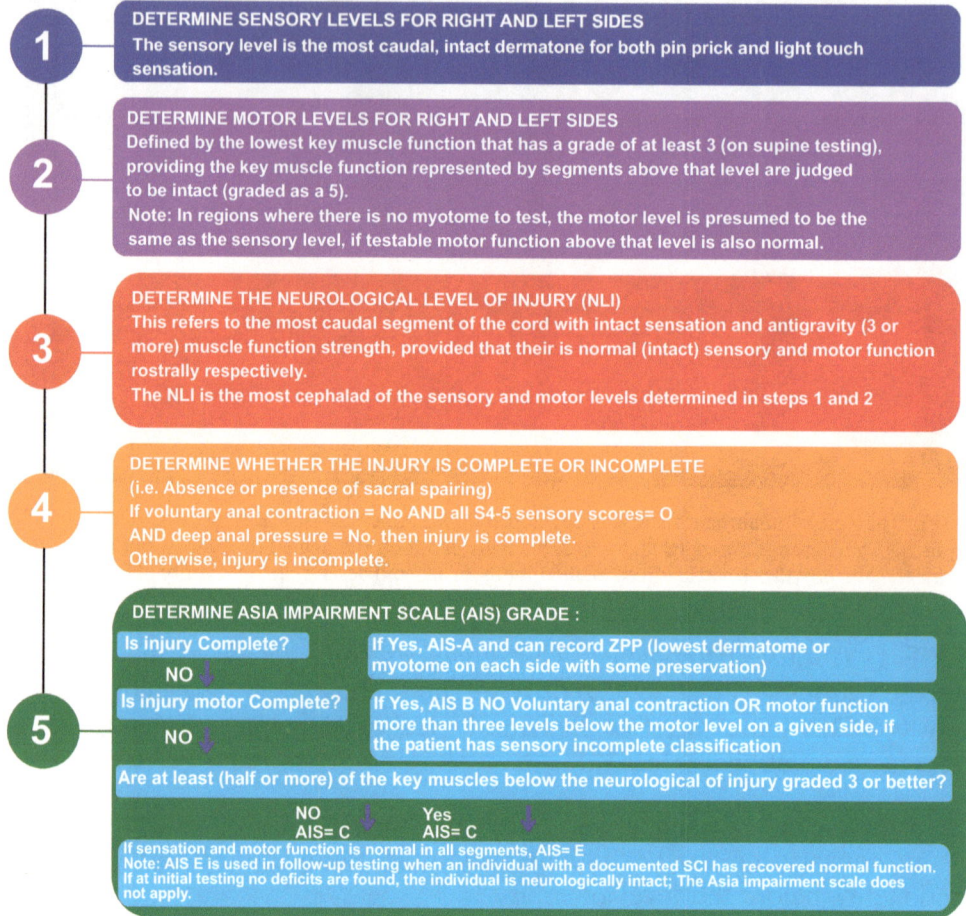

1

DETERMINE SENSORY LEVELS FOR RIGHT AND LEFT SIDES
The sensory level is the most caudal, intact dermatone for both pin prick and light touch sensation.

2

DETERMINE MOTOR LEVELS FOR RIGHT AND LEFT SIDES
Defined by the lowest key muscle function that has a grade of at least 3 (on supine testing), providing the key muscle function represented by segments above that level are judged to be intact (graded as a 5).
Note: In regions where there is no myotome to test, the motor level is presumed to be the same as the sensory level, if testable motor function above that level is also normal.

3

DETERMINE THE NEUROLOGICAL LEVEL OF INJURY (NLI)
This refers to the most caudal segment of the cord with intact sensation and antigravity (3 or more) muscle function strength, provided that their is normal (intact) sensory and motor function rostrally respectively.
The NLI is the most cephalad of the sensory and motor levels determined in steps 1 and 2

4

DETERMINE WHETHER THE INJURY IS COMPLETE OR INCOMPLETE
(i.e. Absence or presence of sacral spairing)
If voluntary anal contraction = No AND all S4-5 sensory scores= O
AND deep anal pressure = No, then injury is complete.
Otherwise, injury is incomplete.

5

DETERMINE ASIA IMPAIRMENT SCALE (AIS) GRADE :

| Is injury Complete? | If Yes, AIS-A and can record ZPP (lowest dermatome or myotome on each side with some preservation) |

NO ↓

| Is injury motor Complete? | If Yes, AIS B NO Voluntary anal contraction OR motor function more than three levels below the motor level on a given side, if the patient has sensory incomplete classification |

NO ↓

Are at least (half or more) of the key muscles below the neurological of injury graded 3 or better?

NO   Yes
AIS= C   AIS= C
↓   ↓

If sensation and motor function is normal in all segments, AIS= E
Note: AIS E is used in follow-up testing when an individual with a documented SCI has recovered normal function. If at initial testing no deficits are found, the individual is neurologically intact; The Asia impairment scale does not apply.

Fig. (2). Infogram showing the clinical steps to be taken when classifying the ASIA grade of spinal cord injury.

1. Elicitation of Comprehensive Anamnesis: A healthcare practitioner is tasked with the acquisition of exhaustive medical historiography, inclusive of the etiological factors precipitating the injury, the symptomatological panorama manifested, and any antecedent pathophysiological conditions that could potentially confound the diagnostic exercise.

2. Execution of Rigorous Somato-Sensory Examination: The healthcare professional conducts an in-depth physical appraisal encompassing evaluations of sensory acuity, neuromotor integrity, and reflexive responses, distal to the lesion site. The procedural aspects incorporate both qualitative and quantitative measures of sensory reception across diverse stimulus modalities, as well as assessments of selective muscle motility.

3. Neurological Test Battery Administration: A suite of specialized neurodiagnostic assays are administered to delineate the intricacies of sensory and motor responsiveness. Methodologies may encompass evaluations of tactile discrimination *via* light touch, nociceptive sensitivity *via* pinprick, proprioceptive acumen in joint positioning, muscular force quantification, and reflexogenic assessments.

4. Ascertainment of Neurological Demarcation: The medical practitioner identifies the most caudal spinal cord segment manifesting unimpaired sensory and motor faculties bilaterally. This demarcation serves as the focal point for designating the "neurological level of injury."

5. Assignment of AIS Taxonomy: A culmination of the preceding evaluations allows the healthcare provider to allocate an appropriate AIS grade (A, B, C, D, or E). This taxonomical classification offers a calibrated reflection of the extent of neurosensory and neuromotor deficits, as well as prognostic indicators for potential functional recuperation.

This structured approach furnishes an invaluable framework for the unambiguous delineation and characterization of SCI, instrumental in both clinical diagnostics and academic research.

Incomplete spinal cord injury (SCI) syndromes manifest as divergent constellations of neurofunctional deficits, attributable to variances in the etiological factors, topographical locale, and severity of spinal lesions [34]. Such syndromes are diagnostically characterized by unique clinical phenotypes, thus providing healthcare providers with germane data for prognosticating and localizing spinal cord lesions. Listed below are prominent syndromes of incomplete spinal cord injuries, further elucidated in Fig. (**3**):

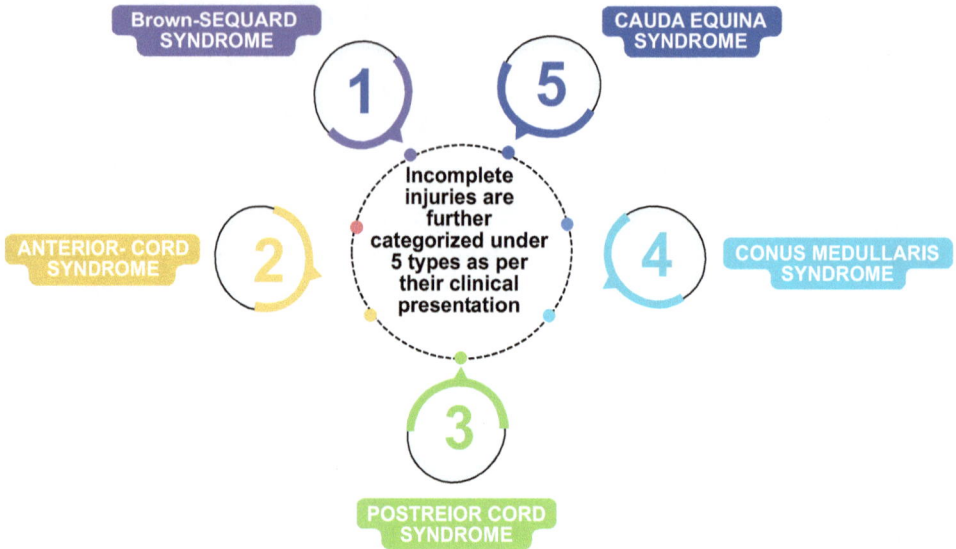

Fig. (3). Infogram characterizing the incomplete spinal cord injury syndromes (SCIs). Correctly classifying patients with incomplete SCIs determines treatment and impacts prognosis.

1. Brown-Séquard Syndrome: This diagnostic category emerges from a hemisection or unilateral insult to the spinal cord, commonly precipitating an ipsilateral decrement in neuromotor activity and proprioceptive acumen. Correspondingly, contralateral diminution in nociceptive and thermosensory perceptions occurs due to the decussation of motor and proprioceptive pathways at the opposite spinal hemisection, while pain and temperature pathways remain ipsilateral.

2. Anterior Cord Syndrome: This syndrome results from a lesion compromising the anterior sector of the spinal cord. It invariably precipitates an impairment in neuromotor faculties and thermosensory-nociceptive perceptions distal to the lesion locus. Conversely, preservation of proprioceptive and tactile sensory modalities is often noted due to the sparing of the dorsal columns responsible for these functionalities.

3. Central Cord Syndrome: This syndrome is typified by disproportionality in motor deficits, more pronounced in the brachial region as opposed to the crural region. Its etiological substratum usually resides in the central spinal cord. Affected individuals may exhibit muscular enfeeblement, dysmetria, and sensory diminution, predominantly in the upper anatomical segments, while the lower compartments remain relatively unscathed.

4. Conus Medullaris Syndrome: This diagnostic category pertains to lesions affecting the terminal region of the spinal cord, known as the conus medullaris. Clinically, it manifests as a compound spectrum of motor and sensory debilitations in the lower extremities, accompanied by detrusor and sphincter dyssynergia. Sexual dysfunction may additionally be a symptomatic component.

5. Cauda Equina Syndrome: This syndrome arises from an insult to the neural roots distal to the spinal cord termination. Etiological factors may range from herniated intervertebral discs to neoplastic or infectious spinal pathologies. It frequently culminates in crural weakness, sensorimotor decrements, and autonomic dysregulation affecting bowel and bladder functionalities.

These syndromes afford clinicians valuable taxonomies for nuanced interpretation of SCI manifestations and offer a framework for guided therapeutic interventions.

Acute Injury Phase

Traumatic spinal cord injury (SCI) encompasses a pathophysiological continuum that can be stratified temporally into acute (<48 hours), subacute (48-336 hours), intermediate (14 days to 6 months), and chronic (>6 months) phases, as delineated in Fig. (**4**) [34]. The etiopathogenesis of acute-phase traumatic SCI is a multifaceted interplay between primary and secondary injuries, each contributing distinctively to the neurostructural damage and resultant functional deficits [30].

The primary injury constitutes the mechanical insult to the spinal cord, inflicted at the moment of traumatic impact. This primary event can result from a variety of mechanistic origins, such as compressive forces, contusive trauma, lacerative damage, or even spinal cord transection. Each of these inciting mechanisms undermines the structural integrity and physiological homeostasis of the spinal cord, culminating in instantaneous neurofunctional impairments. The prevalent mechanisms are categorized as follows:

1. Compressive Etiologies: These induce mechanical strain on the spinal cord or result in its deformation, thereby injuring the neural substrate, compromising hemodynamics, and inhibiting axonal conduction.

2. Contusive Etiologies: Such injuries give rise to localized ecchymosis and hemorrhagic phenomena, potentially impeding vascular perfusion and eliciting intramedullary edema.

3. Lacerative or Transective Etiologies: These involve either a partial or complete severance of spinal cord continuity due to incisive objects, osseous fractures, or

articular dislocations, leading to either total or partial loss of neurofunctional capabilities distal to the lesion site.

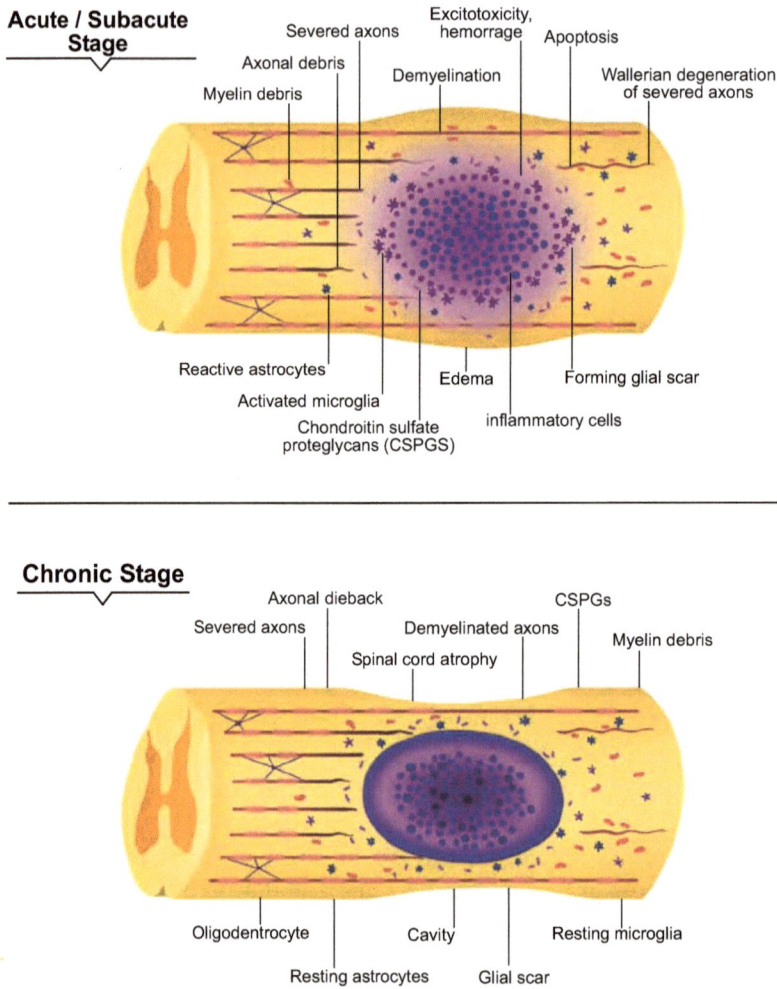

Fig. (4). Schematics illustrating the different stages of spinal cord injury (SCI), which can be categorized as follows: the acute phase (less than 48 hours), the subacute phase (48 hours to 14 days), the intermediate phase (14 days to 6 months), and the chronic phase (over six months). SCI sets off a series of biological and molecular processes. It commences with tissue bruising or tearing caused by mechanical trauma, disrupting nerve fibers and blood vessels, degeneration of nerve and glial cells, ischemia, and tissue swelling. Following SCI, physical forces, metabolic damage, and ischemia contribute to cellular damage. The presence of cellular debris can be harmful. Various mechanisms come into play to balance debris clearance and preservation of neighboring neural tissue that may still have functional potential. In mature chronic SCI lesions, three distinct tissue compartments can be identified, each exhibiting unique cellular characteristics: (a) a central non-neural lesion core (depicted as a deep purple area), often referred to as fibrotic scar, mesenchymal scar, or connective tissue scar; (b) an astroglial scar border surrounding the lesion core; and (c) a surrounding region of viable neural tissue that remains spared and functional, albeit reactive, delineated by the presence of reactive glia [30].

This taxonomy offers a systematic framework for comprehending the immediate causative factors involved in traumatic SCIs, thereby informing both diagnostic and therapeutic strategies.

The secondary phase of spinal cord injury (SCI) involves a complex ensemble of pathological cascades that ensue subsequent to the primary insult, exacerbating the initial neural damage and perpetuating neurofunctional derangements [5]. The mechanistic underpinnings of secondary injury comprise:

1. Ischemic-Hypoxic Events: The primary insult disrupts vascular perfusion to the spinal cord, inducing ischemic and hypoxic conditions. These hemodynamic perturbations not only potentiate neural tissue injury but also instigate a series of intracellular pathological occurrences, including inflammatory activation and cellular apoptosis.

2. Inflammatory Milieu: Post-primary injury, an inflammatory cascade is activated, characterized by the infiltration of immune cells and the release of cytokines and other pro-inflammatory mediators. Uncontrolled or protracted inflammation has the propensity to further exacerbate neural damage.

3. Excitotoxic Phenomena: Subsequent to the primary insult, an abnormal surge in neurotransmitter release, particularly that of glutamate, can occur. Elevated glutamate concentrations can engender neural hyper-excitability, inciting calcium ion influx and initiating cytotoxic pathways culminating in cellular demise.

4. Vasogenic Edema: Fluid accumulation in the spinal cord can augment compression, obstruct vascular flow, and intensify neural tissue damage.

5. Cell Death Pathways: The accentuation of cellular mortality processes, such as apoptosis (programmed cell demise) and necrosis (uncontrolled cell death due to traumatic injury), may occur in the wake of the primary injury, further exacerbating the loss of neural tissue and propagating neurofunctional impairments.

Understanding these secondary mechanisms of injury is pivotal for elucidating the pathological landscape of SCI and informs targeted therapeutic interventions.

History of Cell-based Therapy

Recent strides in cellular biology and the burgeoning field of regenerative medicine have precipitated a paradigm shift in spinal cord injury (SCI) research. Advances in cellular manipulation techniques have enabled the orchestration of differentiation cascades, culminating in the generation of rather homogeneous cellular cohorts derived from multipotent and totipotent progenitors. This scientific watershed carries monumental implications for the remediation and reparative strategies in SCI [35]. *In vivo* models have compellingly illustrated the therapeutic utility of multipotent neural progenitor cells in fostering axonal extension and synaptic architecture. These progenitors possess the plasticity to transdifferentiate into diverse neural lineages, inclusive of neurons and glial elements, thereby serving pivotal roles in neural functional restoration and structural integrity.

Since the advent of the second decade of the 21st century, the application of cellular transplantation methodologies in acute SCI cases has experienced an upswing. Geron Corporation launched an innovative clinical initiative, entailing the transplantation of oligodendrocyte progenitor cells (OPCs) sourced from human embryonic stem cells (ESCs) into the lesioned spinal cord [36]. Oligodendrocytes are specialized myelinogenic cells pivotal for neural insulation and the efficacious propagation of nerve impulses. The introduction of ESC-derived OPCs aims to catalyze remyelination processes and ameliorate signal transduction across the lesion site [37]. Current investigative focus is centered on refining the precision and efficacy of cellular delivery, exploring variables that influence post-transplantation cell survival, tissue integration, and spatial arrangement within the lesion matrix.

Stem Cell Types

Stem cells represent a singular category of cellular entities endowed with the remarkable faculties of pluripotency and self-renewal, permitting differentiation into an array of specialized cellular lineages, as well as the capability for limitless self-propagation [38]. Current clinical work has categorized these cells into various subtypes, notably differentiated by their origin as either autologous or allogeneic (Fig. **5**). The former proffers an immunologically compatible option which avoids eliciting host immune reactions, in contrast to the latter which can potentially trigger immunological responses (Fig. **6**).

Embryonic Stem Cells (ESCs) are procured from the blastocyst phase of embryonic development, approximately 4-5 days subsequent to fertilization. These cells are characterized by their pluripotentiality, denoting their capacity to give rise to cellular components of all three embryonic germ strata: ectoderm, endoderm, and mesoderm. This expansive differentiation repertoire has rendered ESCs the subject of exhaustive scientific scrutiny, reinforcing their potential to provide virtually any specialized cell type inherent to the human organism [5]. Conversely, Induced Pluripotent Stem Cells (iPSCs) result from the epigenetic reversion of differentiated adult somatic cells, such as epidermal or hematopoietic cells, to a pluripotent status [39]. This cellular reprogramming is effected through the introduction of select genetic elements or molecular catalysts.

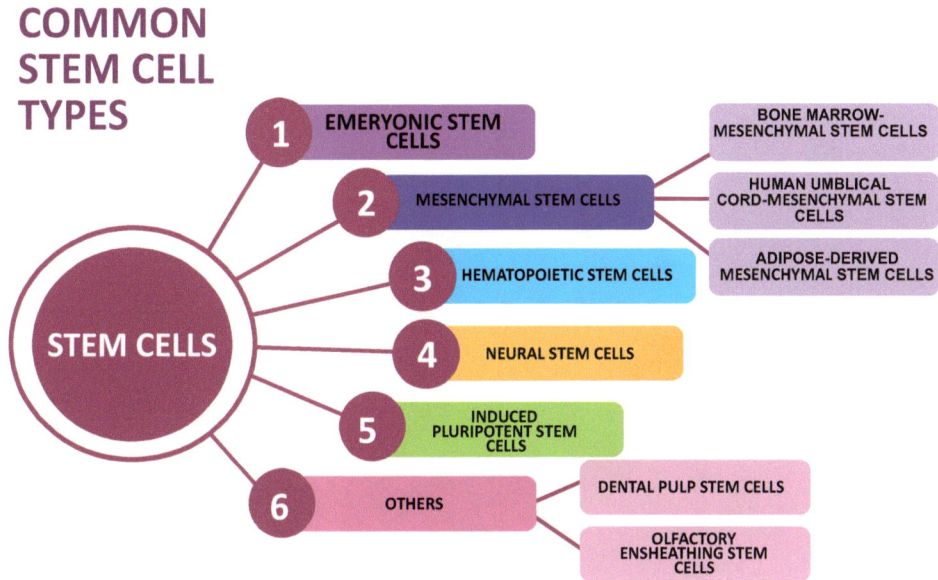

Fig. (5). Infogram characterizing the commonly employed types of stem cells.

Induced pluripotent stem cells are generated by reprogramming adult somatic cells, such as skin or blood cells, back into a pluripotent state. Pluripotent stem cells have the remarkable ability to differentiate into any cell type found in the human body. iPSCs are created by introducing a combination of specific genes or factors into the somatic cells, reprograming them to regain pluripotency, and reverting them to an embryonic-like state. iPSCs closely resemble embryonic stem cells (ESCs) in their characteristics and potential to differentiate into various cell types. This ability makes iPSCs valuable for regenerative medicine, disease modeling, drug discovery, and personalized cell-based therapies. They are relevant to SCI repair.

Analogous to Embryonic Stem Cells (ESCs), Induced Pluripotent Stem Cells (iPSCs) exhibit pluripotentiality, possessing the ability to differentiate into a myriad of specialized cellular phenotypes [40]. These cells hold pronounced therapeutic importance, owing to their autologous origin, which attenuates the immunological impediments often associated with transplantation procedures.

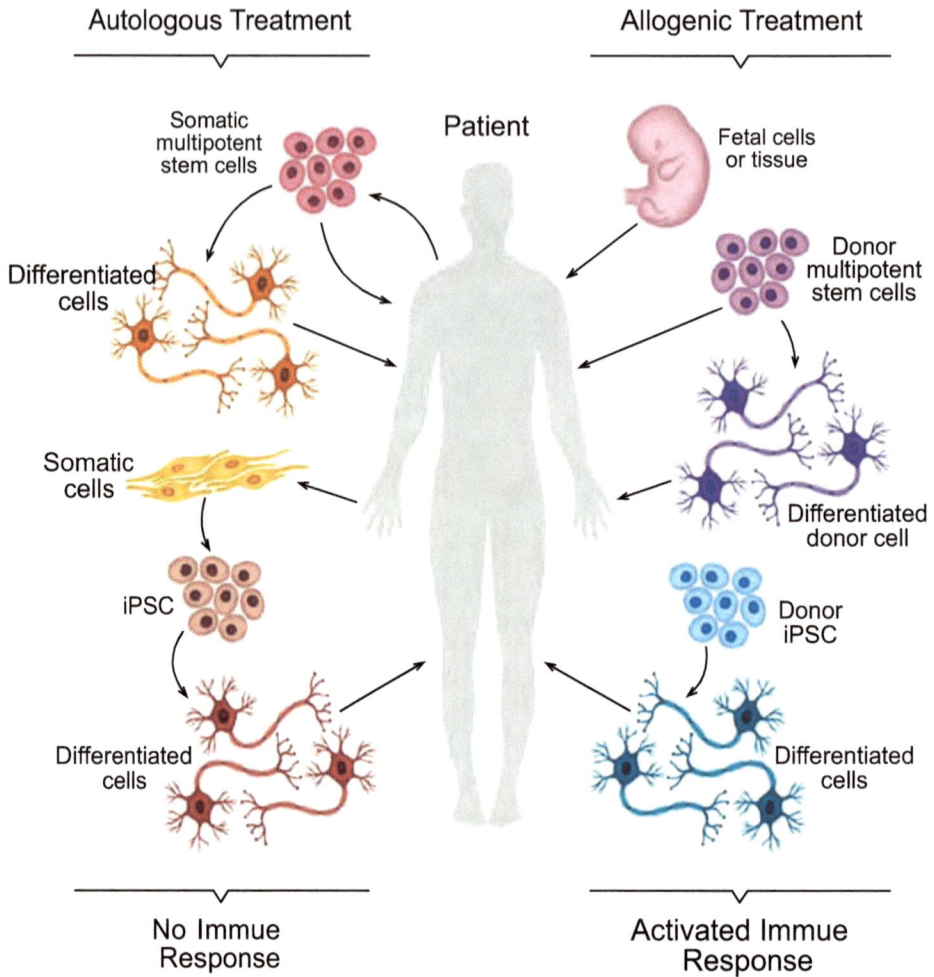

Fig. (6). Autologous stem cells are usually derived from sources such as bone marrow or adipose tissue. Autologous stem cell therapy offers the advantage of avoiding immune rejection and ethical concerns associated with using cells from other individuals. Allogeneic stem cells are typically from healthy donors. Sources include umbilical cord blood, embryonic stem cells, or induced pluripotent stem cells (iPSC). Allogeneic stem cell therapy offers a broader availability of cells and the ability to select specific cell types for therapeutic purposes, but may provoke an immune response.

Somatically-derived stem cells, ubiquitously distributed across diverse anatomical structures, function as innate repositories for tissue homeostasis and regenerative undertakings [5]. These cells customarily manifest multipotency, with archetypes encompassing hematopoietic and mesenchymal stem cells (Fig. **7**).

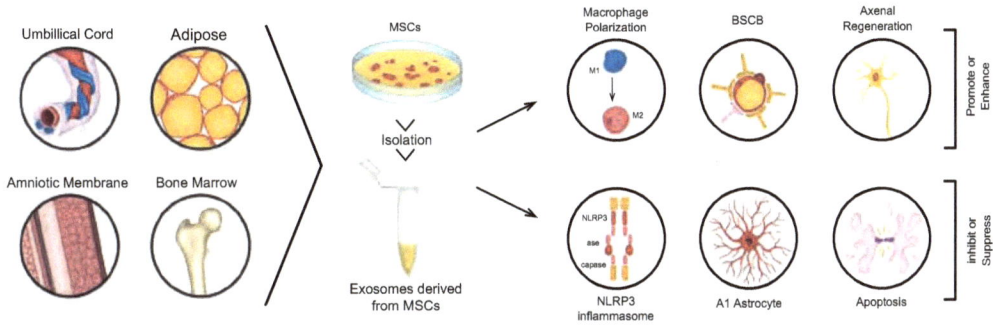

Fig. (7). Sources of commonly employed stem cells. Stem cells hold the potential for neuroprotection, immunomodulation, axon sprouting, regeneration, neuronal relay formation, and myelin regeneration; all of which are mechanisms that could contribute to functional recovery following spinal cord injury (SCI) [41]. The NLRP3 inflammasome is a crucial multiprotein complex that regulates the innate immune system and inflammatory signaling. Promising results have been observed in treating various pathological conditions by targeting the NLRP3 inflammasome pathway using small molecules and biologics to inhibit chronic inflammation [42]. The blood-spinal cord barrier (BSCB) usually acts as a safeguard, preventing the entry of toxins, blood cells, and pathogens into the spinal cord while maintaining the precise chemical balance necessary for proper neural function. Disruption of the BSCB plays a significant role in the primary and secondary injury processes associated with SCI. Following SCI, the breakdown of the BSCB structure leads to direct leakage of blood components and increased permeability. Addressing the disruption of the BSCB could alleviate the pathology associated with SCI [43]. In response to SCI, astrocytes, including inflammatory astrocyte 1 (A1), assume an activated state and perform several vital functions such as necrotic tissue clearance, formation of a protective barrier [44], maintenance of microenvironmental balance, interaction with immune cells, and formation of the glial scar. Targeting new subtypes of astrocytes may hold promise for SCI repair.

In contrast, tissue-restricted progenitor cells, confined to specific biological matrices or organ systems, exhibit a circumscribed differentiation scope relative to their pluripotent counterparts. Such cells support the sustainment and restitution of cellular populations within their native tissues. Noteworthy exemplars comprise neural progenitor cells, useful in the genesis of neurons and glial elements, as well as cutaneous epithelial stem cells important in dermal cell renewal.

Perinatal stem cells, procured from the biological matrices encircling the gestating fetus and neonate, include such variants as umbilical cord hemopoietic cells, amniotic fluid-derived stem cells, and placental stem cells (Fig. **8**). These cells are prized for their profusion, facile retrievability, and reduced ethical entanglements vis-à-vis embryonic stem cell research.

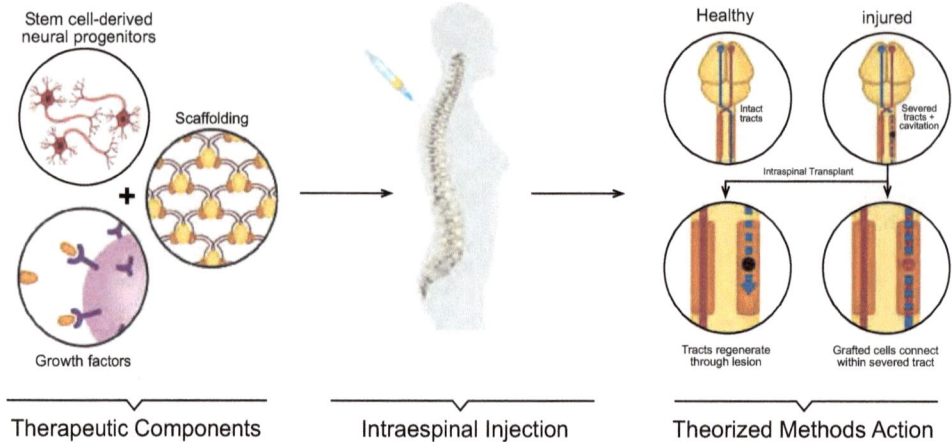

Fig. (8). Schematic of the theorized benefit and mechanism of action of the intraspinal administration of stem cells.

Bone Marrow-derived Mesenchymal Stem Cells

In a pioneering longitudinal study focusing on cervical Spinal Cord Injury (SCI), the intramedullary and intradural administration of Bone Marrow-derived Mesenchymal Stem Cells (BM-MSCs) – harvested and expanded from the patients' own iliac bone – was shown to engender amelioration in functional recuperation [45]. Six-month post-transplantation assessments revealed enhancements in upper-limb motor capacities and magnetic resonance imaging (MRI) alterations in 60% and 70% of the ten participating patients, respectively [46]. Extended longitudinal surveillance exceeding a triennial post-transplantation period corroborated the sustainability of upper-extremity functional improvements, devoid of any observed morbidities, including neoplastic formation [46].

Several ongoing investigations are employing the American Spinal Injury Association (ASIA) graded scale as a metric for evaluating functional gains, and some even amalgamate alternative therapeutic regimens such as exoskeletal neuromodulation and virtual reality interfaces with either intravenous or intranasal applications of BM-MSCs. Notably, these studies are predominantly currently at the stage of Phase I or II clinical trials.

Umbilical Cord MSCs

Mesenchymal Stem Cells (MSCs) derived from adipose tissue and the umbilical cord present viable alternatives for cellular therapies in neuro-regenerative contexts. These particular stem cells manifest the capacity for neural marker expression, thereby approximating morphological and phenotypical attributes reminiscent of fully differentiated neurons, such as bipolar elongations and intricate end-branching patterns [47]. Subsequent investigations have reported additional therapeutic efficacies when Brain-Derived Neurotrophic Factor (BDNF) was co-administered with umbilical cord-derived MSCs (U-MSCs). Immunohistochemical analysis targeting Glial Fibrillary Acidic Protein (GFAP) and Microtubule-Associated Protein 2 (MAP2) validated the MSCs' pluripotent differentiation into both astrocytic and neuronal lineages [48]. Moreover, the application of U-MSCs was associated with a diminution in glial scar tissue accrual and an augmentation in angiogenesis, likely attributable to the upregulation of matrix metalloproteinases [49, 50].

Adipocyte MSCs

Adipose-derived Mesenchymal Stem Cells (AD-MSCs) boast a higher cellular yield and a more facile extraction process compared to their bone marrow-derived counterparts (BM-MSCs). Initial investigations evaluating the safety profile of intravenously administered AD-MSCs reported an absence of adverse events, including tumorigenic manifestations [51]. A contemporary study scrutinized the therapeutic ramifications of intrathecal administration of autologous AD-MSCs in a cohort of 14 spinal cord injury (SCI) patients. Outcome metrics encompassed both the American Spinal Injury Association (ASIA) motor and sensory indices, as well as a range of electrophysiological assessments, such as electromyography and magnetic resonance imaging (MRI). Post-intervention analysis revealed that sensory gains were appreciable in 10 of the 14 subjects, though MRI-determined lesion dimensions remained invariable. Notably, severe adverse sequelae were conspicuously absent across the patient population receiving AD-MSCs, and any minor side-effects that did manifest were adjudged to be unrelated to the stem cell administration [52].

Further, intravenous infusion of AD-MSCs demonstrated an activation of angiogenetic pathways and an upregulation of key kinase proteins, such as Extracellular Signal-Regulated Kinase 1/2 (ERK1/2) and Protein Kinase B (Akt), which are implicated in cellular survival and tissue reparative mechanisms [53]. A number of nascent clinical trials is underway, and their findings will necessitate broader investigative efforts to conclusively delineate the therapeutic efficacy of AD-MSCs in the context of acute SCI.

MSC Transplantation Strategies for Chronic SCI

Intravenous administration, although invasive, does not cause damage to the spinal cord. Animal models suggest that a significant number of cells should be administered for effective results [54]. Neural Stem Cells (NSCs) can be quickly delivered to the central nervous system through this route, where they have the potential to replace damaged cells and differentiate into glial cells and neurons [55]. Ohta *et al.* conducted a study in which adipose tissue-derived mesenchymal stem cells (AD-MSCs) were injected into the veins of rats with spinal cord injury (SCI). It was observed that the cells gradually accumulated at the injury site, improving the rats' motor function [53].

Another potential NSC administration method is intra-arterial administration, which requires further study to ensure its feasibility and convenience. This approach is less commonly used due to concerns such as the risk of blood vessel embolism. Intranasal administration, although less effective than intramedullary injections, has shown some therapeutic effects. Ramalho *et al.* compared the intraperitoneal and intravenous administration of bone marrow-derived mesenchymal stem cells (BMMSCs) and found similar therapeutic effects for both approaches in SCI [56].

Intrathecal inoculations, when juxtaposed against intramedullary injections, offer reduced invasiveness. Nonetheless, preclinical evidence suggests that cellular viability may extend merely to a two-month time frame subsequent to intramedullary introduction, whereas post-intrathecal administration cellular detection remains elusive [57]. Intrathecal infusion exerts a modest influence on spinal cord injury (SCI) *via* a paracrine modality, thereby promoting sustained regenerative processes, a finding corroborated in extant literature [58]. Levi and colleagues conducted an exploration into the safety profile of intramedullary injections in a cohort comprising chronic cervical and thoracic SCI patients, identifying an absence of deleterious effects among the 29 participants [57].

The most efficacious modality for cellular delivery remains a topic under ongoing investigation. Intravenous infusion, although invasive, does not engender spinal cord damage. *In vivo* models corroborate the requirement for a substantial cellular payload to yield therapeutically meaningful results. Neural Stem Cells (NSCs) are amenable to translocation *via* this route to the central nervous system, where they possess the capability to substitute for damaged cellular constituents and undergo differentiation into glial cells and neurons [55]. A study carried out by Ohta and colleagues involved the intravenous instillation of adipose tissue-derived mesenchymal stem cells (AD-MSCs) into a rat model with SCI, observing a gradual accretion of these cells at the lesion locus and noting enhancements in motor function [53].

Alternative routes for NSC introduction include intra-arterial infusion—an avenue warranting additional investigative rigor owing to concerns of vascular embolism—and intranasal application, which, although suboptimal relative to intramedullary injections, exhibits therapeutic promise. Ramalho *et al.* conducted a comparative analysis of intraperitoneal and intravenous administration of bone marrow-derived mesenchymal stem cells (BM-MSCs), discerning comparable therapeutic efficacies between the two methodologies in the context of SCI [56].

MSC Benefit in Chronic SCI

Chang and colleagues performed an investigation which elucidated the anti-inflammatory ramifications resulting from mesenchymal stem cell (MSC) transplantation. This diminution of inflammation was manifested through a noteworthy decrement in neutrophil accumulation and inducible nitric oxide synthase-positive (iNOS+)/mac-2+ cellular presence within the lesioned territory. Concurrently, quantitative transcriptional analyses revealed a substantial reduction in the mRNA expression levels of pro-inflammatory cytokines, namely, tumor necrosis factor-alpha (TNF-α), interleukin-1 beta (IL-1β), interleukin-6 (IL-6), and interleukin-12 (IL-12); in comparison to a control cohort. This suggested an MSC-mediated modulation of inflammatory cell trafficking and consequent inflammation attenuation [59].

Wang and associates conducted an exploratory study focusing on the utility of bone marrow-derived mesenchymal stem cells (BM-MSCs) in conjunction with decellularized spinal cord scaffolds for the remediation of spinal cord hemisection defects. This integrative methodology resulted in the regulated ingress of inflammatory cells, alongside a concomitant diminution in apoptotic processes and secondary inflammatory responses, cumulatively culminating in observable functional recuperation [60].

Establishing a conducive intracellular milieu augmented by the presence of growth factors facilitates the inducement of mesenchymal stem cells (MSCs) to undergo differentiation into glial and neuronal phenotypes, thereby expediting tissue restitution. Zhao and collaborators conducted an experiment wherein mesenchymal stem cells in their nascent state, harvested from human embryonic sources, were introduced into the developing avian central nervous system. These incipient MSCs seamlessly integrated within the neural tube architecture, subsequently coalescing into aggregates that underwent differentiation into neuronal entities. Upon transplantation into lesioned spinal cord sites, these embryonic-origin MSCs exhibited the capability to differentiate into fully mature neurons and glial cells, thereby contributing to the establishment of functional neural circuitry proximal to the site of spinal injury and fostering axonal regeneration [61]. Furthermore, in primate models, temporally deferred transplantation of MSCs into sites of spinal cord injury culminated in their differentiation into astrocytes, neurons, and oligodendrocytes [61].

The process of angiogenesis, which entails the genesis of new vascular networks, is integral to tissue regenerative mechanisms. Investigations corroborate that the engraftment of neural stem cells (NSCs) correlates with an amplification of Vascular Endothelial Growth Factor (VEGF) expression, a pivotal angiogenic modulator, when juxtaposed with control cohorts [62, 63]. This elevation suggests that MSC transplantation could potentiate VEGF synthesis, thereby fostering angiogenesis and ameliorating motor functionality in afflicted extremities. Subsequent rodent-based research in the context of spinal cord injury (SCI) underscores the salutary influence of angiogenic mediators such as VEGF, Angiopoietin-1, and basic Fibroblast Growth Factor (bFGF) on neuroregeneration and neurological competency [57]. These agents stimulate vasculogenesis and encourage axonal resurgence, expediting neurological recovery. Several molecular entities and nutritive factors have been identified as being essential for neural recuperation [64, 65]. The paradigms through which stem cell-mediated interventions for SCI exert their potentially therapeutic effects are iterated in Fig. (9).

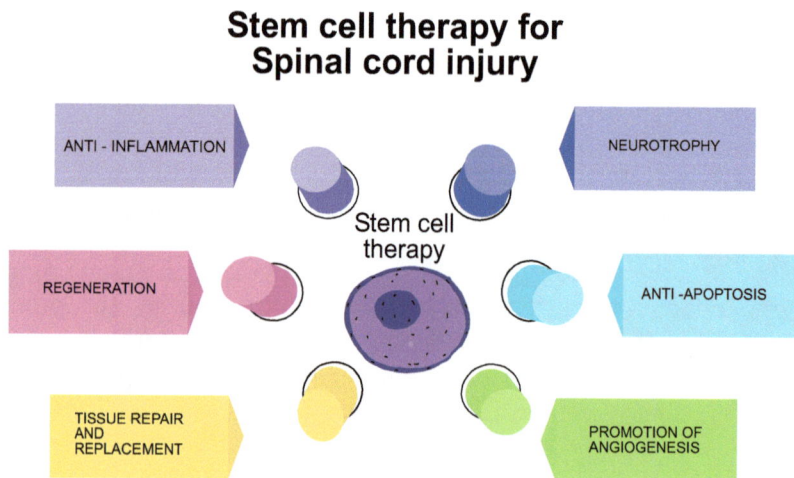

Fig. (9). Illustrative infogram on the target mechanisms of stem cell-based SCI treatments.

Additional benefits may emanate from the anti-apoptotic propensity of stem cells. Investigations reveal that in the milieu of SCI, the regulation of both proapoptotic and antiapoptotic elements, such as Tumor Necrosis Factor-Alpha (TNF-α), p53, and Bcl-2 Associated X Protein (Bax), may be compromised. Stem cell intervention has been shown to elevate the levels of B-cell lymphoma-2 (Bcl2) [66-70]. According to Nicola *et al.*, data indicated a pronounced downregulation of the proapoptotic mediator TNF-α in the stem cell-treated cadre, while conversely elevating the antiapoptotic effector Bcell lymphoma-extra-large (Bcl-xL) in relation to the control group. Collectively, these findings insinuate that stem cell engraftment mitigates early apoptosis, thus contributing to the preservation of neural and tissue integrity and facilitating the revival of neurological function [71].

While therapeutics may present deleterious ramifications, evidence suggests that inordinate introduction of stem cells may precipitate adverse effects such as vascular thrombosis or embolic events. Immune-related reactions also represent potential complications, indicating a possible need for concomitant immunosuppressive strategies [53, 59, 72]. Among the most serious prospective side effects is tumorigenicity. Research by Lida *et al.* discerned that the DNA methylation configurations in NSCs and progenitor cells, sourced from human-induced pluripotent stem cells, exhibit a state of instability. Moreover, instances of malignant cellular metamorphosis have been observed, such as fibrosarcoma, consequent to chromosomal aberrations [73, 74].

Biomaterial Scaffolds and Hydrogels

Advancements in biomaterial science have led to the formulation of innovative scaffolds and hydrogels designed to augment the efficacy of stem cell engraftment and to selectively promote cellular proliferation subsequent to spinal cord injuries (SCIs). These developments are graphically represented in Fig. (**1**). Initial endeavors concentrated on the employment of chitosan-based conduits in tandem with neural progenitor cells (NPCs), formulating a microenvironment conducive to axonal elongation and neural tissue reconstitution. However, current scientific progress in the domains of both biomaterials and stem cell biology has expanded the investigative purview to encompass a more diverse array of cell-biomaterial synergies. Contemporary research has revealed that the administration of a peptide-functionalized hydrogel, synthesized from hyaluronan and methylcellulose, substantially augments the viability and proliferation of oligodendrocyte progenitor cells (OPCs) that are induced from pluripotent stem cells (iPSCs) in rodent models of SCI. Notably, these treated rats exhibited an escalation in OPC migratory activity and a diminution in teratoma incidence when subjected to a regimen combining OPCs and the aforementioned injectable hydrogel. An alternative inquiry found that the incorporation of a gelatin/methyl acrylate hydrogel in conjunction with NPCs mitigates glial scar tissue deposition, attenuates localized inflammatory cascades, and expedites functional recuperation post-SCI [75].

Clinical Application

A plethora of ongoing clinical investigations are deploying an array of cellular permutations, with the majority currently working through Phase I or II developmental stages. One exemplar study carried out by Curtis *et al.* explored the transplantation of human spinal cord-derived neural stem cells (NSCs) in a Phase I clinical trial targeting chronic spinal cord injuries (SCIs) within the T2-T12 segment [76]. This intervention entailed laminectomy, dural incision, and the stereotactic injection of stem cells bilaterally along the midline on six separate occasions. Longitudinal observations spanning 18-27 months post-transplantation corroborated an absence of severe adverse sequelae in all enrollees. Neurological function, gauged *via* the International Standards for Neurological Classification of Spinal Cord Injury (ISNCSCI) scores, revealed functional ameliorations in one to two spinal segments. Concurrently, research by Satti *et al.* scrutinized the safety profile of intrathecally administered autologous bone marrow stromal cells in a cohort of nine SCI sufferers, including six chronic and three subacute cases [77]. Each participant was given two or three injections, each containing a median cellular density of $1:2 \times 10^6$ cells/kg of body mass. The absence of untoward events attributed to the treatment was confirmed during the follow-up period [78]. Mendoza *et al.* conducted a Phase I nonrandomized, controlled clinical trial, incorporating 14 subjects afflicted with chronic traumatic SCI persisting for over six months [79]. These patients received bone marrow-derived mesenchymal stem cell (BM-MSC) injections postoperatively in the impacted spinal cord region. Various diagnostic modalities including somatosensory evoked potentials, magnetic resonance imaging, and urodynamic studies were employed both pre- and post-intervention. Additionally, subjective pain indices were evaluated utilizing the McGill Pain Questionnaire and the Visual Analog Scale. Cumulative data substantiated that autologous BM-MSC transplantation represents a safe and potentially efficacious therapeutic avenue for individuals with complete chronic SCIs, possibly enhancing neurological functionality [79]. Prospective clinical endeavors may opt for a multifaceted approach, amalgamating stem cells, biomaterials, and bioactive molecules for enhanced SCI remediation (Fig. **10**).

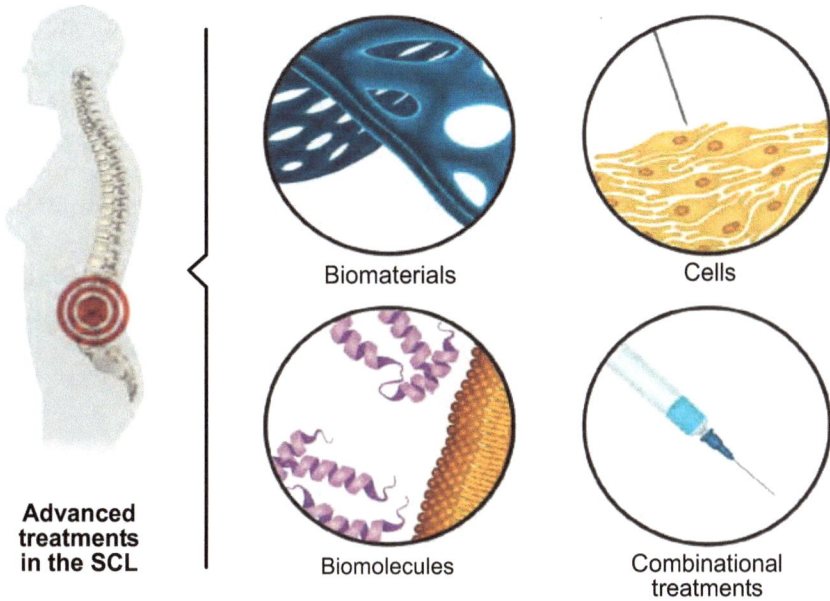

Fig. (10). Potential applications of stem cells, biomaterials, and biomolecules for future clinical use in spinal cord injury (SCI) patients. Stem cells can differentiate into various cell types and potentially regenerate damaged neural tissue. In future clinical treatment of SCI, stem cells may replace damaged cells, promote neuroprotection, stimulate axon regeneration, and enhance functional recovery. Biomaterials may prove crucial in developing scaffolds and matrices that support stem cell delivery and integration into the injured spinal cord. These biomaterials may provide physical support, promote cell adhesion, guide axonal growth, and create a microenvironment conducive to tissue repair and regeneration. Biomolecules may be utilized to modulate the inflammatory response, promote angiogenesis, stimulate neuronal growth, and enhance the survival and differentiation of transplanted cells. Growth factors, cytokines, and small molecules could be delivered locally to the injured site to optimize therapeutic outcomes.

Shin *et al.* ascertained the safety and therapeutic efficacy of human neural stem cell (NSC) transplantation in the context of traumatic cervical spinal cord injuries (SCIs) [78]. Among the 19 patients administered the NSC grafts, none manifested adverse outcomes such as syringomyelia or neoplastic formations, and a subset of eight patients exhibited enhancements in their AIS (American Spinal Injury Association Impairment Scale) scores [78]. Ghobrial *et al.* corroborated these findings, documenting favorable outcomes following the intramedullary injection of human NSCs in a cohort of five individuals suffering from chronic cervical SCIs [80]. Conversely, in Phase III clinical explorations conducted by Oh *et al.*, only 16 SCI patients who were recipients of autologous bone marrow-derived mesenchymal stem cell (BM-MSC) grafts experienced neurological ameliorations [81]. Importantly, these individuals encountered no untoward events linked to the stem cell infusions [81, 82].

Notwithstanding these advancements, clinical endeavors specific to SCI interventions have been sporadically initiated, truncated, or entirely aborted due to an array of limitations such as fiscal constraints, suboptimal patient enrollment, or strategic corporate resolutions. It is imperative to underscore the heterogeneity inherent in these clinical studies, which diverge in multiple parameters including patient sample size, anatomical locus of injury, cellular taxonomy, mode of cellular administration, and dosage; thereby complicating direct comparisons and conclusive interpretations. The need for methodologically rigorous, long-term, expansive, multicenter, standardized, and randomized controlled trials remains salient. Future investigative pursuits are indispensable for elucidating the authentic clinical utility of stem cell-based therapeutics in the management of SCIs [83].

Addressing Ethical Concerns

Ethical conundrums surrounding the utilization of Embryonic Stem Cell (ESC)-centric treatments arise from their embryonic origin. Although the philosophical quandaries concerning the commencement of human life and the embryo's ethical standing lie outside the ambit of this chapter— concentrated on stem cell-mediated interventions for spinal cord lesions—it remains indisputable that the contentious nature of informed consent protocols and the provenance of embryonic stem cells, typically harvested from embryos initially reserved for *In vitro* Fertilization (IVF), warrants further ethical scrutiny. Concurrently, ethical and moral complexities could emerge when refraining from employing potentially curative stem cell interventions for spinal cord injuries, especially when considering the consequent debility and societal ramifications associated with such catastrophic impairments. Thus, alternative cell-based therapies have been explored, incorporating adult stem cells or induced pluripotent stem cells (iPSCs), obviating the need for embryonic destruction. In addition, autologous stem cell modalities serve as another viable avenue, facilitating minimally invasive cell transplantation techniques such as peripheral administration. Such approaches not only mitigate the risks associated with graft rejection and immunogenicity, but also minimize immune system activation attributable to secondary injury phenomena.

The ethical appraisal of emerging technologies is intrinsic to their judicious assimilation into clinical practice. Novel therapeutic innovations mandate rigorous scrutiny through a structured cascade of preclinical investigations, followed by Phase I feasibility assessments and Phase II and III evaluations focused on safety and efficacy parameters (Refer to Fig. **11**). Cellular therapy research, particularly in the stem cell domain, has catalyzed intricate, and occasionally polemical, ethical discourses. Transparent deliberations on these topics are indispensable, and should be dynamically revisited to accommodate diverse societal perspectives and ontological paradigms. Such an iterative dialogue can engender community-endorsed, sustainable frameworks for technology deployment.

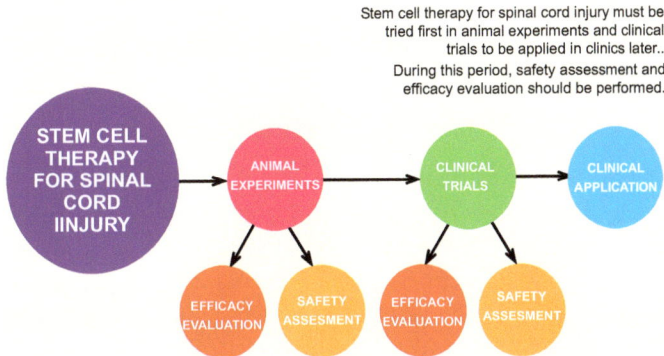

Fig. (11). Illustrative flow-diagram on preclinical and clinical investigation of stem cell-based SCI treatments.

Regrettably, an alarming number of commercial entities globally proffer non-evidence-based cellular therapies, frequently imposing prohibitive financial burdens on patients while neglecting rigorous pre- and post-treatment evaluations. Such providers often promulgate a monolithic therapeutic approach across a spectrum of clinical indications, without substantiating efficacy. Therefore, ongoing scrutiny of technological advances remains essential, framed within the milieu of societal, cultural, and ethical norms. Sustained interdisciplinary dialogue encompassing the ethical, legal, and social dimensions of stem cell research is of paramount importance.

DISCUSSION

The prospective trajectory of stem cell-oriented interventions for acute spinal cord injury (SCI) will be profoundly influenced by the resolution of extant ethical quandaries. The incremental advancements in therapeutic modalities for SCI have been tempered by ethical reservations, particularly concerning Embryonic Stem Cells (ESCs), fiscal logistics, and the nascent state of such therapeutic regimens. Investigations into intrathecal delivery mechanisms are underway to discern optimal therapeutic avenues. Concurrently, burgeoning research in scaffolding technologies, biomaterial applications, and immunomodulatory treatments holds potential for instigating spinal cord regeneration.

Despite the encouraging scientific inroads in cell-based modalities for acute SCI, the transition to robust clinical assessments remains dilatory. There exists a compelling imperative for the initiation of expansive Phase III investigations aimed at ascertaining the clinical efficacy of stem cell transplantation—a delay partly attributable to ethical complexities and budgetary limitations. Historical investigations have often been compromised by mediocre efficacy or suboptimal research design, thereby necessitating further rigorous clinical trials to affirm the therapeutic potential of cell-based interventions for acute SCI.

Current research endeavors predominantly focus on the validation of the safety and efficacy profiles of Mesenchymal Stem Cells (MSCs) in the context of acute SCI clinical trials. Among the nine ongoing studies, a significant 89% are centered around MSC transplantation, eschewing an ESC-centric paradigm. These studies are overwhelmingly oriented towards intrathecal administration of stem cells, although alternative delivery modalities are under scrutiny to comprehensively explore optimal therapeutic techniques. While the majority of these inquiries are in Phase I/II trials, preliminary evaluations deploying predefined neurofunctional scales are expected to provide invaluable insights, paving the way for subsequent late-phase trials designed to conclusively ascertain the therapeutic efficacy of emerging cell-based interventions for acute SCI.

CONCLUSION

The therapeutic potential of stem cell interventions for spinal cord injuries (SCI) is increasingly substantiated, albeit several crucial challenges warrant immediate attention. These encompass ethical dilemmas, conceivable adverse reactions, complications intrinsic to the procedure, immunological rejection risks, the imperatives of cellular purity, and the oncogenic hazards associated with such therapies. These safety concerns are nontrivial and necessitate scrupulous evaluation.

Notwithstanding these obstacles, the elucidation of precise therapeutic modalities and underlying mechanisms is advancing, facilitating more efficacious management of post-transplantation side effects. Moreover, although the extant corpus of research is predominantly founded on animal models, the imperative for additional animal experimentation is diminishing as the clinical applicability of stem cell-based therapies for SCI becomes increasingly feasible.

Emerging strategies, including targeted Embryonic Stem Cell (ESC) utilization and synergistic stem cell amalgamations, offer optimistic prospects for future clinical applications in SCI treatment. Concomitant with ongoing advancements in stem cell technology, the clinical deployment of stem cell-based interventions for SCI is poised for significant progression.

REFERENCES

[1]   International Perspectives on Spinal Cord Injury 2023 [06 28 2023] Available from: https://www.who.int/publications/i/item/international-perspectives-on-spinal-cord-injury 2023.

[2]   Rexed B. A cytoarchitectonic atlas of the spinal coed in the cat. J Comp Neurol 1954; 100(2): 297-379.
[http://dx.doi.org/10.1002/cne.901000205] [PMID: 13163236]

[3]   Ronzano R, Lancelin C, Bhumbra GS, Brownstone RM, Beato M. Proximal and distal spinal neurons innervating multiple synergist and antagonist motor pools. eLife 2021; 10e70858
[http://dx.doi.org/10.7554/eLife.70858] [PMID: 34727018]

[4]   Frara N, Giaddui D, Braverman AS, *et al.* Nerve transfer for restoration of lower motor neuron-lesioned bladder function. Part 1: attenuation of purinergic bladder smooth muscle contractions. Am J Physiol Regul Integr Comp Physiol 2021; 320(6): R885-96.
[http://dx.doi.org/10.1152/ajpregu.00299.2020] [PMID: 33759578]

[5]   Ackery A, Tator C, Krassioukov A. A global perspective on spinal cord injury epidemiology. J Neurotrauma 2004; 21(10): 1355-70.
[http://dx.doi.org/10.1089/neu.2004.21.1355] [PMID: 15672627]

[6]   Rowland JW, Hawryluk GWJ, Kwon B, Fehlings MG. Current status of acute spinal cord injury pathophysiology and emerging therapies: promise on the horizon. Neurosurg Focus 2008; 25(5)E2
[http://dx.doi.org/10.3171/FOC.2008.25.11.E2] [PMID: 18980476]

[7]   Zhang N, Yin Y, Xu SJ, Wu YP, Chen WS. Inflammation & apoptosis in spinal cord injury. Indian J Med Res 2012; 135(3): 287-96.
[PMID: 22561613]

[8]   Silva NA, Sousa N, Reis RL, Salgado AJ. From basics to clinical: A comprehensive review on spinal cord injury. Prog Neurobiol 2014; 114: 25-57.
[http://dx.doi.org/10.1016/j.pneurobio.2013.11.002] [PMID: 24269804]

[9]   Grossman SD, Rosenberg LJ, Wrathall JR. Relationship of altered glutamate receptor subunit mRNA expression to acute cell loss after spinal cord contusion. Exp Neurol 2001; 168(2): 283-9.
[http://dx.doi.org/10.1006/exnr.2001.7629] [PMID: 11259116]

[10]   Beattie MS, Li Q, Bresnahan JC. Cell death and plasticity after experimental spinal cord injury. Prog Brain Res 2000; 128: 9-21.
[http://dx.doi.org/10.1016/S0079-6123(00)28003-5] [PMID: 11105665]

[11]   Blight AR. Spinal cord injury models: neurophysiology. J Neurotrauma 1992; 9(2): 147-50.
[http://dx.doi.org/10.1089/neu.1992.9.147] [PMID: 1404430]

[12]   Vismara I, Papa S, Rossi F, Forloni G, Veglianese P. Current Options for Cell Therapy in Spinal Cord Injury. Trends Mol Med 2017; 23(9): 831-49.
[http://dx.doi.org/10.1016/j.molmed.2017.07.005] [PMID: 28811172]

[13]   Fehlings MG, Nakashima H, Nagoshi N, Chow DSL, Grossman RG, Kopjar B. Rationale, design and critical end points for the Riluzole in Acute Spinal Cord Injury Study (RISCIS): a randomized, double-blinded, placebo-controlled parallel multi-center trial. Spinal Cord 2016; 54(1): 8-15.
[http://dx.doi.org/10.1038/sc.2015.95] [PMID: 26099215]

[14]   Hayta E, Elden H. Acute spinal cord injury: A review of pathophysiology and potential of non-steroidal anti-inflammatory drugs for pharmacological intervention. J Chem Neuroanat 2018; 87: 25-31.
[http://dx.doi.org/10.1016/j.jchemneu.2017.08.001] [PMID: 28803968]

[15]   Gazdic M, Volarevic V, Harrell C, *et al.* Stem Cells Therapy for Spinal Cord Injury. Int J Mol Sci 2018; 19(4): 1039.
[http://dx.doi.org/10.3390/ijms19041039] [PMID: 29601528]

[16]   Garcia E, Aguilar-Cevallos J, Silva-Garcia R, Ibarra A. Cytokine and Growth Factor Activation *In Vivo* and *In Vitro* after Spinal Cord Injury. Mediators Inflamm 2016; 2016: 1-21.
[http://dx.doi.org/10.1155/2016/9476020] [PMID: 27418745]

[17]   Papa S, Caron I, Erba E, *et al.* Early modulation of pro-inflammatory microglia by minocycline loaded nanoparticles confers long lasting protection after spinal cord injury. Biomaterials 2016; 75: 13-24.
[http://dx.doi.org/10.1016/j.biomaterials.2015.10.015] [PMID: 26474039]

[18]   Shechter R, Schwartz M. Harnessing monocyte-derived macrophages to control central nervous system pathologies: no longer 'if' but 'how'. J Pathol 2013; 229(2): 332-46.
[http://dx.doi.org/10.1002/path.4106] [PMID: 23007711]

[19]   David S, López-Vales R, Wee Yong V. Harmful and beneficial effects of inflammation after spinal cord injury. Handb Clin Neurol 2012; 109: 485-502.
[http://dx.doi.org/10.1016/B978-0-444-52137-8.00030-9] [PMID: 23098732]

[20]   Fournier AE, GrandPre T, Strittmatter SM. Identification of a receptor mediating Nogo-66 inhibition of axonal regeneration. Nature 2001; 409(6818): 341-6.
[http://dx.doi.org/10.1038/35053072] [PMID: 11201742]

[21]   GrandPré T, Nakamura F, Vartanian T, Strittmatter SM. Identification of the Nogo inhibitor of axon regeneration as a Reticulon protein. Nature 2000; 403(6768): 439-44.
[http://dx.doi.org/10.1038/35000226] [PMID: 10667797]

[22]   Schwab ME. Nogo and axon regeneration. Curr Opin Neurobiol 2004; 14(1): 118-24.
[http://dx.doi.org/10.1016/j.conb.2004.01.004] [PMID: 15018947]

[23]   Schwab ME, Strittmatter SM. Nogo limits neural plasticity and recovery from injury. Curr Opin Neurobiol 2014; 27: 53-60.
[http://dx.doi.org/10.1016/j.conb.2014.02.011] [PMID: 24632308]

[24]   Yuan YM, He C. The glial scar in spinal cord injury and repair. Neurosci Bull 2013; 29(4): 421-35.
[http://dx.doi.org/10.1007/s12264-013-1358-3] [PMID: 23861090]

[25]   Snow DM, Beller JA. Proteoglycans: road signs for neurite outgrowth. Neural Regen Res 2014; 9(4): 343-55.
[http://dx.doi.org/10.4103/1673-5374.128235] [PMID: 25206822]

[26]   Correa MD, López MR. Alternative macrophage activation: the diversity of one cell involved in innate immunity in response to its environmental complexity. Inmunologia 2007; 26(2): 73-86.

[27]   Sabin KZ, Jiang P, Gearhart MD, Stewart R, Echeverri K. AP-1$^{cFos/JunB}$/miR-200a regulate the pro-regenerative glial cell response during axolotl spinal cord regeneration. Commun Biol 2019; 2(1): 91.
[http://dx.doi.org/10.1038/s42003-019-0335-4] [PMID: 30854483]

[28]   van Niekerk EA, Tuszynski MH, Lu P, Dulin JN. Molecular and Cellular Mechanisms of Axonal Regeneration After Spinal Cord Injury. Mol Cell Proteomics 2016; 15(2): 394-408.
[http://dx.doi.org/10.1074/mcp.R115.053751] [PMID: 26695766]

[29]   Tran AP, Warren PM, Silver J. The Biology of Regeneration Failure and Success After Spinal Cord Injury. Physiol Rev 2018; 98(2): 881-917.
[http://dx.doi.org/10.1152/physrev.00017.2017] [PMID: 29513146]

[30]   O'Shea TM, Burda JE, Sofroniew MV. Cell biology of spinal cord injury and repair. J Clin Invest

2017; 127(9): 3259-70.
[http://dx.doi.org/10.1172/JCI90608] [PMID: 28737515]

[31] Kirshblum S, Botticello A, Benedetto J, *et al.* A Comparison of Diagnostic Stability of the ASIA Impairment Scale Versus Frankel Classification Systems for Traumatic Spinal Cord Injury. Arch Phys Med Rehabil 2020; 101(9): 1556-62.
[http://dx.doi.org/10.1016/j.apmr.2020.05.016] [PMID: 32531222]

[32] Gündoğdu İ, Akyüz M, Öztürk EA, Çakcı FA. Can spinal cord injury patients show a worsening in ASIA impairment scale classification despite actually having neurological improvement? The limitation of ASIA Impairment Scale Classification. Spinal Cord 2014; 52(9): 667-70.
[http://dx.doi.org/10.1038/sc.2014.89] [PMID: 24891005]

[33] Capaul M, Zollinger H, Satz N, Dietz V, Lehmann D, Schurch B. Analyses of 94 consecutive spinal cord injury patients using ASIA definition and modified Frankel score classification. Paraplegia 1994; 32(9): 583-7.
[PMID: 7997337]

[34] Zheng R, Fan Y, Guan B, *et al.* A critical appraisal of clinical practice guidelines on surgical treatments for spinal cord injury. Spine J 2023; 23(12): 1739-49.
[http://dx.doi.org/10.1016/j.spinee.2023.06.385] [PMID: 37339698]

[35] Manley NC, Priest CA, Denham J, Wirth ED III, Lebkowski JS. Human Embryonic Stem Cell-Derived Oligodendrocyte Progenitor Cells: Preclinical Efficacy and Safety in Cervical Spinal Cord Injury. Stem Cells Transl Med 2017; 6(10): 1917-29.
[http://dx.doi.org/10.1002/sctm.17-0065] [PMID: 28834391]

[36] Priest CA, Manley NC, Denham J, Wirth ED III, Lebkowski JS. Preclinical safety of human embryonic stem cell-derived oligodendrocyte progenitors supporting clinical trials in spinal cord injury. Regen Med 2015; 10(8): 939-58.
[http://dx.doi.org/10.2217/rme.15.57] [PMID: 26345388]

[37] Li Y, Gautam A, Yang J, *et al.* Differentiation of oligodendrocyte progenitor cells from human embryonic stem cells on vitronectin-derived synthetic peptide acrylate surface. Stem Cells Dev 2013; 22(10): 1497-505.
[http://dx.doi.org/10.1089/scd.2012.0508] [PMID: 23249362]

[38] Cofano F, Boido M, Monticelli M, *et al.* Mesenchymal Stem Cells for Spinal Cord Injury: Current Options, Limitations, and Future of Cell Therapy. Int J Mol Sci 2019; 20(11): 2698.
[http://dx.doi.org/10.3390/ijms20112698] [PMID: 31159345]

[39] Islam SMR, Maeda T, Tamaoki N, *et al.* Reprogramming of Tumor-reactive Tumor-infiltrating Lymphocytes to Human-induced Pluripotent Stem Cells. Cancer Research Communications 2023; 3(5): 917-32.
[http://dx.doi.org/10.1158/2767-9764.CRC-22-0265] [PMID: 37377887]

[40] Yu H, Yang S, Li H, Wu R, Lai B, Zheng Q. Activating Endogenous Neurogenesis for Spinal Cord Injury Repair: Recent Advances and Future Prospects. Neurospine 2023; 20(1): 164-80.
[http://dx.doi.org/10.14245/ns.2245184.296] [PMID: 37016865]

[41] Ashammakhi N, Kim HJ, Ehsanipour A, *et al.* Regenerative Therapies for Spinal Cord Injury. Tissue Eng Part B Rev 2019; 25(6): 471-91.
[http://dx.doi.org/10.1089/ten.teb.2019.0182] [PMID: 31452463]

[42] Blevins HM, Xu Y, Biby S, Zhang S. The NLRP3 Inflammasome Pathway: A Review of Mechanisms and Inhibitors for the Treatment of Inflammatory Diseases. Front Aging Neurosci 2022; 14879021
[http://dx.doi.org/10.3389/fnagi.2022.879021] [PMID: 35754962]

[43] Jin LY, Li J, Wang KF, *et al.* Blood–Spinal Cord Barrier in Spinal Cord Injury: A Review. J Neurotrauma 2021; 38(9): 1203-24.
[http://dx.doi.org/10.1089/neu.2020.7413] [PMID: 33292072]

[44] Hou J, Bi H, Ge Q, *et al.* Heterogeneity analysis of astrocytes following spinal cord injury at single-cell resolution. FASEB J 2022; 36(8)e22442
[http://dx.doi.org/10.1096/fj.202200463R] [PMID: 35816276]

[45] Huang LY, Sun X, Pan HX, Wang L, He CQ, Wei Q. Cell transplantation therapies for spinal cord injury focusing on bone marrow mesenchymal stem cells: Advances and challenges. World J Stem Cells 2023; 15(5): 385-99.
[http://dx.doi.org/10.4252/wjsc.v15.i5.385] [PMID: 37342219]

[46] Jeon SR, Park JH, Lee JH, Kim DY, Kim HS, Sung IY, *et al.* Treatment of spinal cord injury with bone marrowderived, cultured autologous mesenchymal stem cells. Tissue Eng Regen Med 2010; 7(3): 316-22.

[47] Goodwin HS, Bicknese AR, Chien S-N, *et al.* Multilineage differentiation activity by cells isolated from umbilical cord blood: Expression of bone, fat, and neural markers. Biol Blood Marrow Transplant 2001; 7(11): 581-8.
[http://dx.doi.org/10.1053/bbmt.2001.v7.pm11760145] [PMID: 11760145]

[48] Kuh SU, Cho YE, Yoon DH, Kim KN, Ha Y. Functional recovery after human umbilical cord blood cells transplantation with brain-derived neutrophic factor into the spinal cord injured rat. Acta Neurochir (Wien) 2005; 147(9): 985-92.
[http://dx.doi.org/10.1007/s00701-005-0538-y] [PMID: 16010451]

[49] Ning G, Tang L, Wu Q, *et al.* Human umbilical cord blood stem cells for spinal cord injury: early transplantation results in better local angiogenesis. Regen Med 2013; 8(3): 271-81.
[http://dx.doi.org/10.2217/rme.13.26] [PMID: 23627822]

[50] Veeravalli KK, Dasari VR, Tsung AJ, *et al.* Human umbilical cord blood stem cells upregulate matrix metalloproteinase-2 in rats after spinal cord injury. Neurobiol Dis 2009; 36(1): 200-12.
[http://dx.doi.org/10.1016/j.nbd.2009.07.012] [PMID: 19631747]

[51] Blum B, Bar-Nur O, Golan-Lev T, Benvenisty N. The anti-apoptotic gene survivin contributes to teratoma formation by human embryonic stem cells. Nat Biotechnol 2009; 27(3): 281-7.
[http://dx.doi.org/10.1038/nbt.1527] [PMID: 19252483]

[52] Hur JW, Cho TH, Park DH, Lee JB, Park JY, Chung YG. Intrathecal transplantation of autologous adipose-derived mesenchymal stem cells for treating spinal cord injury: A human trial. J Spinal Cord Med 2016; 39(6): 655-64.
[http://dx.doi.org/10.1179/2045772315Y.0000000048] [PMID: 26208177]

[53] Ohta Y, Hamaguchi A, Ootaki M, *et al.* Intravenous infusion of adipose-derived stem/stromal cells improves functional recovery of rats with spinal cord injury. Cytotherapy 2017; 19(7): 839-48.
[http://dx.doi.org/10.1016/j.jcyt.2017.04.002] [PMID: 28478920]

[54] Shimizu K, Mitsuhara T, Maeda Y, *et al.* Impact of intravenously administered cranial bone-derived mesenchymal stem cells on functional recovery in experimental spinal cord injury. Neurosci Lett 2023; 799137103
[http://dx.doi.org/10.1016/j.neulet.2023.137103] [PMID: 36738956]

[55] Takeuchi H, Natsume A, Wakabayashi T, *et al.* Intravenously transplanted human neural stem cells migrate to the injured spinal cord in adult mice in an SDF-1- and HGF-dependent manner. Neurosci Lett 2007; 426(2): 69-74.
[http://dx.doi.org/10.1016/j.neulet.2007.08.048] [PMID: 17884290]

[56] Martinez AMB, Ramalho BS, Almeida FM, Sales CM, de Lima S. Injection of bone marrow mesenchymal stem cells by intravenous or intraperitoneal routes is a viable alternative to spinal cord injury treatment in mice. Neural Regen Res 2018; 13(6): 1046-53.
[http://dx.doi.org/10.4103/1673-5374.233448] [PMID: 29926832]

[57] Levi AD, Okonkwo DO, Park P, *et al.* Emerging safety of intramedullary transplantation of human neural stem cells in chronic cervical and thoracic spinal cord injury. Neurosurgery 2018; 82(4): 562-

75.
[http://dx.doi.org/10.1093/neuros/nyx250] [PMID: 28541431]

[58]   Amemori T, Ruzicka J, Romanyuk N, Jhanwar-Uniyal M, Sykova E, Jendelova P. Comparison of intraspinal and intrathecal implantation of induced pluripotent stem cell-derived neural precursors for the treatment of spinal cord injury in rats. Stem Cell Res Ther 2015; 6(1): 257.
[http://dx.doi.org/10.1186/s13287-015-0255-2] [PMID: 26696415]

[59]   Yousefifard M, Rahimi-Movaghar V, Nasirinezhad F, *et al.* Neural stem/progenitor cell transplantation for spinal cord injury treatment; A systematic review and meta-analysis. Neuroscience 2016; 322: 377-97.
[http://dx.doi.org/10.1016/j.neuroscience.2016.02.034] [PMID: 26917272]

[60]   Wang YH, Chen J, Zhou J, Nong F, Lv JH, Liu J. Reduced inflammatory cell recruitment and tissue damage in spinal cord injury by acellular spinal cord scaffold seeded with mesenchymal stem cells. Exp Ther Med 2017; 13(1): 203-7.
[http://dx.doi.org/10.3892/etm.2016.3941] [PMID: 28123490]

[61]   Zhao J, Sun W, Cho HM, *et al.* Integration and long distance axonal regeneration in the central nervous system from transplanted primitive neural stem cells. J Biol Chem 2013; 288(1): 164-8.
[http://dx.doi.org/10.1074/jbc.M112.433607] [PMID: 23155053]

[62]   Li Z, Guo GH, Wang GS, Guan CX, Yue L. Influence of neural stem cell transplantation on angiogenesis in rats with spinal cord injury. Genet Mol Res 2014; 13(3): 6083-92.
[http://dx.doi.org/10.4238/2014.August.7.23] [PMID: 25117366]

[63]   Yahata K, Kanno H, Ozawa H, *et al.* Low-energy extracorporeal shock wave therapy for promotion of vascular endothelial growth factor expression and angiogenesis and improvement of locomotor and sensory functions after spinal cord injury. J Neurosurg Spine 2016; 25(6): 745-55.
[http://dx.doi.org/10.3171/2016.4.SPINE15923] [PMID: 27367940]

[64]   Yu S, Yao S, Wen Y, Wang Y, Wang H, Xu Q. Angiogenic microspheres promote neural regeneration and motor function recovery after spinal cord injury in rats. Sci Rep 2016; 6(1): 33428.
[http://dx.doi.org/10.1038/srep33428] [PMID: 27641997]

[65]   Seo JH, Cho SR. Neurorestoration induced by mesenchymal stem cells: potential therapeutic mechanisms for clinical trials. Yonsei Med J 2012; 53(6): 1059-67.
[http://dx.doi.org/10.3349/ymj.2012.53.6.1059] [PMID: 23074102]

[66]   Han D, Chen S, Fang S, Liu S, Jin M, Guo Z, *et al.* The neuroprotective effects of muscle-derived stem cells via brain-derived neurotrophic factor in spinal cord injury model. BioMed Research International 2017.

[67]   Wang C, Shi D, Song X, Chen Y, Wang L, Zhang X. Calpain inhibitor attenuates ER stress-induced apoptosis in injured spinal cord after bone mesenchymal stem cells transplantation. Neurochem Int 2016; 97: 15-25.
[http://dx.doi.org/10.1016/j.neuint.2016.04.015] [PMID: 27137651]

[68]   Wang Y, Liu H, Ma H. Intrathecally transplanting mesenchymal stem cells (MSCs) activates ERK1/2 in spinal cords of ischemia-reperfusion injury rats and improves nerve function. Med Sci Monit 2016; 22: 1472-9.
[http://dx.doi.org/10.12659/MSM.896503] [PMID: 27135658]

[69]   Wu SH, Huang SH, Lo YC, *et al.* Autologous adipose-derived stem cells attenuate muscular atrophy and protect spinal cord ventral horn motor neurons in an animal model of burn injury. Cytotherapy 2015; 17(8): 1066-75.
[http://dx.doi.org/10.1016/j.jcyt.2015.03.687] [PMID: 26139546]

[70]   Sabelström H, Stenudd M, Réu P, *et al.* Resident neural stem cells restrict tissue damage and neuronal loss after spinal cord injury in mice. Science 2013; 342(6158): 637-40.
[http://dx.doi.org/10.1126/science.1242576] [PMID: 24179227]

[71]   Nicola FC, Marques MR, Odorcyk F, *et al.* Neuroprotector effect of stem cells from human exfoliated deciduous teeth transplanted after traumatic spinal cord injury involves inhibition of early neuronal apoptosis. Brain Res 2017; 1663: 95-105.
[http://dx.doi.org/10.1016/j.brainres.2017.03.015] [PMID: 28322752]

[72]   Wang L, Wang Q, Zhang X-M. [Progress on bone marrow mesenchymal stem cells transplantation for spinal cord injury]. Zhongguo Gu Shang 2014; 27(5): 437-40.
[PMID: 25167680]

[73]   Xu P, Yang X. The efficacy and safety of mesenchymal stem cell transplantation for spinal cord injury patients: a meta-analysis and systematic review. Cell Transplant 2019; 28(1): 36-46.
[http://dx.doi.org/10.1177/0963689718808471] [PMID: 30362373]

[74]   Piltti KM, Salazar DL, Uchida N, Cummings BJ, Anderson AJ. Safety of human neural stem cell transplantation in chronic spinal cord injury. Stem Cells Transl Med 2013; 2(12): 961-74.
[http://dx.doi.org/10.5966/sctm.2013-0064] [PMID: 24191264]

[75]   Shin JE, Jung K, Kim M, *et al.* Brain and spinal cord injury repair by implantation of human neural progenitor cells seeded onto polymer scaffolds. Exp Mol Med 2018; 50(4): 1-18.
[http://dx.doi.org/10.1038/s12276-018-0054-9] [PMID: 29674624]

[76]   Curtis E, Martin JR, Gabel B, *et al.* A First-in-Human, Phase I Study of Neural Stem Cell Transplantation for Chronic Spinal Cord Injury. Cell Stem Cell 2018; 22(6): 941-950.e6.
[http://dx.doi.org/10.1016/j.stem.2018.05.014] [PMID: 29859175]

[77]   Satti HS, Waheed A, Ahmed P, *et al.* Autologous mesenchymal stromal cell transplantation for spinal cord injury: A Phase I pilot study. Cytotherapy 2016; 18(4): 518-22.
[http://dx.doi.org/10.1016/j.jcyt.2016.01.004] [PMID: 26971680]

[78]   Shin JC, Kim KN, Yoo J, *et al.* Clinical Trial of Human Fetal Brain-Derived Neural Stem/Progenitor Cell Transplantation in Patients with Traumatic Cervical Spinal Cord Injury. Neural Plast 2015; 2015: 1-22.
[http://dx.doi.org/10.1155/2015/630932] [PMID: 26568892]

[79]   Mendonça MVP, Larocca TF, de Freitas Souza BS, *et al.* Safety and neurological assessments after autologous transplantation of bone marrow mesenchymal stem cells in subjects with chronic spinal cord injury. Stem Cell Res Ther 2014; 5(6): 126.
[http://dx.doi.org/10.1186/scrt516] [PMID: 25406723]

[80]   Ghobrial GM, Anderson KD, Dididze M, Martinez-Barrizonte J, Sunn GH, Gant KL, *et al.* Human Neural Stem Cell Transplantation in Chronic Cervical Spinal Cord Injury: Functional Outcomes at 12 Months in a Phase II Clinical Trial. Neurosurgery 2017; 64(CN_suppl_1)

[81]   Oh SK, Choi KH, Yoo JY, Kim DY, Kim SJ, Jeon SR. A Phase III Clinical Trial Showing Limited Efficacy of Autologous Mesenchymal Stem Cell Therapy for Spinal Cord Injury. Neurosurgery 2016; 78(3): 436-47.
[http://dx.doi.org/10.1227/NEU.0000000000001056] [PMID: 26891377]

[82]   El-Kheir WA, Gabr H, Awad MR, *et al.* Autologous bone marrow-derived cell therapy combined with physical therapy induces functional improvement in chronic spinal cord injury patients. Cell Transplant 2014; 23(6): 729-45.
[http://dx.doi.org/10.3727/096368913X664540] [PMID: 23452836]

[83]   Gao L, Peng Y, Xu W, *et al.* Progress in Stem Cell Therapy for Spinal Cord Injury. Stem Cells Int 2020; 2020: 1-16.
[http://dx.doi.org/10.1155/2020/2853650] [PMID: 33204276]

CHAPTER 7

Ultrasound-Guided and Single Portal Endoscopic Carpal Tunnel Release

Morgan P. Lorio[1,*] and **Paul Paterson**[2]

[1] *Advanced Orthopedics, 499 East Central Parkway, Altamonte Springs, FL 32701, USA*

[2] *Vero Orthopedics, 3955 Indian River Dr, Vero Beach, FL 32960, USA*

Abstract: As surgeons evolve to minimize morbidity and maximize outcomes or return-to-work (RTW) in the treatment of carpal tunnel syndrome (CTS), so have both single portal neuro-endoscopy and ultrasound-guided (US) technical applications procedurally in the safe, effective, and complete release/transection of the transverse carpal ligament (TCL). The chapter is intended as an independent complete go-to content-repository for surgeons desiring to revisit/review a relevant topic or area of thought without needing to reread the entirety of the same prior to a surgical case as a quick refresher. For those surgeons who have either mastered neuro-endoscopy or remain a novice, US techniques may offer patients new possibilities through the simple overlay of novel instruments and instructions over one's accumulated past experience.

Keywords: Carpal tunnel syndrome, Carpal tunnel release, Endoscopy, Ultrasound.

INTRODUCTION

Learmonth described the first open surgical release of the TCL in 1933 [1]. Brain and Phalen, respectively, defined idiopathic CTS from both clinical and anatomopathological points of view [2, 3]. SPECTR (Single Portal Endoscopic Carpal Tunnel Release) and USCTR (Ultrasound Guided Carpal Tunnel Release) are two modern surgical techniques that have emerged as advancements in the treatment of CTS. While they share the common goal of alleviating pressure on the median nerve, their historical origins and overlap in development have distinctive characteristics. Open procedures utilize extensile exposure to protect vital structures during surgery. However, open-approach techniques create surgical morbidity in normal tissues. Over time, surgeons have sought to minimize morbidity, leveraging technological advances to create minimally inva-

---

* **Corresponding author Morgan P. Lorio:** Advanced Orthopedics, 499 East Central Parkway, Altamonte Springs, FL 32701, USA; E-mail: mloriomd@gmail.com

Kai-Uwe Lewandrowski & William Omar Contreras López (Eds.)

sive solutions without sacrificing safety or efficacy. The result has been to reduce patient recovery times and complications inherent in open techniques. The origins of SPECTR can be traced back to the introduction of endoscopic techniques in the late 1980s. Until recently, surgeons have been traditionally divided into three main camps: standard open/extensile (34%), mini-open (46%), and endoscopic (20%) (See Fig. **1**) [4]. In 1989, Chow *et al.* technically reported a dual-portal endoscopic carpal tunnel release (ECTR) [5]. After that, in 1992, Agee *et al.* detailed his SPECTR technique in a prospective randomized control trial (PRCT) using a transverse incision in the area of the proximal wrist crease [6]. This pistol-shaped 3M® Agee device evolution led to the birth of SPECTR, with the primary objective of providing enhanced visualization and reduced tissue trauma. MicroAire® Surgical Instruments later purchased the 3M® Agee device. A subsequent PRCT in 2002 by Trumble and Diao *et al.*demonstrated an equally safe and faster recovery (faster RTW) with SPECTR compared to open release [7]. Both co-authors of this book chapter were blessed to have been orthopedic residents in training within SUNY-Buffalo, a Beta-site for Agee's Hand Biomechanics Lab; both have 30 years of experience with SPECTR. The development of specialized instrumentation and improved surgical techniques have contributed to the refinement of SPECTR over the years with a proliferation of devices, including the Arthrex® Centerline ECTR, which shares a very similar ergonomic profile with USCTR paralleling the longitudinal axis of the forearm and wrist while using direct neuro-endoscopic visualization in the former and ultrasound visualization in the latter. In 2010, Arthrex® settled a patent infringement spat with MicroAire®, and now MicroAire® licenses its patented ECTR technology to Arthrex® with both companies agreeing to "maintain Microaire's practice of requiring surgeon training for the procedure" [8].

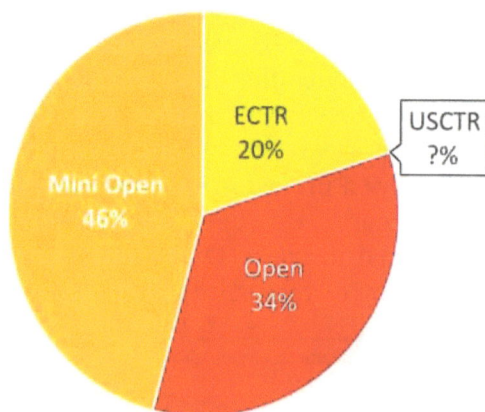

Fig. (1). Treatment of CTS (adapted from a 2012 survey of the American Association of Hand Surgery).

Although SPECTR and USCTR have distinct historical origins, there is an overlap in their evolution and technological advancements. Both techniques aim to minimize invasiveness and improve outcomes in the surgical treatment of CTS. They demonstrate the ongoing efforts within the surgical community to refine and optimize procedures to benefit patients. The development of specialized instrumentation, improved imaging modalities, and the integration of minimally invasive principles have contributed to the evolution and overlap of SPECTR and USCTR as valuable personalized precision treatment options for CTS. This chapter will attempt to describe both techniques simultaneously to avoid redundancy and expound where it is necessary to differentiate the distinctly different characteristics and nuances of each when appropriate.

Expectations

Two prominent techniques have gained recognition in the realm of minimally invasive surgical options for CTS: SPECTR and USCTR. With the increasing demand for less invasive approaches, patients and surgeons alike are eager to understand the expectations associated with the procedures. SPECTR offers the advantage of enhanced direct and familiar visualization with precise surgical intervention within the carpal tunnel, leading to potentially improved outcomes with Level I Evidence [9]. On the other hand, USCTR provides a guided and controlled release of the TCL, with minimal incision and potential for faster recovery. This chapter explores the innovations associated with these innovative techniques, highlighting their respective benefits, limitations, and anticipated outcomes, ultimately aiding clinicians and patients in making informed decisions regarding the optimal approach for CTR.

The anatomic expectation of either procedure is a complete release of the TCL, thereby releasing compression on the carpal tunnel contents, specifically the median nerve. In 1994, using advanced MRI techniques, Ablove *et al.* at SUNY-Buffalo validated that both SPECTR and a dual-portal subcutaneous CTR morphologically produced a marked increase in canal volume and median nerve cross-sectional area, suggesting equivalence to open release [10]. After that, in 1996, Ablove *et al.* found that pressures decreased in both the carpal tunnel and Guyon's canal (GC) after both endoscopic and open release, suggesting that CTR alone may be sufficient to relieve symptomatic carpal and ulnar tunnel syndromes [11]. Recently, Peters *et al.*, in 2021, using an MRI protocol, confirmed no significant morphologic differences between Agee SPECTR and open release, with both resulting in a significant increase in the AP dimensions of the carpal tunnel and GC, respectively [12]. Likewise, Occam's razor or the 'law of parsimony' would suggest that a successful USCTR would have similar results.

The functional expectation for SPECTR and USCTR is for the resolution of palmar pain, diminution of numbness, improved function, and a speedy recovery with RTW or ADLs. However, specific expectations and outcomes may vary depending on individual patient factors and the surgeon's expertise. A relatively recent Cochrane review regarding SPECTR cited a slight increase in popularity partly due to an alignment of personalized medicine (quality-of-life), reduced scarring and work absence, and subjective well-being. Although CRPS (chronic regional pain syndrome) is equally associated with open release and SPECTR [13], it is valuable to note that treating unilateral traumatic CRPS may respond therapeutically to CTR as median nerve transmitted sympathomimetics are decompressed [14]. A minimally invasive approach to carpal tunnel release, as with USCTR, should have similar results for the abovementioned reasons. SPECTR does not influence median nerve excursion regardless of wrist position [15]. USCTR would be expected to perform similarly. Anecdotally, palmar pain may be reported with either SPECTR or USCTR. However, the patient may not be able to correlate pillar pain as an etiology as they might with open release. The rationale is that the wrist incision is proximal to the pillars and thus may be confounding from a personalized sensory homunculus perspective.

Indications

When considering the optimal surgical approach for CTS, assessing the indications for SPECTR and USCTR is crucial. These innovative techniques offer distinct advantages and considerations that may make them suitable for specific patient populations. SPECTR excels in cases where enhanced visualization and precise surgical intervention within the carpal tunnel are desired, allowing for effective median nerve decompression. USCTR can be used in any CTR environment as ultrasonic imaging provides clear visualization of the TCL and all vital structures, much like an open extensile exposure. Open CTR is the historical standard and provides symptom relief at the expense of increased recovery time [16].

The clinical indications for CTR are otherwise generally agnostic procedurally after a patient with mild CTS has failed six months of pre-operative conservative treatment by 1) neutral wrist immobilization and 2) steroid injections, both of which have received a strong level of recommendation through the best evidence synthesis by an AAOS Guideline in 2016 [17]. While these treatments ameliorate CTS symptoms, they rarely resolve them entirely. The AAOS guideline recognizes only one Grade A recommendation to resolve CTS symptoms, and that is surgery. That same AAOS Guideline provides a strong level of recommendation that both BMI and high hand/wrist repetition rate are associated with CTS development [17]. A recent literature review in UpToDate adds moderate-to-severe CTS with axonal loss or denervation on electrodiagnostic testing as an obvious additional indication for CTR [18]. A 2019 commissioned NHS Policy [19] recommends CTS referral for surgical intervention without conservative steroid treatment first if:

1. EMG and NCS demonstrate nerve damage,
2. Symptoms are severe and constant,
3. Severe sensory disturbance and thenar motor weakness are present,
4. Progressive motor or sensory deficit is present (*Not commissioned is pregnancy-associated CTS).

Contraindications

When contemplating minimally invasive surgical approaches for CTR, it is crucial to identify the contraindications associated with SPECTR and USCTR. While these techniques offer numerous benefits, specific patient factors and clinical scenarios may render them unsuitable or present potential challenges. Relative contraindications for SPECTR may include:

1. Severe CTS with significant nerve damage,
2. Previous failed carpal tunnel surgery,
3. Anatomical variations that limit visualization,
4. Accessibility within the carpal tunnel,
5. Patients with complex anatomical variations,
6. Significant scarring from previous surgeries,
7. Unusual anomalous deformities of the medial border of the carpal tunnel, *i.e.*, the hook of the hamate [20].

The co-authors have used both SPECTR and USCTR in complex revision strategies, including scar. Early in the launch of SPECTR in the 1990s, there was concern that trauma-induced bloody fluid within the osseofibrous canal of the volar wrist would preclude visualization with this dry technique. As surgeon experience has grown, routine release of the TCL concomitantly with fracture fixation has been performed with SPECTR to reduce the incidence of postoperative median nerve dysfunction. Although USCTR is still in a relative phase of infancy relative to surgeon adoption, it is clear that ultrasound visualization with a trained eye can and will easily obviate these same concerns relative to traumatic blood or an atraumatic 'wet' forearm/wrist due to synovitis or edema. Absolute contraindications for both SPECTR and USCTR include the following:

1. Uncorrected coagulopathy,
2. Internal neurolysis requiring an operating microscope,
3. A mass,
4. Tuberculosis (mycobacterium) or rheumatoid arthritis (RA) induced CTS requiring radical flexor tenosynovectomy.

Special Considerations

SPECTR and USCTR techniques offer unique advantages and considerations requiring careful assessment to ensure optimal patient outcomes. Special considerations for SPECTR include requiring specialized equipment and surgical expertise and appropriate patient positioning and access to the carpal tunnel. Surgeons must also be proficient in endoscopic techniques and thoroughly understand the anatomy and variations within the carpal tunnel. Sometimes the endoscope must be canted ulnarward to avoid iatrogenic injury of an encroaching ulnar border of the median nerve. During the surgical release of the TCL with SPECTR, the TCL underside must be continuously visualized while the release is performed retrograde, from distal to proximal. Inexperience with SPECTR is circumvented with a keen utilization of fundamental topographic palmar wrist landmarks to improve outcomes and avoid complications [21]. Great care to not go beyond the overlying topographic skin landmark of Kaplan's cardinal line is necessary with SPECTR to avoid iatrogenic, catastrophic injury to the superficial palmar arch (SPA). Other topographic landmarks and anatomic considerations avoid incomplete TCL release and accidental entry into GC, which places the ulnar neurovascular bundle at risk. False entry is negated by palpating the radial border of the hook of the hamate during tactile blunt probe dilation and parallel-exchange scope entry. An adequate and gratifying TCL release is discerned indirectly by palpation and increased transillumination of the skin and further confirmed directly by visual loop inspection and endoscopic visualization of a wide diastasis created between the radial and ulnar leaves of the TCL.

Conversely, USCTR necessitates skill in ultrasound imaging and needle placement, as well as a more comprehensive understanding of the following: 1) the pinpoint targeted location of the TCL relative to adjacent structures; and 2) the precise locale of safe zones in both transverse and longitudinal axes. The terminus of the longitudinal safe zone is distinct from the sagittal view offered by USCTR, avoiding the SPA by a measured distance. USCTR represents a real-time confirmation for complete transection of the TCL by dynamically illustrating adequacy of release with a visualized probe prodding through the palmar roof of the TCL, thus demonstrating loss of TCL integrity as viewed in the axial transverse view and safe zone. Using ultrasound guidance, entry into GC is avoided by direct visualization of the carpal and ulnar tunnel simultaneously during instrument placement. Additionally, patient factors such as obesity, anatomical variations, or underlying medical conditions may present challenges or necessitate modifications in the surgical approach. This section explores these special considerations in detail, aiding surgeons in making informed decisions and optimizing SPECTR and USCTR procedures.

When comparing the diagnostic accuracy of Magnetic Resonance Imaging (MRI) and ultrasound (US) in evaluating CTS, both imaging modalities offer valuable insights, although they differ in sensitivity and specificity. The role of a nerve conduction study (NCS) as a historical standard in diagnosing CTS is being challenged as MRI and US are complementary in evaluating patients with electro-negative NCS and patients either undergoing surgical planning or experiencing recurrent symptoms after CTR [22]. MRI provides detailed anatomical images and can assess the structures within the carpal tunnel, including the median nerve and surrounding tissues. It offers high sensitivity in detecting structural abnormalities and can aid in ruling out alternative diagnoses. However, MRI may lack specificity as it can identify nerve enlargement without necessarily correlating it with clinical symptoms and is expensive. On the other hand, ultrasound provides real-time imaging, allowing evaluation of the median nerve size and carpal tunnel during various wrist positions. Ultrasound demonstrates sensitivity and specificity in detecting nerve compression and can assess the median nerve's mobility, cross-sectional area, and bowing during provocative maneuvers. Ultrasound's ability to directly visualize the nerve and assess its function in real-time enhances its utility in diagnosing CTS. The US accomplishes this in the convenient setting of the treating physician's office at a much lower cost. Ultimately, the choice between MRI and US for diagnosing CTS depends on factors such as availability, expertise, and specific clinical scenarios, with each modality contributing unique advantages to the diagnostic evaluation of CTS.

The translation of in-office diagnosis confirmation and visualization of CTS has revolutionized the management and treatment of this condition, enabling same-day USCTR. Using the US as a first-line exam, surgeons can accurately diagnose CTS by measuring the cross-sectional area of the nerve within the carpal tunnel [23]. Median nerve enlargement and the exclusion of structural abnormality contributing to CTS symptoms may be an indication to proceed with in-office USCTR *via* informed consent, provided that coagulopathy is absent. This in-office confirmation allows for a more streamlined approach, as eligible patients can undergo USCTR on the same day as an alternative to what was traditionally considered either high-risk or a contraindication for open CTR or SPECTR. Anatomic variants of the flexors and palmaris longus may-by their mass effect, anomalous connections, or friction-affect symptoms consistent with a dynamic CTS or tenosynovitis mimicking the same. Identifying these variants by the surgeon-ultrasound operator is crucial as the US provides an opportunity for their debridement on open exploration, affecting pathogenesis and their therapy [24]. The ability to perform USCTR immediately following diagnostic confirmation provides numerous benefits, including reduced wait times, improved patient convenience, and potentially faster relief of symptoms sustained at one-year follow-up [25]. By harnessing the power of in-office US visualization and incorporating it into the surgical management of CTS, clinicians can offer a more efficient and patient-centered approach with USCTR, ensuring timely intervention and enhancing the overall patient experience.

Special Instructions, Position and Anesthesia

Performing SPECTR requires specific instructions, patient positioning, and anesthesia considerations to ensure successful surgical outcomes. In SPECTR, surgeons should provide patients with preoperative instructions regarding avoiding blood-thinning medications and needing to fast before the procedure. Positioning the patient typically involves supine positioning with the affected hand extended, providing optimal access to the carpal tunnel. General or regional anesthesia, such as brachial plexus block, is commonly employed to ensure patient comfort and immobility during the procedure. The entire upper extremity is best prepped out free to allow the best access to that ipsilateral involved limb while working with the endoscope and potentially allowing access for multiple coordinated procedures for the multi-involved appendage. A tourniquet is best applied to the proximal upper arm. However, it may also be applied on the proximal forearm for IV access in trauma (although not ideal) and when it is necessary to minimize tourniquet pain when anesthesia is light. Attention to minimizing the bulk in the layered drapes will aid access within the field of work when the tourniquet is on the forearm. Local lidocaine is best avoided with SPECTR as the technique is technically dry and hindered to some degree by fluid, which may extravasate within the tunnel during local lidocaine infiltration, compromising visualization. It is customary to ensure that the ipsilateral digits demonstrate adequate perfusion by capillary refill assessment after the tourniquet is let down and that the wound is dry before dressings are applied.

USCTR utilizes the Wide-awake Local Anesthesia No Tourniquet (WALANT) technique. Patients do not need to fast. Patient anticoagulant status is not usually a consideration, and a tourniquet is not required. This is due to the minimally invasive technique and the vasoconstrictive effect of epinephrine in the local anesthetic that make bleeding complications rare. Patient positioning can be seated or supine with the arm abducted and the forearm supinated, allowing for proper ultrasound visualization of the carpal tunnel anatomy. USCTR anesthesia uses 10 ccs of lidocaine with epinephrine and sodium bicarbonate. A subcutaneous anesthetic is injected superficially into the TCL and distal antebrachial fascia along the ulnar aspect of the wrist and hand. A free-access arm and hand surgery table eases both SPECTR and USCTR. The routine use of prophylactic antibiotics is generally not indicated with CTR, regardless of technique, even in diabetics [26]. USCTR wounds are usually closed with an adhesive strip. The light postoperative dressing is removed in 48 hours. The 2016 AAOS Guideline regarding CTS shows strong evidence that postop immobilization has no benefits [17]. The first author, however, has anecdotally seen that neutral splints (that leave the thumb free) and temporary sling elevation/immobilization maintain postoperative dressings intact and minimize needless postoperative concerns of patients while reinforcing compliance with a standard postoperative regimen until their postoperative follow-up with the surgeon and/or Certified Hand Therapist (CHT). Greater than 90% of USCTR patients require no postop follow-up. Special instructions, patient positioning, and anesthesia considerations play crucial roles in the success of both SPECTR and USCTR. Adherence to these expert opinions ensures patient safety, optimal surgical exposure, and effective pain management, ultimately contributing to favorable surgical outcomes and improved patient satisfaction.

Tips and Pearls

As surgeons gain experience in performing SPECTR and USCTR, valuable tips, pearls, and lessons learned emerge, contributing to enhanced surgical outcomes and improved patient care. General tips include meticulous preoperative planning, *i.e.*

1. advanced imaging if appropriate;
2. surgical marking and palpation of topographic landmarks with SPECTR;
3. precise portal placement proximal to wrist crease--in line with the radial border of the ring ray and ulnar to palmaris longus if present;
4. Identify and protect the median nerve and surrounding structures during either SPECTR or USCTR.

SPECTR and USCTR may be incorporated elegantly as adjuncts to more complex reconstructive procedures. The potential for irreversible damage from median nerve compromise from radial fracture repair [27], radial osteotomy [28], and open wrist arthrodesis [29] necessitates briefly mentioning the utility of prophylactic CTR to lessen compression. Minimizing the surgical impact of CTR by either SPECTR or USCTR fits well within the Hippocratic schema to 'first do no harm' while functionally diminishing physician work. Implementing the elective CTR work process within the initial phase of workflow functionally ensures that this measure is technically feasible, not forgotten as an add-on step while keeping the workspace tidy and organized as the specialized instruments for SPECTR or USCTR can be removed from the operative field and/or terminally cleansed if appropriate as soon as this interventional step is completed. Volar plate prominence, *i.e.*, hardware mass effect, distraction with corrective opening wedge osteotomy and grafting, alterations within the post-traumatic or degenerative morphologic relationships of the carpal tunnel contents, and immobility induced by wrist arthrodesis have all been implicated in the multi-factorial etiology for CTS.

These accumulated tips, pearls, and lessons learned are vital in refining SPECTR and USCTR. Sharing and implementing these insights can improve surgical proficiency, reduce complications, and improve patient outcomes, ultimately benefiting surgeons and individuals seeking relief from CTS.

SPECTR Tips

A small hemostat placed into the osseofibrous canal post-SPECTR should be used to palpate residual bands distally that might otherwise preclude separation of the TCL unless they are blunted and disrupted by the controlled, gentle spread of the hemostat. Pearls of wisdom include meticulous hemostasis to minimize the risk of complications. One should be willing to hold pressure for an adequate time post-TCL release and then reevaluate as necessary, possibly instilling a 'liquid hemostat' *via* a cannulated installation as an added measure and placing a mini-vessel loop through the incision to allow for indirect fluid egression, avoiding hematoma. Lessons learned revolve around the importance of surgeon proficiency in SPECTR, maintaining a clear visualization of the surgical field, and adapting to anatomical variations encountered during the procedure. Suppose there is any doubt concerning the adequacy of the SPECTR. In that case, it should be either converted to a dual-portal incision working between the incisions or opened for direct inspection and a further chance to continue lifelong learning.

USCTR Tips

Obese patients' thick, soft tissue envelopes can make positioning the blade against the TCL challenging. Moving the incision 5mm proximal improves the approach angle and allows safe blade placement against the TCL. Hydro-dissection is a valuable technique to expand safe zones that might be only 2 mm wide. Typically, 2-5 cc of anesthetic injected into the safe zone will push the median nerve radially 4-7 mm. US imaging makes it easy to ensure the blade is in the safe zone along the entire TCL, proximal to the distal. Therefore, median nerve injury is unlikely. However, the third common digital nerve (TCDN) can be injured if the blade is deployed too distal. Imaging this nerve can be challenging. An aid to finding the nerve is to image the ulnar artery from proximal to distal. The first ulnar branch of the SPA is the third common digital artery. The artery corresponds to the location of the nerve. Thus, keeping the distal tip of the device proximal to the pulsing third common digital artery (TCDA) will prevent TCDN injury. Lessons learned to encompass the importance of continuous skill development in ultrasound-guided procedures include understanding the US of carpal tunnel and recognizing potential challenges, such as patients with deep-set ligaments or scar tissue.

Difficulties

Either SPECTR or USCTR can present particular challenges that surgeons must be prepared to overcome. In SPECTR, difficulties may arise due to limited visualization of the carpal tunnel anatomy, especially in cases of extensive scarring or anatomical variations or with bleeding despite a tourniquet. Letting the tourniquet back down and re-applying an Esmarch with elevation after checking the competence of the blood pressure cuff may prove immensely helpful in providing a dry operative field with improved visualization. Maintaining pressure on the scaphoid tubercle by an assistant during surgery or by the non-device hand may add significantly to maintaining surgeon orientation by keeping the palm and wrist horizontal to the floor, allowing for completion of the SPECTR. Surgeons must visually navigate with utmost care to avoid injury and adequately visualize the surgical area in which they work. The endoscopic function of SPECTR is performed dry without infusing fluid. A 'wet' carpal tunnel due to bleeding, increased tenosynovitis, or edema is problematic for viewing. However, it can be remedied by disconnecting the arthroscope base from the disposable integrated blade retractor and simply suctioning the exposed opening of the disposable. Alternatively, the scope can be removed in toto, and a Q tip carefully introduced into the osseofibrous canal so as to not leave a cotton-tipped foreign body while attempting to dry the same. The Q tip is withdrawn in toto. Finally, a smooth-tipped metal Frazier cannula tip can be introduced gently into the osseofibrous canal and then connected to suction. An anti-fog agent for endoscopic camera lenses is also available on the market but may not be formulary at some facilities despite being inexpensive. A very thick working man's hand may present one with technical difficulties; the TCL may require multiple repasses with the surgical blade to accomplish complete transection.

Similarly, USCTR may need help identifying the TCL and ensuring instrument placement. Patients with deep-set ligaments, obesity, or anatomical variations can pose challenges in achieving a successful release. Incomplete or inadequate release may occur, requiring additional interventions or a conversion to an alternative surgical technique. Recognizing these potential difficulties and developing strategies to address them is crucial for surgeons performing SPECTR and USCTR, requiring continuous skill development, adapting techniques based on individual patient characteristics, and having a comprehensive understanding of the anatomical variations and potential complications that may be encountered. By anticipating and managing these difficulties, surgeons can enhance their surgical proficiency and improve patient outcomes in the treatment of CTS. It has been shown that there is indeed a learning curve with SPECTR [30]. The co-authors are unaware of any *In vivo* study as yet on the learning curve with USCTR, but less experienced junior radiologists have demonstrated a rapid learning curve during *In vitro* simulation in a cadaveric study [31].

SPECTR Procedural Steps

1. Patient positioning: Place the patient supine with the affected arm extended and secured appropriately, preferably with a dedicated hand table. [A rolled surgical towel placed under the extended wrist is helpful during steps 3-7 for controlled hand/wrist positioning and visualization.] The arthroscopy tower is placed ergonomically across from the surgeon.
2. Anesthesia: Administer general or regional anesthesia, such as brachial plexus block, to ensure patient comfort and immobility during the procedure. The limb is then elevated and exsanguinated with Esmarch, and a tourniquet is put up to 250 mm Hg or 100 mm Hg above systolic in a pediatric patient.
3. Portal placement: After landmarks are identified and delineated with a surgical marker, make a small transverse incision at the appropriate site for the single portal entry, typically 1 cm proximal to the volar distal wrist ulnar to palmaris longus. Opposing retraction is obtained with a 5 mm double prong Joseph sharp skin hooks. A distally based stump is created sharply from the underlying antebrachial fascia and gently retracted distally using an additional 2 mm double prong Joseph sharp skin hook. The larger Joseph is then removed.
4. 'Spatula' or Tenosynovial Elevator (Fig. **2**): The instrument is introduced into the osseofibrous canal and clears the overlying TCL until it reveals a 'washboard surface."
5. Serial Dilation (progressive, mechanical push-type) follows with Dilator palpation followed by Endoscope insertion (Fig. **2**): Insert a small-diameter retractor endoscope through the portal, providing enhanced visualization of the carpal tunnel and its contents.
6. TCL Release: Use the Arthrex® Centerline to visualize the terminal aspect of the TCL (Fig. **3**) and then engage the blade (See Fig. **4**), pulling it from distal to proximal while maintaining gentle pressure down over the raised blade, which is canted upwards towards the volar roof of TCL to completely release the TCL, thereby relieving compression on the median nerve. A repass may be required on endoscopic inspection. The scope is rolled from side to side to visualize the TCL's transected and retracted ulnar and radial leaves. A junior Ragnell retractor may be introduced to lift the encroaching palmar fat pad

upwards after release. This maneuver allows for either a re-introduction of the scope or direct inspection under loupe magnification. A hemostat is introduced and used to palpate the release and identify residual tethering bands released while receiving audible 'pops' and tactile 'give' or loss of TCL integrity. Confirmation of adequate release is further suggested by increased transillumination. The distal forearm fascia is then released proximal to the skin incision *via* the portal with tenotomy scissors under direct loupe visualization to prevent a possible constriction band compromise of median nerve function.

7. Hemostasis and closure: Ensure meticulous hemostasis is achieved, usually with gentle pressure applied for a few minutes. Bipolar is applied as necessary, avoiding injury to the median nerve or other vital structures. Close the portal incision with sutures and adhesive strips as necessary.

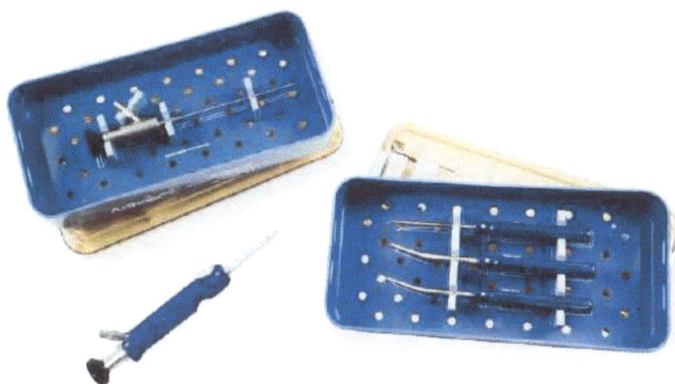

Fig. (2). Arthrex® Centerline ECTR Instrument Tray, including Endoscope with Disposable Blade (Left), Tenosynovial Elevator (Top Right), and Dilators (Bottom Right), respectively. Courtesy with permission Arthrex®.

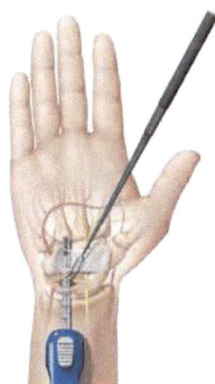

Fig. (3). Arthrex® Centerline ECTR 3D Multi-Layer Longitudinal View. Courtesy with permission Arthrex®.

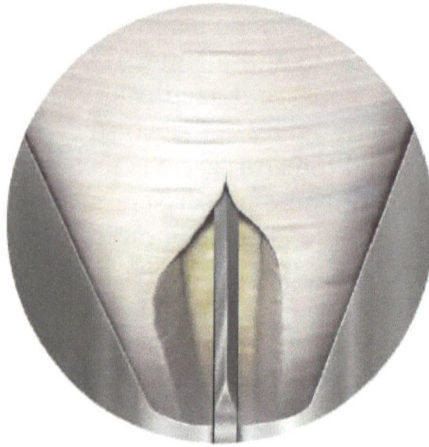

Fig. (4). Arthrex® Centerline Partial TCL Release View. Courtesy with permission Arthrex®.

SPECTR Bailout Procedure

During SPECTR, certain situations that require bailout, rescue, or salvage procedures to address unexpected complications or difficulties encountered during the surgery may arise. These procedures aim to mitigate potential adverse outcomes and optimize patient safety and outcomes.

1. Conversion to open CTR: In cases with limited visualization, excessive bleeding, or unanticipated anatomical variations, it may be necessary to convert the procedure to an open CTR. This conversion involves making a larger incision to gain better access and visualization of the carpal tunnel, allowing for the safe release of the TCL and decompression of the median nerve. A noncontiguous mini-open incision or an extensile approach, possibly incorporating the prior incision to provide a plastic closure ultimately, is generally performed in this instance.
2. Hemostasis and vessel control: Excessive bleeding during SPECTR may require additional measures for hemostasis—application of Bipolar and/or hemostatic agents to adequately control bleeding vessels within the surgical field.

USCTR Procedural Steps

1. Patient positioning: Usually seated with the hand resting in a supinated position of a sterile Mayo stand. Patients prone to fainting or significant anxiety are placed in the supine position. Field sterility is created with multiple sterile towels. A rolled towel helps to extend the wrist, providing a better device approach angle. The Ultrasound machine is positioned across the table from the

surgeon (Fig. **5**). One hand holds the ultrasound probe while the other controls the surgical instruments. The US probe hand helps control the hand position and assists in triangulating the device hand (Fig. **6**).

2. Anesthesia: Administer local anesthesia, such as lidocaine, at the wrist to provide anesthesia and facilitate the procedure.
3. Ultrasound-guided identification: Use US imaging to precisely locate the TCL, median nerve, and TCDN/A and confirm the pathology of CTS (Fig. **7**).
4. Hydro-dissection: Insert a 22 gauge, 1.5-inch needle into the ulnar volar forearm between the ulnar artery and median nerve using transverse ultrasound imaging. Inject 2-5 ccs of anesthetic to widen the safe zone. Place a 5 mm longitudinal stab incision at the needle entry site. Then pass a Freer elevator into the CT to release any soft tissues adherent to the TCL. Like the endoscopic technique, the 'washboard' haptics confirm proper instrument placement.
5. TCL Release: Coordinated balloon dilatation (Stealth MicroGuards®️ deployment) (Figs. **8 & 9**) is followed by protected TCL Blade®️ advancement into the wound directly, under the TCL, and within the safe zone. Release of the TCL is distal to proximal (retrograde transection) as with SPECTR.

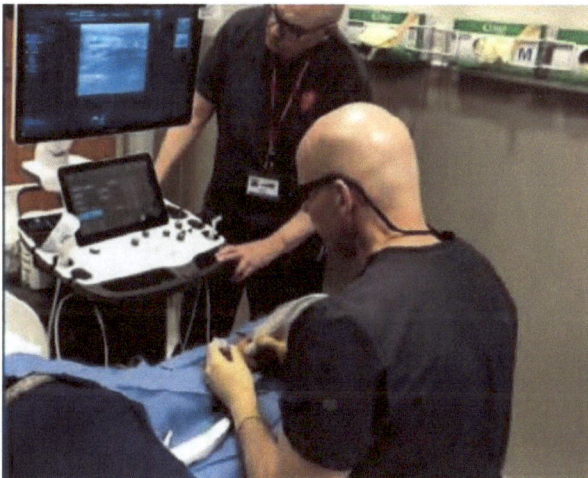

Fig. (5). Typical USCTR Setup -- US machine is positioned directly across from the surgeon [this example illustrates Hydro-dissection]. Note field sterility obtained *via* sterile towels used for draping. Image courtesy of the second author.

1. Confirmation and closure: Confirm the complete release of TCL using US imaging (Fig. **10**). Balloon deflation follows the inactivation of the TCL Blade®️ with the removal of the Sonex®️ UltraGuide CTR device (Fig. **11**).
2. Obtain hemostasis with direct pressure; close the wound with adhesive strips; and apply a light, dry sterile dressing.
3. These key procedural steps (above) outline the actions involved in SPECTR

and USCTR. Certain variations and techniques may exist among different surgeons and institutions, and procedural steps may be modified based on individual patient characteristics and surgeon preferences.

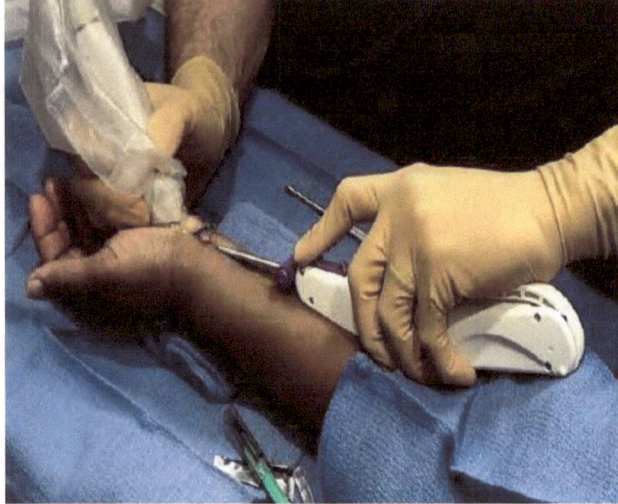

Fig. (6). Hand Position – Hand position used for USCTR. Sterile rolled towel behind the wrist extends the hand. The US probe hand keeps the patient's hand positioned and helps to triangulate the Sonex® UltraGuide CTR device during TCL release. Image courtesy of the second author.

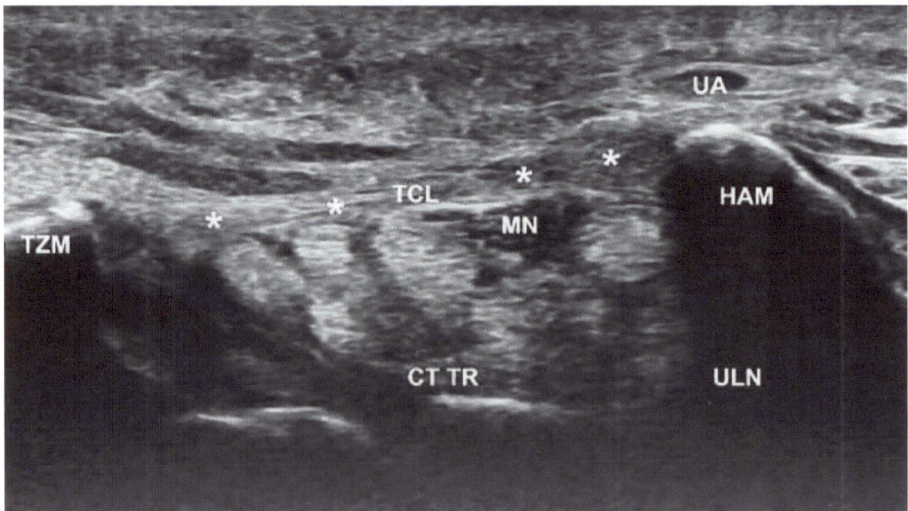

Fig. (7). Transverse view at distal extent of carpal tunnel. UA – ulnar artery, MN – median nerve, TZM – Trapezium, HAM – Hook of the Hamate, ULN -, CT TR -, TCL – Transverse Carpal ligament. * marks course of TCL from TZM to HAM. Note UA volar to HAM. Safe zone defined by interval between MN and HAM.

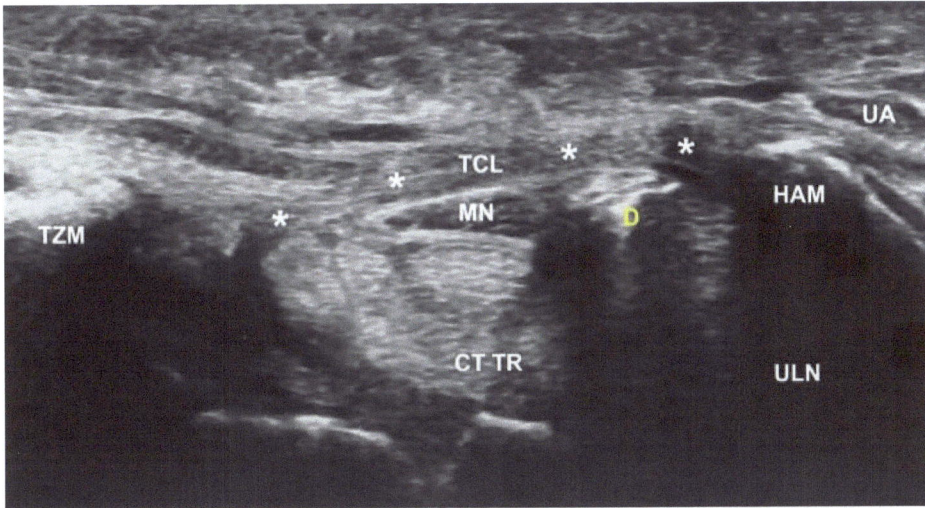

Fig. (8). Transverse view at distal extent of carpal tunnel with device (D) positioned in the safe zone between the MN and HAM. UA – ulnar artery, MN – median nerve, TZM – Trapezium, HAM – Hook of the Hamate, ULN -, CT TR -, TCL – Transverse Carpal ligament. * Marks course of TCL from TZM to HAM. Note UA volar to HAM.

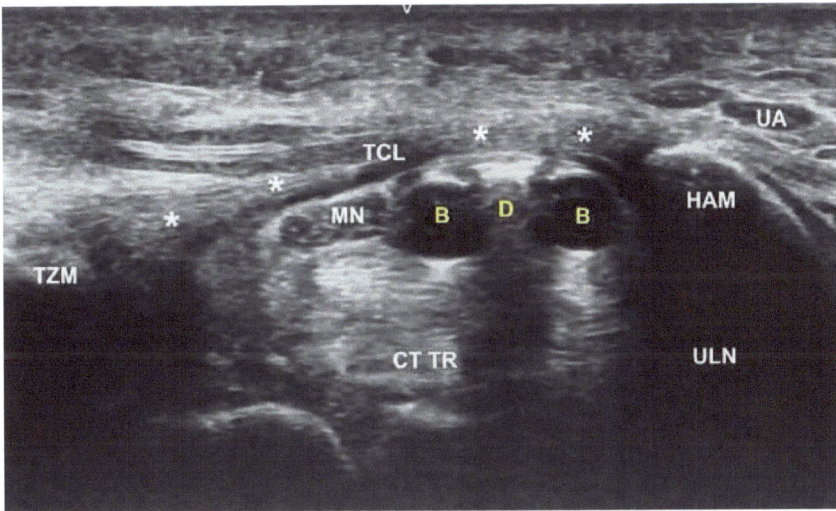

Fig. (9). Transverse view at the distal extent of carpal tunnel with device (D) positioned in the safe zone between the MN and HAM. Device balloons have been deployed, effectively expanding the safe zone. UA – ulnar artery, MN – median nerve, TZM – Trapezium, HAM – Hook of the Hamate, ULN -, CT TR -, TCL – Transverse Carpal ligament. * Marks course of TCL from TZM to HAM. Note UA volar to HAM.

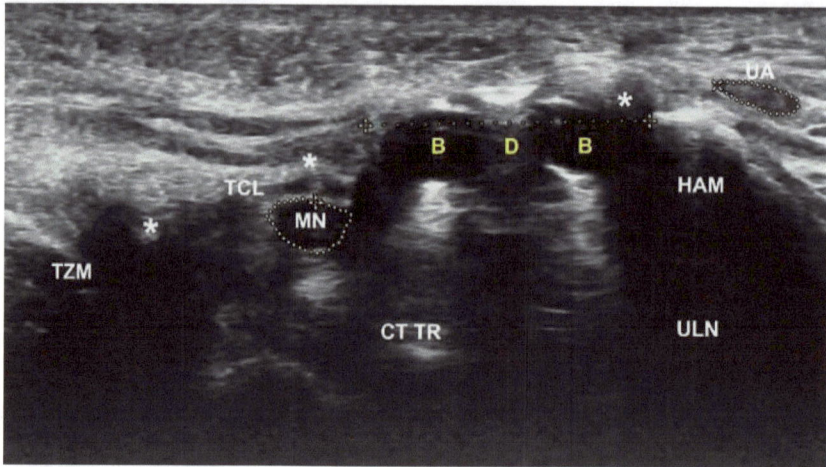

Fig. (10). Transverse view at the distal extent of the carpal tunnel after TCL transection. Device (D) with balloons (B) deployed is now volar to the MN, HAM, and TCL, indicating complete TCL transection. UA – ulnar artery, MN – median nerve, TZM – Trapezium, HAM – Hook of the Hamate, ULN -, CT TR -, TCL – Transverse Carpal ligament. * Marks course of TCL from TZM to HAM. Note UA volar to HAM.

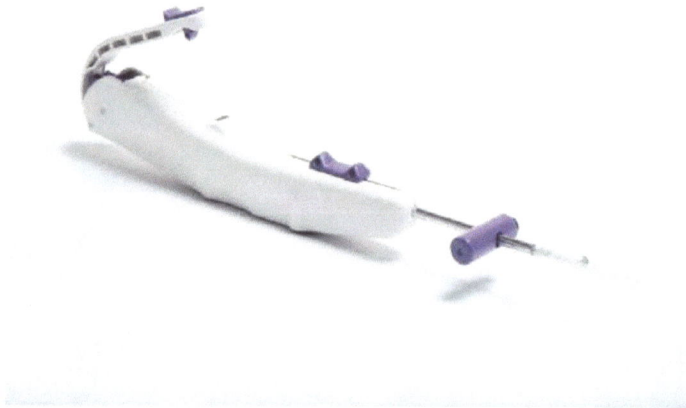

Fig. (11). Sonex® UltraGuide Carpal Tunnel Release device. Courtesy with permission Sonex® (UltraGuide CTR Side View).

USCTR Bailout Procedure

During USCTR, specific situations may necessitate bailout, rescue, or salvage procedures to manage unexpected complications or challenges encountered during the surgery. These procedures aim to address difficulties and optimize patient safety and outcomes.

1. Instrument repositioning or redirection: In cases where instrument placement is

challenging or incomplete release of the TCL is suspected, the instrument can be repositioned or redirected under ultrasound guidance. This maneuver helps ensure optimal ligament release and decompression of the median nerve.

2. Conversion to alternative techniques: If the USCTR procedure encounters significant difficulties or complications that prevent successful completion, conversion to an open carpal tunnel release may be considered. This conversion allows for the appropriate treatment of CTS and relief of median nerve compression.

DISCUSSION

Endoscopic release of symptomatic CTS offers patients shorter recovery times, reduced postoperative pain, and improved cosmetic outcomes. Open CTR has traditionally been the gold standard treatment for CTS. However, further advancements in technology have led to the development of USCTR, which has the advantage of minimized trauma and scarring, improved visualization with ultrasound guidance, less postoperative pain, and faster recovery. Many such procedures are being performed in an ambulatory surgery center and/or in-office setting with decreased healthcare costs and improved patient outcomes because of lower complication rates.

These procedures require mastering a learning curve(s)—other challenges are related to the need for the surgeon to have expertise in endoscopic techniques and ultrasound imaging. Surgeons must acquire proficiency in both aspects to ensure safe and effective procedures. The learning curve may pose a challenge during the initial stages of implementation—another common implementation hurdle may be equipment costs. Adopting this technological approach requires investment in specialized endoscopic instruments and/or ultrasound equipment. While the long-term benefits may outweigh the initial costs, they can be a barrier for some healthcare facilities or surgeons. Patient selection criteria are also being redefined since not all patients with carpal tunnel syndrome are suitable candidates for the endoscopic procedure. An accurate preoperative assessment is crucial to identify individuals who would most benefit from such a minimally invasive procedure. Patients with severe CTS or anatomical variations, previous surgery, and other relative/absolute contraindications may require an alternative approach. Some of the relative contraindications may not be relevant to some surgeons with high skill levels or those who can implement technological advances quickly.

Bailout, rescue, and salvage procedures are contingency measures to address unexpected complications or challenges that may arise during SPECTR and USCTR. Surgeons must be prepared to employ these procedures when necessary, prioritizing patient safety and optimal outcomes. Surgeons must have the necessary skills, experience, and resources to execute these procedures effectively to ensure the best possible results. Revision CTR incidence has not been tracked in general as there is no specific Current Procedural Terminology or CPT® Code for the same. As aforementioned, many revision CTRs can be handled either by SPECTR or USCTR, depending on surgeon preference, mainly if there is incomplete resection or regrowth of the flexor retinaculum. Open conversion is recommended if the recurrence is due to the median nerve being encased in a scar (fibrous proliferation) and abnormally transposed by scar, flexor tenosynovitis, or extrinsic compression due to muscle belly or cyst. A native hypothenar-pedicled fat flap or a less morbid amnion allograft wrap-conduit for improved local bed biology should be considered for these open revision scenarios.

CONCLUSION

Ongoing research and development efforts should further improve the effectiveness and safety of endoscopic or ultrasound-guided carpal tunnel release procedures. Advancements in instrumentation, imaging technology, and surgical techniques will likely enhance outcomes and expand the application(s). Both technologies and procedures, SPECTR and USCTR, significantly advance the treatment of CTS. Comparative studies evaluating the long-term outcomes against open CTR have been published, and the efficacy and advantages over traditional approaches have been validated. However, the substantial high-grade evidence base does not diminish the importance of mastering the operation(s), which may be one of the most significant hurdles to widespread adoption. Prospects may include the integration of robotic assistance.

ACKNOWLEDGMENTS

The co-authors would like to acknowledge Dr. Owen J. Moy's kind review.

REFERENCES

[1]   Learmonth J. The principle of decompression in the treatment of certain diseases of peripheral nerves. Surg Clin North Am 1933; 13: 905-13.

[2]   Russell Brain W, Dickson Wright A, Wilkinson M. Spontaneous compression of both median nerves in the carpal tunnel; six cases treated surgically. Lancet 1947; 249(6443-6445): 277-82. [http://dx.doi.org/10.1016/S0140-6736(47)90093-7] [PMID: 20287146]

[3]   Phalen GS, Gardner WJ, Wilkinson M, La Londe AA. Nfuropathy of the median nerve due to compression beneath the transverse carpal ligament. JBJS 1950; 32(1): 109-12. [http://dx.doi.org/10.2106/00004623-195032010-00011]

[4]   Shin EK, Bachoura A, Jacoby SM, Chen NC, Osterman AL. Treatment of carpal tunnel syndrome by members of the American Association for Hand Surgery. Hand (N Y) 2012; 7(4): 351-6. [http://dx.doi.org/10.1007/s11552-012-9455-8] [PMID: 24294152]

[5]   Chow JCY. Endoscopic release of the carpal ligament: A new technique for carpal tunnel syndrome. Arthroscopy 1989; 5(1): 19-24.

[http://dx.doi.org/10.1016/0749-8063(89)90085-6] [PMID: 2706047]

[6]   Agee JM, McCarroll HR, Tortosa RD, Berry DA, Szabo RM, Peimer CA. Endoscopic release of the carpal tunnel: A randomized prospective multicenter study. J Hand Surg Am 1992; 17(6): 987-95. [http://dx.doi.org/10.1016/S0363-5023(09)91044-9] [PMID: 1430964]

[7]   Trumble TE, Diao E, Abrams RA, Gilbert-Anderson MM. Single-portal endoscopic carpal tunnel release compared with open release : a prospective, randomized trial. J Bone Joint Surg Am 2002; 84(7): 1107-15. [http://dx.doi.org/10.2106/00004623-200207000-00003] [PMID: 12107308]

[8]   Staff M. MicroAire and Arthrex settle patent spat 2010. Available from: https://www.massdevice.com/microaire-and-arthrex-settle-patent-spat/

[9]   Thoma A, Veltri K, Haines T, Duku E. A meta-analysis of randomized controlled trials comparing endoscopic and open carpal tunnel decompression. Plast Reconstr Surg 2004; 114(5): 1137-46. [http://dx.doi.org/10.1097/01.PRS.0000135850.37523.D0] [PMID: 15457025]

[10]   Ablove RH, Peimer CA, Diao E, Oliverio R, Kuhn JP, Buffalo NY. Morphologic changes following endoscopic and two-portal subcutaneous carpal tunnel release. J Hand Surg Am 1994; 19(5): 821-6. [http://dx.doi.org/10.1016/0363-5023(94)90194-5] [PMID: 7806811]

[11]   Ablove RH, Moy OJ, Peimer CA, Wheeler DR, Diao E. Pressure changes in Guyon's canal after carpal tunnel release. J Hand Surg [Br] 1996; 21(5): 664-5. [http://dx.doi.org/10.1016/S0266-7681(96)80155-0] [PMID: 9230958]

[12]   Peters BR, Martin AM, Memauri BF, *et al.* Morphologic Analysis of the Carpal Tunnel and Median Nerve Following Open and Endoscopic Carpal Tunnel Release. Hand (N Y) 2021; 16(3): 310-5. [http://dx.doi.org/10.1177/1558944719861711] [PMID: 31331208]

[13]   Mertz K, Trunzter J, Wu E, Barnes J, Eppler SL, Kamal RN. National Trends in the Diagnosis of CRPS after Open and Endoscopic Carpal Tunnel Release. J Wrist Surg 2019; 8(3): 209-14. [http://dx.doi.org/10.1055/s-0039-1678674] [PMID: 31192042]

[14]   del Piñal F. Outcomes of Carpal Tunnel Release in Complex Regional Pain Syndrome/Reflex Sympathetic Dystrophy/Sudeck Disease Patients. Plast Reconstr Surg 2022; 150(1): 93-101. [http://dx.doi.org/10.1097/PRS.0000000000009243] [PMID: 35536771]

[15]   Tuzuner S, Özkaynak S, Acikbas C, Yildirim A. Median nerve excursion during endoscopic carpal tunnel release. Neurosurgery 2004; 54(5): 1155-61. [http://dx.doi.org/10.1227/01.NEU.0000119232.57668.98] [PMID: 15113471]

[16]   Rojo-Manaute JM, Capa-Grasa A, Chana-Rodríguez F, *et al.* Ultra☐Minimally Invasive Ultrasound☐Guided Carpal Tunnel Release. J Ultrasound Med 2016; 35(6): 1149-57. [http://dx.doi.org/10.7863/ultra.15.07001] [PMID: 27105949]

[17]   Management of Carpal Tunnel Sundrome: Evidence-Based Clinical Practice Guidelines: American Academy of Orthopaedic Surgeons Board of Directors; 2016. Available from: https://www.aaos.org/globalassets/quality-and-practice-resources/car-al-tunnel/management-of-carpal-tunnel-syndrome-7-31-19.pdf

[18]   Alice A, Hunter M, Barry P, Simmons M. Surgery for carpal tunnel syndrome 2023.Available from: https://www.uptodate.com/contents/surgery-for-carpal-tunnel-syndrome#H2UpToDate.com

[19]   Great Manchester EUR Policy Statement on: Surgical Interventions for Carpal Tunnel Syndrome 2019.   Available   from: http://northwestcsu.nhs.uk/BrickwallResource/GetResource/ca466296-cc1f-49d6-860a-e00ab0e0486a

[20]   Jebson PJL, Agee JM. Carpal tunnel syndrome: Unusual contraindications to endoscopic release. Arthroscopy 1996; 12(6): 749-51. [http://dx.doi.org/10.1016/S0749-8063(96)90182-6] [PMID: 9115567]

[21]   Cobb TK, Knudson GA, Cooney WP. The use of topographical landmarks to improve the outcome of

agee endoscopic carpal tunnel release. Arthroscopy 1995; 11(2): 165-72.
[http://dx.doi.org/10.1016/0749-8063(95)90062-4] [PMID: 7794428]

[22]   Kasundra GM, Sood I, Bhargava AN, *et al.* Carpal tunnel syndrome: Analyzing efficacy and utility of clinical tests and various diagnostic modalities. J Neurosci Rural Pract 2015; 6(4): 504-10.
[http://dx.doi.org/10.4103/0976-3147.169867] [PMID: 26752893]

[23]   Lange J. Carpal tunnel syndrome diagnosed using ultrasound as a first-line exam by the surgeon. J Hand Surg Eur Vol 2013; 38(6): 627-32.
[http://dx.doi.org/10.1177/1753193412469581] [PMID: 23232332]

[24]   Presazzi A, Bortolotto C, Zacchino M, Madonia L, Draghi F. Carpal tunnel: Normal anatomy, anatomical variants and ultrasound technique. J Ultrasound 2011; 14(1): 40-6.
[http://dx.doi.org/10.1016/j.jus.2011.01.006] [PMID: 23396809]

[25]   Kamel SI, Freid B, Pomeranz C, Halpern EJ, Nazarian LN. Minimally Invasive Ultrasound-Guided Carpal Tunnel Release Improves Long-Term Clinical Outcomes in Carpal Tunnel Syndrome. AJR Am J Roentgenol 2021; 217(2): 460-8.
[http://dx.doi.org/10.2214/AJR.20.24383] [PMID: 32876476]

[26]   Harness NG, Inacio MC, Pfeil FF, Paxton LW. Rate of infection after carpal tunnel release surgery and effect of antibiotic prophylaxis. J Hand Surg Am 2010; 35(2): 189-96.
[http://dx.doi.org/10.1016/j.jhsa.2009.11.012] [PMID: 20141890]

[27]   Medici A, Meccariello L, Rollo G, *et al.* Does routine carpal tunnel release during fixation of distal radius fractures improve outcomes? Injury 2017; 48 (Suppl. 3): S30-3.
[http://dx.doi.org/10.1016/S0020-1383(17)30654-X] [PMID: 29025606]

[28]   Gary C, Shah A, Kanouzi J, *et al.* Carpal Tunnel Syndrome Following Corrective Osteotomy for Distal Radius Malunion: A Rare Case Report and Review of the Literature. Hand (N Y) 2017; 12(5): NP157-61.
[http://dx.doi.org/10.1177/1558944717708053] [PMID: 28511570]

[29]   Hastings H II, Weiss APC, Quenzer D, Wiedeman GP, Hanington KR, Strickland JW. Arthrodesis of the wrist for post-traumatic disorders. J Bone Joint Surg Am 1996; 78(6): 897-902.
[http://dx.doi.org/10.2106/00004623-199606000-00013] [PMID: 8666608]

[30]   Beck JD, Deegan JH, Rhoades D, Klena JC. Results of endoscopic carpal tunnel release relative to surgeon experience with the Agee technique. J Hand Surg Am 2011; 36(1): 61-4.
[http://dx.doi.org/10.1016/j.jhsa.2010.10.017] [PMID: 21193127]

[31]   Dekimpe C, Andreani O, Camuzard O, *et al.* Ultrasound-guided percutaneous release of the carpal tunnel: comparison of the learning curves of a senior *versus* a junior operator. A cadaveric study. Skeletal Radiol 2019; 48(11): 1803-9.
[http://dx.doi.org/10.1007/s00256-019-03207-y] [PMID: 31114970]

CHAPTER 8

Ozone and PRP Injections for Symptomatic Lumbar Herniated Disc

Luis Miguel Duchén Rodríguez[1], Jorge Felipe Ramírez León[2,3,4], Tania Arancibia Baspineiro[5], Stephan Knoll[6], Álvaro Dowling[7], William Omar Contreas López[8] and Kai-Uwe Lewandrowski[9,10,11,*]

[1] *Center for Neurological Diseases and Public University of El Alto, La Paz, Bolivia*

[2] *Minimally Invasive Spine Center. Bogotá, D.C., Colombia*

[3] *Reina Sofía Clinic. Bogotá, D.C., Colombia*

[4] *Fundación Universitaria Sanitas. Bogotá, D.C., Colombia*

[5] *Center for Neurological Diseases, La Paz, Bolivia*

[6] *Biological Therapies Center, La Paz, Bolivia*

[7] *Department of Orthopaedic Surgery, USP, Ribeirão Preto, Brazil*

[8] *Clínica Foscal Internacional, Autopista Floridablanca - Girón, Km 7, Floridablanca, Santander, Colombia*

[9] *Center for Advanced Spine Care of Southern Arizona and Surgical Institute of Tucson, Tucson, AZ, USA*

[10] *Departmemt of Orthopaedics, Fundación Universitaria Sanitas, Bogotá, D.C., Colombia*

[11] *Department of Neurosurgery in the Video-Endoscopic Postgraduate Program at the Universidade Federal do Estado do Rio de Janeiro - UNIRIO, Rio de Janeiro, Brazil*

Abstract: Low back pain from arthritic lumbar facet joints and painful degenerative lumbar discs is widespread and one of the world's most disabling diseases, consuming significant health care resources. In this chapter, the authors report using autologous platelet-rich plasma (PRP) and ozone spinal injections into arthritic lumbar facet joints and painful lumbar degenerative discs to treat inflammatory pain. A prospective observational cohort study from January 2016 to March 2020 was performed at an outpatient clinic of a single academic medical center to assess these injections' safety and therapeutic effectiveness in conjunction with epidural transforaminal epidural steroid injections. Results indicated functional improvements measured by Oswestry Disability Index (ODI) and modified MacNab criteria and pain measured by visual analog scale leg pain (VAS) at rest and during flexion. Although our study was limited in scope, and by the observational nature of our research and the lack of randomized

* **Corresponding author Kai-Uwe Lewandrowski:** Center for Advanced Spine Care of Southern Arizona and Surgical Institute of Tucson, Tucson, AZ, USA; Departmemt of Orthopaedics, Fundación Universitaria Sanitas, Bogotá, D.C., Colombia and Department of Neurosurgery in the Video-Endoscopic Postgraduate Program at the Universidade Federal do Estado do Rio de Janeiro - UNIRIO, Rio de Janeiro, Brazil; E-mail: migueleduchen@hotmail.com

and double-blinding, our work suggests that rapid pain reduction and functional gains may materialize in patients with low back pain due to herniated disc after spinal injections with ozone and activated PRP.

Keywords: Low back pain, Ozone, Autologous platelet-rich plasma, Spinal injection.

INTRODUCTION

Chronic lumbar pain predominantly arises from intervertebral disc degeneration. In contrast, acute episodes of severe pain in the lower back and leg, resembling sciatica, usually result from herniated lumbar discs, adversely impacting patients' daily life and productivity. Such conditions pose a significant medical challenge. Lumbar degenerative disc disease has emerged as a pressing global concern, particularly prevalent among the aging population [1, 2]. Current treatments encompass conservative methods: anti-inflammatory medication, physical therapy, and microdiscectomy. Yet, the surgical route might expedite degeneration, potentially demanding further interventions [3 - 7].

In the 1980s, chymopapain, a cysteine protease from papaya latex, was a popular choice for chemical nucleolysis in patients with persistent herniated disc symptoms. Due to complications, its use was discontinued [8]. In the same decade, intradiscal oxygen/ozone injections for symptomatic lumbar herniations were introduced [9]. Numerous studies [9 - 22] and select randomized trials [12, 13, 23 - 26] have since underscored the efficacy of ozone therapy, either standalone or combined with steroids and other inflammation-reducing agents. Techniques, such as periradicular and intraforaminal injections, have proven beneficial in managing lumbar herniated disc pain [21, 23, 25, 27 - 32].

Ozone's primary modus operandi is believed to be chemonucleolysis, as it interacts with proteoglycan GAGs that help retain intradiscal osmotic balance, causing them to decompose. This leads to the nucleus pulposus dehydrating, thereby reducing disc volume. Moreover, ozone's inherent antimicrobial properties negate the need for preventive antibiotics [33]. Interactions with intradiscal cytokines may further produce an anti-inflammatory effect, diminishing pain levels, as supported by animal studies [34, 35]. Imaging analyses, including CT and MRI scans, have confirmed the reduced size of ozone-treated herniated lumbar discs [26, 36 - 39].

Platelet Rich Plasma (PRP)

Platelet Rich Plasma (PRP), derived from autologous sources, has shown promise in alleviating pain associated with symptomatic lumbar herniated and degenerative black discs [40]. PRP is essentially a concentrated blend of platelets suspended in a minimal volume of plasma. Its therapeutic potential arises from its capacity to promote extracellular matrix synthesis, which in turn may catalyze wound repair and intradiscal regeneration [41]. On a molecular front, PRP appears to modulate cytokine secretion, promoting the release of anti-inflammatory agents while suppressing pro-inflammatory cytokines. This modulation doesn't trigger immune reactions due to the autologous origin of the PRP [42].

Mirroring ozone's properties, PRP possesses anti-inflammatory and anti-microbial characteristics, thus potentially minimizing infection risks post-spinal injections [4, 5]. Several in vitro studies have confirmed the multifaceted advantages of PRP on degenerative disc tissues [6]. Notably, PRP has been associated with the rejuvenation of denatured discs by enhancing glycosaminoglycan concentrations [43]. Contemporary clinical findings indicate PRP's efficacy in pain mitigation related to lumbar disc conditions. However, concrete evidence verifying structural and functional enhancements remains elusive [44].

In the referenced prospective observational cohort study, the authors delve into the synergistic effects of ozone combined with activated PRP, aiming to optimize therapeutic outcomes for patients suffering from painful lumbar herniated discs.

Ozone Therapy

Ozone $[O_{(2)}\text{-}O_{(3)}]$ has been applied in the treatment of herniated discs. It also is believed to have therapeutic effects. Chemically, ozone is a highly reactive form of oxygen. It has been employed in the treatment of painful lumbar disc herniations. In addition to anti-inflammatory effects, it has been proposed to have analgesic properties [22]. The latter property was attributed to alleviating pain stemming from acute lumbar disc herniations by modulating the pain signaling pathways, reducing inflammation, and inhibiting the release of pain-inducing substances in the affected area. Ozone therapy may promote also cause shrinkage or dissolution of the herniated disc material by inducing oxidation. The resulting breakdown of diseased disc material [16, 17, 24] has been instrumental in patients with sciatica-type back and leg symptoms from extruded herniated discs. The resultant volumetric reduction in disc volume and subsequent indirect decompression of lumbar nerve roots [35] are therapeutically beneficial when managing patients with this painful and disabling disease.

Ozone also enhances oxygenation and blood flow [33] to the damaged areas in the annulus and nucleus. It may support the metabolic needs of the disc cells, improve tissue healing, and stimulate tissue regeneration. Additional benefits are its antimicrobial properties, lowering the risk of discitis and infection of the surrounding structures, particularly when surgical or interventional treatment is indicated.

The exact mechanisms of action of ozone therapy for herniated discs are still under investigation. However, its benefits have led to its clinical application as a minimally invasive interventional alternative to traditional surgical spine care with open incisions [9, 10, 12, 18, 32, 34]. Besides its solitary use during interventional procedures, it has also been employed with PRP. In the following, the authors report on their observational clinical study to explain the preparation of ozone and PRP, illustrate the procedural steps, review the clinical indications by describing the inclusion and exclusion criteria and reviewing the clinical outcomes that can be obtained in patients with acutely painful lumbar disc herniations with this interventional pain management strategy.

MRI Changes after Intradiscal Ozone Injection

A study by Bruno *et al.* performed a long-term imaging follow-up [39]. Patients were treated with intradiscal ozone injection three years later to achieve chemo-dialysis. The disc volume and appearance changes, rated according to Pfirrmann and Modic endplate, were analyzed and compared to a control group with sham injections. The authors of the Bruno study observed stable volumetric reduction of the disc herniation in the interventional versus the control group. Imaged-based grading of the MRI appearance of the lumbar motion segment did not show any statistically significant changes in the Pfirrmann appearance or the endplate changes, according to Modic. While ozone dialysis led to a considerable shrinkage of the disc herniation, a regenerative effect was not observed at the final three-year follow-up. Based on MRI criteria, the Bruno study was unable to determine whether biomechanical changes of the intervertebral disc in response to the ozone injection were able to halt the acceleration of the disc degeneration process in comparison to the natural history of the underlying degenerative disease.

Another study evaluated the shrinkage of the herniated disc following intradiscal ozone injection using the T2-shine through effect in diffusion-weighted imaging (DWI) [38]. A total of 154 patients suffering from lumbar radiculopathy refractory to conservative care measures, including 89 men and 65 women with an age range of 23-62 years, were included. The analyzed MRI image series included FSE-T2 and T2-fat, SE-T1, and DWI sequences. In this study, patients were randomly assigned to either the control group (70 patients) with conservative treatment with analgesic transforaminal epidural steroid injection or the interventional group (77 patients) who had the same treatment with the addition of oxygen-ozone. MRI follow-up at six months post-intervention analyzing the identical sequences allowed an intervertebral disc volumetric analysis (IDVA) and a DWI signal score calculation. These results were correlated with clinical outcomes. Chi-square testing and further statistical analysis with Student's t-test showed 58 of the 77 patients had a successful outcome. The DWI T2-shine through effect was noted in 53 of 77 responder patients at six months follow-up (p < 0.05), suggesting a statistically significant morphological and volumetric disc reduction. The author's study indicated that DWI T2-shine through effect is a predictive sign of response to oxygen-ozone treatment.

Clinical Indication for ozone-PRP disc therapy

Patients presenting with sciatica-like symptoms due to lumbar disc herniation are the primary candidates for this therapeutic intervention. To optimize treatment outcomes, candidates should meet the subsequent inclusion criteria:

1. A confirmed diagnosis of acute lumbar disc herniation between L1 and S1 levels.

2. Persistent low back pain for a duration of no less than six weeks, accompanied by a leg pain VAS score exceeding 5.

3. Ineffectiveness of conservative treatment after six weeks.

4. Age bracket: 18 to 65 years.

5. A Body Mass Index (BMI) below 40.

6. Dermatomal pain pattern that aligns with radiographic imaging results.

7. Retained disc height, which is a minimum of 50% compared to adjacent discs.

8. MRI T2-weighted sequences displaying a herniated disc signal intensity either matching or surpassing that of the remaining nucleus pulposus.

Conversely, patients with multifaceted spinal pathologies, including degenerative conditions or discernible spinal malformations, are not suitable candidates for intradiscal ozone injection. The advised exclusion criteria are:

1. Presence of metabolic diseases impacting disc health or other comorbidities.

2. History or signs of infections, malignancies, trauma, or spondylolisthesis.

3. Symptoms of radiculopathy or claudication due to bony stenosis, either foraminal, lateral, or central.

4. Non-contiguous disc fragment herniations or those extending beyond the facet

joint.

5. Dysfunction of bowel or bladder systems.

6. Detectable motor strength reduction in the lower limbs.

7. Recent lumbar epidural steroid injection, specifically within the last fortnight.

8. Previous lumbar surgeries such as discectomy, fusion, or arthroplasty.

9. Manifestations of sacroiliac joint pathology.

10. Prospective pregnancy or current pregnancy in female participants.

11. History of fibromyalgia, over three months of recent sick leave, or both.

12. Confirmed substance misuse or documented psychiatric or emotional disorders.

Oxygen-Ozone Preparation and PRP Methodology

Utilizing the Evozone Basic Plus system (Reutlingen, Germany), a precise gas mixture is generated. This apparatus employs a sterile syringe cartridge alongside a console, ensuring accurate calibration of the oxygen-ozone within the pre-sterilized syringe integrated with a gas filter cartridge. Notably, oxygen is directly transformed into ozone within the syringe, obviating potential dilution or contamination risks associated with transferring from an unsterilized generator. The components of this system are specifically designed to withstand oxygen-ozone, and are silicon-lubricated to prevent degradation or the emergence of unwanted byproducts. The resultant oxygen-ozone gas is maintained at a consistent concentration of 40 µg/mL, the integrity of which is confirmed using an ultraviolet photometer.

Preferred Autologous PRP Protocol

For optimal results, patients undergo preliminary laboratory evaluations including CBC, PT, PTT, INR, glucose, creatinine, blood and Rh-typing, and HIV tests. Employing the authors' favored methodology, 300 cc of venous blood is meticulously drawn. Upon centrifugation at 3000 rpm for 8 minutes, the resultant PRP is isolated under sterile conditions in a laminar flow hood, then activated with an 80 µg/mL ozone concentration.

Injection Technique of Choice

Patients are strategically positioned in a lateral decubitus alignment, cushioned by a lumbar pad. Ensuring unobstructed fluoroscopic visualization of the lumbosacral region, patients' legs remain flexed at the abdomen. The targeted area is then thoroughly sanitized with chlorhexidine (Refer Fig. **1**).

A 20F Chiba needle is then introduced to the intervertebral disc through the oblique transforaminal approach for the intradiscal injection under conscious sedation and local anesthesia with 2% lidocaine. Approximately 3 to 5 ml of the oxygen-ozone mixture at a concentration of 40 µg/mL is injected, followed by three ccs of the activated platelet-rich plasma. The intraarticular facet injections can also be done in the prone position. A 22 G spinal needle (Spinocam®) is introduced to the zygoapophyseal joint to inject 2 ml of the oxygen-ozone PRP mixture. The exact same amount is injected through the sacral hiatus and transforaminal into the neuroforamina of the symptomatic level. After the procedure, patients are monitored for any adverse events for one hour after the interventional procedure. Typically, they can be sent home with acetaminophen 500mg every eight hours for 24 hours and instructed to avoid bending, twisting, and any weight lifting more than over 10 lbs for two weeks after the procedure.

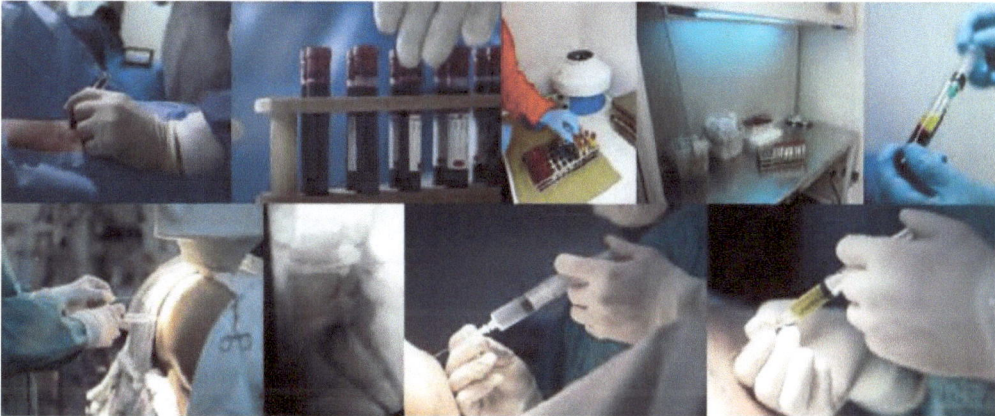

Fig. (1). Procedure for Ozone and PRP Administration in Lumbar Herniated Disc Treatment: Using an ozone concentrator, ozone was meticulously generated. Concurrently, from 350 cc of peripheral venous blood, PRP was isolated within a laminar flow hood through centrifugation. For the transforaminal intradiscal administration of the PRP activated with oxygen-ozone, patients were strategically aligned in a lateral decubitus position, with the 20F Chiba needle poised for injection. To ensure patient comfort, conscious sedation was employed alongside a local anesthetic – 2% lidocaine. Subsequently, around 3 ml of the oxygen-ozone concoction, calibrated to a 40 µg/mL concentration, was infused into the herniated disc. This was succeeded by the introduction of three cc of the activated PRP.

Clinical Outcomes Following Ozone & PRP Treatment

From the designated inclusion and exclusion criteria, 55 patients were chosen for the study, conducted from December 2017 to November 2018 at the Center for Neurological Diseases, La Paz Bolivia. This cohort encompassed 24 females

(44%) and 31 males (56%), averaging 48.63 ± 13.54 years in age and a follow-up duration of 25.84 ± 10.94 months. A statistical power assessment deemed this sample ample for evaluating the safety and clinical ramifications of using ozone and activated PRP for degenerative disc ailments.

Efficacy of the treatment was gauged using the modified McNab criteria [15], VAS for lower back pain [16], and the Oswestry Disability Index (ODI) [17]. These criteria, being patient-reported outcome measures (PROMs), aptly correlate with post-treatment MRI evaluations of lumbar disc recuperation. Clinical assessments occurred at 3, 6, 12, and 24 months post-intervention. Within our cohort, 10 out of 55 underwent post-procedure MRI scanning 4 and 12 weeks after treatment. Evaluation tools encompassed the VAS for pain, the ODI for functional capabilities, and the modified MacNab criteria. Additionally, post-treatment check-ups were conducted to detect any complications or undesired effects, while treatment efficacy was gauged by the absence of any further interventions at the treated disc site. MRI scans were appraised for disc herniation volume reduction and potential annular tear healing. Data analyses were conducted using SPSS™ version 27, applying the paired T-test for statistical significance.

There were zero complications post-treatment. Of the cohort, 22% reported isolated axial back pain, whereas 78% displayed both sciatica-type pain and dermatomal pain, consistent with their MRI scans. Distribution of treated lumbar levels was: L4-L5 (7%), L5-S1 (18%), both L4-L5 & L5-S1 (51%), and more than two levels (24%). The VAS leg pain score plummeted from 7.98 ± 1.65 pre-intervention to 2.72 ± 2.06 within a week (p < 0.001). This pain alleviation persisted throughout the 96-week follow-up, with the VAS score persistently low: 2.85 ± 2.12 (12 weeks), 2.76 ± 2.17 (24 weeks), 2.58 ± 2.25 (48 weeks), and 2.52 ± 2.35 (96 weeks). Initial ODI values diminished from 72.65 ± 11.15 pre-procedure to 30.29 ± 15.67 post-procedure, showcasing a marked 68.3% reduction. Functional enhancements were evident within a week post-treatment. MacNab assessments post-treatment were: excellent (36.4%), good (49.1%), fair (9.1%), and poor (5.4%), with 85.5% reporting favorable outcomes.

10 out of the 55 patients underwent surveillance MRI up to 12 weeks post-intervention. The scans illustrated a discernible reduction in herniated disc volume post spinal injections with oxygen-ozone and activated PRP. Notably, these structural MRI changes were delayed compared to the rapid symptom relief observed, predominantly within the first week post-treatment.

DISCUSSION

The conventional approach to treating lumbar herniated disc-induced acute pain syndromes predominantly revolves around epidural steroid injections. While a spectrum of percutaneous techniques, from radiofrequency [45] to non-visualized disc tissue removal [46 - 49], is available, many of these remain outside the typical training regimen of several acute spine pain management specialists [50, 51]. The nascent realm of interventional pain surgery is poised to bridge this chasm between conventional pain management and the standard microdiscectomy [52 - 55]. Presently, a significant cohort of patients reluctant to undergo spinal surgery grapple with insufficient or ineffective therapeutic interventions [56] (Fig. **2**).

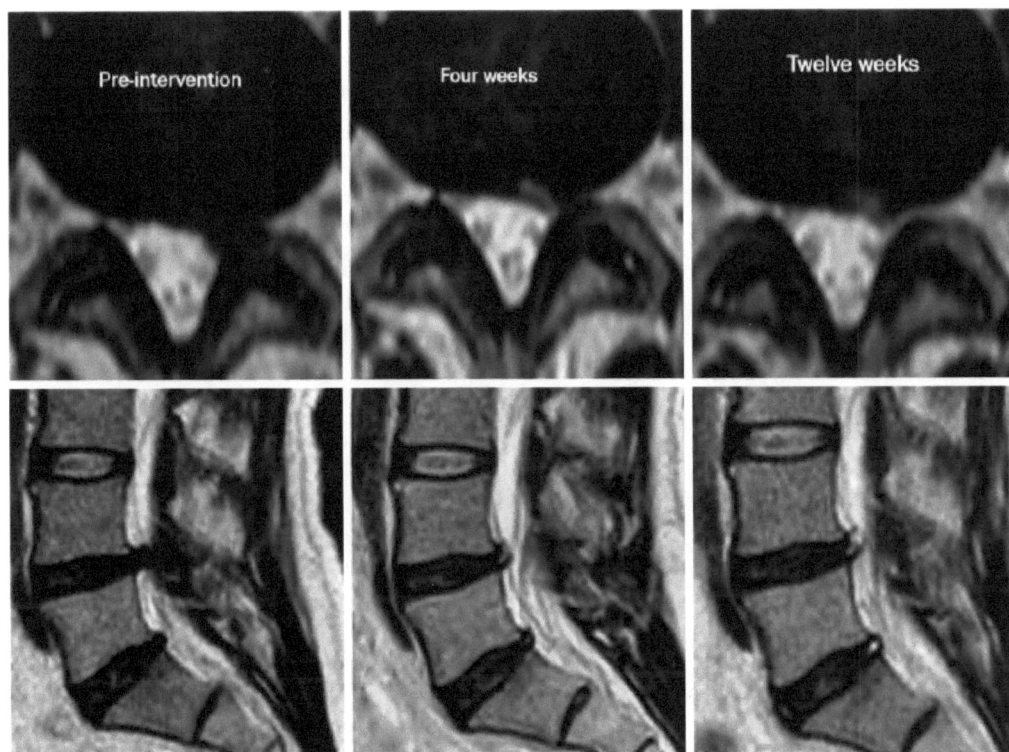

Fig. (2). Post-intervention MRI assessments were conducted on a subset of the 55 participants. Following spinal administrations of oxygen-ozone and activated PRP, there was an evident decrement in the herniated disc volume, as discerned from T2-weighted sequences using a 1.5T MRI, spanning from pre-treatment to the 4th and 12th post-treatment weeks. Notably, while MRI-detectable structural adaptations developed over weeks, symptomatic alleviation manifested predominantly within a week post-procedure.

Although regenerative medicine targeting lumbar intervertebral disc ailments is in its preliminary stages [42, 44, 57 - 65], robust clinical evidence from double-blinded, randomized trials does underscore the regenerative and anti-inflammatory capabilities of both ozone and PRP at the cellular stratum [12, 13, 23 - 25, 31, 63, 66]. Meta-analyses of contemporary clinical findings indicate a lack of unambiguous support for functional enhancement via PRP monotherapy [44]. Subsequent inquiries comparing PRP with other agents, such as steroids [12], and explorations into its regenerative potential have been advocated [44]. This study's primary focus lies in evaluating the efficaciousness of oxygen-ozone and activated PRP injections in ameliorating symptoms of acute lumbar herniated discs [44].

Our study offers compelling evidence that injections of ozone and activated PRP into the afflicted intervertebral disc can usher in rapid amelioration in patient functionality and pain relief, discernible within a week for most participants. Recognizing that acute herniated disc-induced pain is multifaceted [67 - 72], we amalgamated intradiscal injections with facet joint, sacral hiatus, and transforaminal periradicular interventions. Such injections are well-validated in medical literature and backed by rigorous clinical trials [9, 10, 23, 25, 27 - 30]. While discerning the specific source of relief—whether from intradiscal or other injections—is clinically immaterial, MRI analyses do provide robust evidence of lumbar herniated disc reduction post-oxygen-ozone interventions [17, 26, 37 - 39, 73]. Preliminary MRI insights from our study cohort mirror this, revealing a pronounced reduction in herniated disc volume, devoid of overarching disc dehydration. A meticulous MRI-centric exploration of disc volume post-injection remains an avenue for future research.

However, our study is not devoid of limitations. Identifying the paramount contributor within our intervention protocol remains elusive. Potential biases, including proceduralist-driven patient selection [74] and retrospective patient reporting [75], might influence outcomes. Still, the pronounced alleviation in pain and functional enhancement within a week fortifies the practicality of our methodology. To rigorously validate these findings, comprehensive double-blinded, randomized trials are imperative.

CONCLUSION

Our investigation delineates the promising potential of oxygen-ozone and activated PRP spinal injections in alleviating pain and enhancing functionality in acute lumbar herniated disc patients. The synergy of ozone and PRP seems pivotal, possibly due to ozone-mediated disc reduction. Complementary injections, including those in the foramina and sacral hiatus, appear instrumental in bolstering relief. To refine the therapeutic protocols, exhaustive studies, ideally double-blinded randomized trials, centered on varied ozone and PRP dosages are paramount.

REFERENCES

[1]   Ravindra VM, Senglaub SS, Rattani A, *et al.* Degenerative Lumbar Spine Disease: Estimating Global Incidence and Worldwide Volume. Global Spine J 2018; 8(8): 784-94.
[http://dx.doi.org/10.1177/2192568218770769] [PMID: 30560029]

[2]   Smith JS, Shaffrey CI, Baldus CR, *et al.* Orthopedic disease burden in adult patients with symptomatic lumbar scoliosis: results from a prospective multicenter study. J Neurosurg Spine 2021; 35(6): 743-51.
[http://dx.doi.org/10.3171/2021.1.SPINE201911] [PMID: 34416734]

[3]   Leggett LE, Soril LJJ, Lorenzetti DL, *et al.* Radiofrequency ablation for chronic low back pain: a systematic review of randomized controlled trials. Pain Res Manag 2014; 19(5): e146-53.
[http://dx.doi.org/10.1155/2014/834369] [PMID: 25068973]

[4]   Burgstaller JM, Steurer J, Gravestock I, *et al.* Long-term Results After Surgical or Nonsurgical Treatment in Patients With Degenerative Lumbar Spinal Stenosis. Spine 2020; 45(15): 1030-8.
[http://dx.doi.org/10.1097/BRS.0000000000003457] [PMID: 32675604]

[5]   Yee TJ, Terman SW, La Marca F, Park P. Comparison of adjacent segment disease after minimally invasive or open transforaminal lumbar interbody fusion. J Clin Neurosci 2014; 21(10): 1796-801.
[http://dx.doi.org/10.1016/j.jocn.2014.03.010] [PMID: 24880486]

[6]   Zhu H, Wang G, Zhou Z, Fan S. Prospective Study of Long□term Effect between Multifidus Muscle Bundle and Conventional Open Approach in One□level Posterior Lumbar Interbody Fusion. Orthop Surg 2018; 10(4): 296-305.
[http://dx.doi.org/10.1111/os.12402] [PMID: 30402963]

[7]   Zigler JE, Glenn J, Delamarter RB. Five-year adjacent-level degenerative changes in patients with single-level disease treated using lumbar total disc replacement with ProDisc-L versus circumferential fusion. J Neurosurg Spine 2012; 17(6): 504-11.
[http://dx.doi.org/10.3171/2012.9.SPINE11717] [PMID: 23082849]

[8]   Sussman BJ. Inadequacies and hazards of chymopapain injections as treatment for intervertebral disc disease. J Neurosurg 1975; 42(4): 389-96.
[http://dx.doi.org/10.3171/jns.1975.42.4.0389] [PMID: 123576]

[9]   Hosseini B, Taheri M, Sheibani K. Comparing the results of intradiscal ozone injection to treat different types of intervertebral disc herniation based on MSU classification. Interv Neuroradiol 2019; 25(1): 111-6.
[http://dx.doi.org/10.1177/1591019918800458] [PMID: 30227808]

[10]   Rahimzadeh P, Imani F, Ghahremani M, Faiz SHR. Comparison of percutaneous intradiscal ozone injection with laser disc decompression in discogenic low back pain. J Pain Res 2018; 11: 1405-10.
[http://dx.doi.org/10.2147/JPR.S164335] [PMID: 30104895]

[11]   Kılıç M, Erçalık T. The Effect of Lumbar Spinal Surgery History on Intradiscal O_2-O_3 Treatment Results in Patients with Lumbar Disk Herniation. Sisli Etfal Hastan Tip Bul 2019; 53(2): 148-53.
[PMID: 32377074]

[12]   Ercalik T, Kilic M. Efficacy of Intradiscal Ozone Therapy with or without Periforaminal Steroid Injection on Lumbar Disc Herniation: A Double-Blinded Controlled Study. Pain Physician 2020; 5(23): 477-84.
[http://dx.doi.org/10.36076/ppj.2020/23/477] [PMID: 32967390]

[13]   Elawamy A, Kamel EZ, Hassanien M, Wahba OM, Amin SE. Implication of Two Different Doses of Intradiscal Ozone-Oxygen Injection upon the Pain Alleviation in Patients with Low Back Pain: A Randomized, Single-Blind Study. Pain Physician 2018; 21(1): E25-31.
[PMID: 29357333]

[14]   Ozcan S, Muz A, Yildiz Altun A, Onal SA. Intradiscal ozone therapy for lumbar disc herniation. Cell Mol Biol 2018; 64(5): 52-5.
[http://dx.doi.org/10.14715/cmb/2018.64.5.8] [PMID: 29729693]

[15]   Muto M, Ambrosanio G, Guarnieri G, *et al.* Low back pain and sciatica: treatment with intradiscal-

intraforaminal O2-O3 injection. Our experience. Radiol Med (Torino) 2008; 113(5): 695-706.
[http://dx.doi.org/10.1007/s11547-008-0302-5] [PMID: 18594765]

[16]   Kilic M, Ercalik T, Ozdemir B, *et al.* Lumbar Intradiscal Ozone Chemonucleolysis Applied Together with the Epidural Steroid Treatment. Sisli Etfal Hastan Tip Bul 2021; 55(2): 203-9.
[PMID: 34349597]

[17]   Bruno F, Carboni N, Palumbo P, *et al.* O$_2$–O$_3$ chemodiscolysis: How much, how long? Retrospective outcome evaluation of different treatment sessions in partially-responder patients. Interv Neuroradiol 2022; 28(4): 433-8.
[http://dx.doi.org/10.1177/15910199211039914] [PMID: 34516319]

[18]   Migliorini F, Maffulli N, Eschweiler J, Bestch M, Tingart M, Baroncini A. Ozone injection therapy for intervertebral disc herniation. Br Med Bull 2020; 136(1): 88-106.
[http://dx.doi.org/10.1093/bmb/ldaa032] [PMID: 33128379]

[19]   Crockett MT, Moynagh M, Long N, *et al.* Ozone-augmented percutaneous discectomy: A novel treatment option for refractory discogenic sciatica. Clin Radiol 2014; 69(12): 1280-6.
[http://dx.doi.org/10.1016/j.crad.2014.08.008] [PMID: 25240564]

[20]   Ezeldin M, Leonardi M, Princiotta C, *et al.* Percutaneous ozone nucleolysis for lumbar disc herniation. Neuroradiology 2018; 60(11): 1231-41.
[http://dx.doi.org/10.1007/s00234-018-2083-4] [PMID: 30206674]

[21]   Gallucci M, Limbucci N, Zugaro L, *et al.* Sciatica: treatment with intradiscal and intraforaminal injections of steroid and oxygen-ozone versus steroid only. Radiology 2007; 242(3): 907-13.
[http://dx.doi.org/10.1148/radiol.2423051934] [PMID: 17209164]

[22]   Zhang Y, Ma Y, Jiang J, Ding T, Wang J. Treatment of the lumbar disc herniation with intradiscal and intraforaminal injection of oxygen-ozone. J Back Musculoskeletal Rehabil 2013; 26(3): 317-22.
[http://dx.doi.org/10.3233/BMR-130386] [PMID: 23893147]

[23]   Sucuoğlu H, Soydaş N. Does paravertebral ozone injection have efficacy as an additional treatment for acute lumbar disc herniation? A randomized, double-blind, placebo-controlled study. J Back Musculoskeletal Rehabil 2021; 34(5): 725-33.
[http://dx.doi.org/10.3233/BMR-200194] [PMID: 33843663]

[24]   Kelekis A, Bonaldi G, Cianfoni A, *et al.* Intradiscal oxygen-ozone chemonucleolysis versus microdiscectomy for lumbar disc herniation radiculopathy: a non–inferiority randomized control trial. Spine J 2022; 22(6): 895-909.
[http://dx.doi.org/10.1016/j.spinee.2021.11.017] [PMID: 34896609]

[25]   Paoloni M, Di Sante L, Cacchio A, *et al.* Intramuscular oxygen-ozone therapy in the treatment of acute back pain with lumbar disc herniation: a multicenter, randomized, double-blind, clinical trial of active and simulated lumbar paravertebral injection. Spine 2009; 34(13): 1337-44.
[http://dx.doi.org/10.1097/BRS.0b013e3181a3c18d] [PMID: 19478653]

[26]   Perri M, Grattacaso G, di Tunno V, *et al.* T2 shine-through phenomena in diffusion-weighted MR imaging of lumbar discs after oxygen–ozone discolysis: a randomized, double-blind trial with steroid and O2–O3 discolysis versus steroid only. Radiol Med (Torino) 2015; 120(10): 941-50.
[http://dx.doi.org/10.1007/s11547-015-0519-z] [PMID: 25743238]

[27]   Özcan Ç, Polat Ö, Çelik H, Uçar BY. The Effect of Paravertebral Ozone Injection in the Treatment of Low Back Pain. Pain Pract 2019; 19(8): 821-5.
[http://dx.doi.org/10.1111/papr.12812] [PMID: 31228871]

[28]   Vanni D, Galzio R, Kazakova A, *et al.* Intraforaminal ozone therapy and particular side effects: preliminary results and early warning. Acta Neurochir (Wien) 2016; 158(3): 491-6.
[http://dx.doi.org/10.1007/s00701-015-2545-y] [PMID: 26293228]

[29]   Biazzo A, Corriero AS, Confalonieri N. Intramuscular oxygen-ozone therapy in the treatment of low back pain. Acta Biomed 2018; 89(1): 41-6.

[PMID: 29633741]

[30] Yalçın Ü. Paravertebral intramuscular ozone therapy in lumbar disc hernia: A comprehensive retrospective study. J Back Musculoskeletal Rehabil 2021; 34(4): 597-604.
[http://dx.doi.org/10.3233/BMR-200129] [PMID: 33523038]

[31] Lu W, Li YH, He XF. Treatment of large lumbar disc herniation with percutaneous ozone injection *via* the posterior-lateral route and inner margin of the facet joint. World J Radiol 2010; 2(3): 109-12.
[http://dx.doi.org/10.4329/wjr.v2.i3.109] [PMID: 21160944]

[32] Sconza C, Braghetto G, Respizzi S, Morenghi E, Kon E, Di Matteo B. Ultrasound-guided periradicular oxygen-ozone injections as a treatment option for low back pain associated with sciatica. Int Orthop 2021; 45(5): 1239-46.
[http://dx.doi.org/10.1007/s00264-021-04975-w] [PMID: 33629173]

[33] Wei CJ, Li YH, Chen Y, *et al.* [Percutaneous intradiscal oxygen-ozone injection for lumbar disc herniation: no need of perioperative antibiotic prophylaxis]. Nan Fang Yi Ke Da Xue Xue Bao 2007; 27(3): 384-6. [Percutaneous intradiscal oxygen-ozone injection for lumbar disc herniation: no need of perioperative antibiotic prophylaxis].
[PMID: 17426000]

[34] Murphy K, Elias G, Steppan J, *et al.* Percutaneous Treatment of Herniated Lumbar Discs with Ozone: Investigation of the Mechanisms of Action. J Vasc Interv Radiol 2016; 27(8): 1242-1250.e3.
[http://dx.doi.org/10.1016/j.jvir.2016.04.012] [PMID: 27363296]

[35] Wang J, Wu M, Lin X, Li Y, Fu Z. Low-Concentration Oxygen/Ozone Treatment Attenuated Radiculitis and Mechanical Allodynia via PDE2A-cAMP/cGMP-NF- κ B/p65 Signaling in Chronic Radiculitis Rats. Pain Res Manag 2018; 2018: 1-8.
[http://dx.doi.org/10.1155/2018/5192814] [PMID: 30651902]

[36] Niu XK, Bhetuwal A, Yang HF. Diffusion-Weighted Imaging for Pretreatment Evaluation and Prediction of Treatment Effect in Patients Undergoing CT-Guided Injection for Lumbar Disc Herniation. Korean J Radiol 2015; 16(4): 874-80.
[http://dx.doi.org/10.3348/kjr.2015.16.4.874] [PMID: 26175588]

[37] Bruno F, Palumbo P, Tommasino E, *et al.* Evaluation of intervertebral disc using T2 mapping sequences in patients undergoing O_2–O_3 chemiodiscolysis: an instrumental study with clinical correlation. Neuroradiology 2020; 62(1): 55-61.
[http://dx.doi.org/10.1007/s00234-019-02308-8] [PMID: 31760440]

[38] Perri M, Grattacaso G, Di Tunno V, *et al.* MRI DWI/ADC signal predicts shrinkage of lumbar disc herniation after O2–O3 discolysis. Neuroradiol J 2015; 28(2): 198-204.
[http://dx.doi.org/10.1177/1971400915576658] [PMID: 25923680]

[39] Bruno F, Smaldone F, Varrassi M, *et al.* MRI findings in lumbar spine following O_2–O_3 chemiodiscolysis: A long-term follow-up. Interv Neuroradiol 2017; 23(4): 444-50.
[http://dx.doi.org/10.1177/1591019917703784] [PMID: 28485657]

[40] Wang S, Chang Q, Lu J, Wang C. Growth factors and platelet-rich plasma: promising biological strategies for early intervertebral disc degeneration. Int Orthop 2015; 39(5): 927-34.
[http://dx.doi.org/10.1007/s00264-014-2664-8] [PMID: 25653173]

[41] Masuda K. Biological repair of the degenerated intervertebral disc by the injection of growth factors. Eur Spine J 2008; 17(4): 441-51.
[http://dx.doi.org/10.1007/s00586-008-0749-z]

[42] Tavakoli J, Diwan AD, Tipper JL. Advanced Strategies for the Regeneration of Lumbar Disc Annulus Fibrosus. Int J Mol Sci 2020; 21(14): 4889.
[http://dx.doi.org/10.3390/ijms21144889] [PMID: 32664453]

[43] Khalaf K, Nikkhoo M, Kuo Y-W, *et al.* Recovering the mechanical properties of denatured intervertebral discs through Platelet-Rich Plasma therapy. Annu Int Conf IEEE Eng Med Biol Soc

2015; 2015: 933-6.
[http://dx.doi.org/10.1109/EMBC.2015.7318516] [PMID: 26736416]

[44]   Muthu S, Jeyaraman M, Chellamuthu G, Jeyaraman N, Jain R, Khanna M. Does the Intradiscal Injection of Platelet Rich Plasma Have Any Beneficial Role in the Management of Lumbar Disc Disease? Global Spine J 2022; 12(3): 503-14.
[http://dx.doi.org/10.1177/2192568221998367] [PMID: 33840260]

[45]   Kim N, Hong Y, Lee SH. Two-year clinical outcomes of radiofrequency focal ablation using a navigable plasma disc decompression device in patients with lumbar disc herniation: efficacy and complications. J Pain Res 2018; 11: 2229-37.
[http://dx.doi.org/10.2147/JPR.S170704] [PMID: 30349349]

[46]   Freeman BJC, Mehdian R. Intradiscal electrothermal therapy, percutaneous discectomy, and nucleoplasty: What is the current evidence? Curr Pain Headache Rep 2008; 12(1): 14-21.
[http://dx.doi.org/10.1007/s11916-008-0004-7] [PMID: 18417018]

[47]   Quigley MR, Maroon JC, Shih T, Elrifai A, Lesiecki ML. Laser Discectomy. Spine 1994; 19(3): 319-22.
[http://dx.doi.org/10.1097/00007632-199402000-00011] [PMID: 8171364]

[48]   Hoogland T, Scheckenbach C. Low-dose chemonucleolysis combined with percutaneous nucleotomy in herniated cervical disks. J Spinal Disord 1995; 8(3): 228-32.
[http://dx.doi.org/10.1097/00002517-199506000-00009] [PMID: 7670215]

[49]   Kopchok GE, White RA, Mueller M, Cavaye D. Percutaneous laser discectomy. J Clin Laser Med Surg 1992; 10(2): 79-82.
[http://dx.doi.org/10.1089/clm.1992.10.79] [PMID: 10149904]

[50]   Yeung AT, Roberts A, Shin P, Rivers E, Paterson A, Paterson A. Suggestions for a Practical and Progressive Approach to Endoscopic Spine Surgery Training and Privileges. J Spine 2018; 7(2)
[http://dx.doi.org/10.4172/2165-7939.1000414]

[51]   Lewandrowski KU, Soriano-Sánchez JA, Zhang X, *et al.* Surgeon training and clinical implementation of spinal endoscopy in routine practice: results of a global survey. J Spine Surg 2020; 6(S1) (Suppl. 1): S237-48.
[http://dx.doi.org/10.21037/jss.2019.09.32] [PMID: 32195431]

[52]   Hussain I, Yeung AT, Wang MY. Challenges in Spinal Endoscopy. World Neurosurg 2022; 160: 132-7.
[http://dx.doi.org/10.1016/j.wneu.2021.11.082] [PMID: 35364671]

[53]   Butler AJ, Alam M, Wiley K, Ghasem A, Rush AJ III, Wang JC. Endoscopic Lumbar Surgery: The State of the Art in 2019. Neurospine 2019; 16(1): 15-23.
[http://dx.doi.org/10.14245/ns.1938040.020] [PMID: 30943703]

[54]   Xiu P, Zhang X. Endoscopic spine surgery in China: its evolution, flourishment, and future opportunity for advances. J Spine Surg 2020; 6(S1) (Suppl. 1): S49-53.
[http://dx.doi.org/10.21037/jss.2019.07.01] [PMID: 32195415]

[55]   Mayer HM. A History of Endoscopic Lumbar Spine Surgery: What Have We Learnt? BioMed Res Int 2019; 2019: 1-8.
[http://dx.doi.org/10.1155/2019/4583943] [PMID: 31139642]

[56]   Yeung A, Lewandrowski KU. Early and staged endoscopic management of common pain generators in the spine. J Spine Surg 2020; 6(S1) (Suppl. 1): S1-5.
[http://dx.doi.org/10.21037/jss.2019.09.03] [PMID: 32195407]

[57]   Gelalis ID, Christoforou G, Charchanti A, *et al.* Autologous platelet-rich plasma (PRP) effect on intervertebral disc restoration: an experimental rabbit model. Eur J Orthop Surg Traumatol 2019; 29(3): 545-51.
[http://dx.doi.org/10.1007/s00590-018-2337-1] [PMID: 30370433]

[58] Lutz C, Cheng J, Prysak M, Zukofsky T, Rothman R, Lutz G. Clinical outcomes following intradiscal injections of higher-concentration platelet-rich plasma in patients with chronic lumbar discogenic pain. Int Orthop 2022; 46(6): 1381-5.
[http://dx.doi.org/10.1007/s00264-022-05389-y] [PMID: 35344055]

[59] Buser Z, Chung AS, Abedi A, Wang JC. The future of disc surgery and regeneration. Int Orthop 2019; 43(4): 995-1002.
[http://dx.doi.org/10.1007/s00264-018-4254-7] [PMID: 30506089]

[60] Huang YC, Urban JPG, Luk KDK. Intervertebral disc regeneration: do nutrients lead the way? Nat Rev Rheumatol 2014; 10(9): 561-6.
[http://dx.doi.org/10.1038/nrrheum.2014.91] [PMID: 24914695]

[61] Akeda K, Ohishi K, Masuda K, *et al.* Intradiscal Injection of Autologous Platelet-Rich Plasma Releasate to Treat Discogenic Low Back Pain: A Preliminary Clinical Trial. Asian Spine J 2017; 11(3): 380-9.
[http://dx.doi.org/10.4184/asj.2017.11.3.380] [PMID: 28670405]

[62] Navani A, Manchikanti L, Albers SL, *et al.* Responsible, Safe, and Effective Use of Biologics in the Management of Low Back Pain: American Society of Interventional Pain Physicians (ASIPP) Guidelines. Pain Physician 2019; 22(1S): S1-S74.
[PMID: 30717500]

[63] Zielinski MA, Evans NE, Bae H, *et al.* Safety and Efficacy of Platelet Rich Plasma for Treatment of Lumbar Discogenic Pain: A Prospective, Multicenter, Randomized, Double-blind Study. Pain Physician 2022; 25(1): 29-34.
[PMID: 35051141]

[64] Gou S, Oxentenko SC, Eldrige JS, *et al.* Stem cell therapy for intervertebral disk regeneration. Am J Phys Med Rehabil 2014; 93(11) (Suppl. 3): S122-31.
[http://dx.doi.org/10.1097/PHM.0000000000000152] [PMID: 25122106]

[65] Cheng J, Santiago KA, Nguyen JT, Solomon JL, Lutz GE. Treatment of symptomatic degenerative intervertebral discs with autologous platelet-rich plasma: follow-up at 5-9 years. Regen Med 2019; 14(9): 831-40.
[http://dx.doi.org/10.2217/rme-2019-0040] [PMID: 31464577]

[66] Tuakli-Wosornu YA, Terry A, Boachie-Adjei K, *et al.* Lumbar Intradiskal Platelet☐Rich Plasma (PRP) Injections: A Prospective, Double☐Blind, Randomized Controlled Study. PM R 2016; 8(1): 1-10.
[http://dx.doi.org/10.1016/j.pmrj.2015.08.010] [PMID: 26314234]

[67] Ruschel LG, Agnoletto GJ, Aragão A, Duarte JS, de Oliveira MF, Teles AR. Lumbar disc herniation with contralateral radiculopathy: a systematic review on pathophysiology and surgical strategies. Neurosurg Rev 2021; 44(2): 1071-81.
[http://dx.doi.org/10.1007/s10143-020-01294-3] [PMID: 32281018]

[68] Beattie PF, Meyers SP, Stratford P, Millard RW, Hollenberg GM. Associations between patient report of symptoms and anatomic impairment visible on lumbar magnetic resonance imaging. Spine 2000; 25(7): 819-28.
[http://dx.doi.org/10.1097/00007632-200004010-00010] [PMID: 10751293]

[69] Kim SH, Choi SS, Lee MK, Kin JE. Complex Regional Pain Syndrome Caused by Lumbar Herniated Intervertebral Disc Disease. Pain Physician 2016; 19(6): E901-4.
[PMID: 27454281]

[70] den Boer JJ, Oostendorp RAB, Beems T, Munneke M, Evers AWM. Continued disability and pain after lumbar disc surgery: The role of cognitive-behavioral factors. Pain 2006; 123(1): 45-52.
[http://dx.doi.org/10.1016/j.pain.2006.02.008] [PMID: 16563624]

[71] Jensen RK, Kjaer P, Jensen TS, Albert H, Kent P. Degenerative Pathways of Lumbar Motion

Segments - A Comparison in Two Samples of Patients with Persistent Low Back Pain. PLoS One 2016; 11(1): e0146998.
[http://dx.doi.org/10.1371/journal.pone.0146998] [PMID: 26807697]

[72]   Lebow R, Parker SL, Adogwa O, *et al.* Microdiscectomy improves pain-associated depression, somatic anxiety, and mental well-being in patients with herniated lumbar disc. Neurosurgery 2012; 70(2): 306-11.
[http://dx.doi.org/10.1227/NEU.0b013e3182302ec3.] [PMID: 22251975]

[73]   Buric J, Rigobello L, Hooper D. Five and ten year follow-up on intradiscal ozone injection for disc herniation. Int J Spine Surg 2014; 8: 17.
[http://dx.doi.org/10.14444/1017] [PMID: 25694935]

[74]   Zwaan L, Monteiro S, Sherbino J, Ilgen J, Howey B, Norman G. Is bias in the eye of the beholder? A vignette study to assess recognition of cognitive biases in clinical case workups. BMJ Qual Saf 2017; 26(2): 104-10.
[http://dx.doi.org/10.1136/bmjqs-2015-005014] [PMID: 26825476]

[75]   Henriksen K, Kaplan H. Hindsight bias, outcome knowledge and adaptive learning. Qual Saf Health Care 2003; 12(90002) (Suppl. 2): 46ii-50.
[http://dx.doi.org/10.1136/qhc.12.suppl_2.ii46] [PMID: 14645895]

CHAPTER 9

Allogeneic Stem Cell Therapy for Painful Intermediate Lumbar Degenerative Discs

Álvaro Dowling[1], Juan Carlos Vera[2], Jorge Felipe Ramírez León[3,4,5], William Omar Contreras López[6], Morgan P. Lorio[7] and Kai-Uwe Lewandrowski[8,9,10,*]

[1] *Orthopaedic Spine Surgeon, Director of Endoscopic Spine Clinic, Santiago, Chile*

[2] *Universidad de Chile, Santiago, Chile*

[3] *Minimally Invasive Spine Center. Bogotá, D.C., Colombia*

[4] *Reina Sofía Clinic. Bogotá, D.C., Colombia*

[5] *Fundación Universitaria Sanitas. Bogotá, D.C., Colombia*

[6] *Clínica Foscal Internacional, Autopista Floridablanca - Girón, Km 7, Floridablanca, Santander, Colombia*

[7] *Advanced Orthopedics, 499 East Central Parkway, Altamonte Springs, FL 32701, USA*

[8] *Center for Advanced Spine Care of Southern Arizona and Surgical Institute of Tucson, Tucson, AZ, USA*

[9] *Departmemt of Orthopaedics, Fundación Universitaria Sanitas, Bogotá, D.C., Colombia*

[10] *Department of Neurosurgery in the Video-Endoscopic Postgraduate Program at the Universidade Federal do Estado do Rio de Janeiro - UNIRIO, Rio de Janeiro, Brazil*

Abstract: The management of mid-stage degenerative disc disease presenting with pain remains contentious, attributed in part to the scarcity of conclusive clinical trials. Allogeneic mesenchymal stem cells (MSCs), procured from donors, emerge as a viable alternative to autologous stem cell therapy. These MSCs are characterized by their accessibility and the streamlined administration process suitable for procedure-room settings, particularly for addressing discogenic lumbar pain. Within this manuscript, the authors delineate their proprietary protocol involving allogeneic MSC application, detailing the efficacy, safety, and clinical implications post-infusion into symptomatic lumbar intervertebral discs. Their clinical series encompassed 32 subjects, 14 females and 18 males, averaging 47.6 years of age, with a mean follow-up duration of 26.88 months. Two-year post-treatment evaluations revealed notable decrements in both ODI and VAS scores for lumbar pain. Evaluating Macnab outcomes, 11 participants (33.3%) showcased excellent results, 19 (57.6%) reported good outcomes, and a mere 3 (9.1%) indicated fair results. Notably, none necessitated supplementary interventions at

* **Corresponding author Kai-Uwe Lewandrowski:** Center for Advanced Spine Care of Southern Arizona and Surgical Institute of Tucson, Tucson, AZ, USA; Departmemt of Orthopaedics, Fundación Universitaria Sanitas, Bogotá, D.C., Colombia and Department of Neurosurgery in the Video-Endoscopic Postgraduate Program at the Universidade Federal do Estado do Rio de Janeiro - UNIRIO, Rio de Janeiro, Brazil; E-mail: adowling@dws.cl

the MSC-treated disc level. Despite the study's constraints, such as its observational nature, potential selection and hindsight biases, and modest participant count, the authors' findings substantiate the potential of intradiscal allogeneic MSC injections in managing mid-stage painful degenerative disc afflictions. To fortify these preliminary insights, future research endeavors should encompass a more regimented structure, potentially incorporating a placebo cohort or a natural progression study group.

Keywords: Allogeneic, Mesenchymal stem cells, Low back pain, Degenerative intervertebral disc disease.

INTRODUCTION

The dawn of the 21st century heralded significant strides in biotechnology, ushering in transformative therapeutic modalities that have markedly elevated patient care and outcomes. Predominantly, regenerative medicine has spearheaded this metamorphosis, encompassing novel techniques like cell therapy, gene therapy, and tissue engineering [1 - 4]. Forefront interventions in this arena include the deployment of platelet-enriched plasma [5 - 8], stem cells [3, 9], and the derivatives procured from their culture. These interventions, in many cases, have not only ameliorated symptoms but also proffered potential cures [10 - 12].

A meticulous review by Sanapati *et al.* probed into the therapeutic efficacy of mesenchymal stem cells (MSCs) and platelet-rich plasma (PRP) for conditions including discogenic low back pain, radicular pain, and sacroiliac joint pain, among others [13]. The outcomes showcased a spectrum of evidentiary support for the therapeutic promise of MSCs and PRP for these pain manifestations.

In contemporary research, allogeneic stem cell transplantation has surfaced as a compelling counterpart to autologous bone marrow transplants [14 - 17]. Its preeminence is accentuated by its capacity to curtail functional discrepancies through the employment of multi-donor cell aggregates housed in a central repository. Notably, MSCs exhibit an inherent aptitude for allogeneic transplantation with a negligibly low rejection proclivity [18]. Within this discourse, the authors delineate their modus operandi for deploying allogeneic stem cell interventions for degenerative disc disease (DDD)-induced pain. The overarching endeavor is to interrogate the therapeutic safety profile of MSCs and their potential to mitigate chronic low back pain (CLBP) symptoms, thereby optimizing patient functionality. This exploration aims to set the stage for ensuing inquiries into the merits and safety considerations of allogeneic stem cell interventions for back pain and varying stages of DDD.

This chapter's focus is the safety appraisal of a solitary allogeneic MSC injection in a clinical setting, targeting a symptomatic lumbar disc, and concurrently gauging the ensuing therapeutic ramifications in patients grappling with CLBP linked to moderate DDD.

Allogeneic Mesenchymal Stem Cells (MSCs)

The increase of allogeneic mesenchymal stem cells (MSCs) in regenerative medicine positions them as an attractive counterpart to autologous transplants. Sourced from external donors, these cells stand out due to their simplified procurement process, stellar safety record, and demonstrated efficacy in addressing myriad medical and musculoskeletal maladies. Typically extracted from bone marrow, peripheral blood, or umbilical cord blood, allogeneic MSCs present diminished risks associated with contamination, mutation, and graft rejection compared to their autologous counterparts. These multipotent cells, endowed with the ability for differentiation into diverse cell types and self-renewal, also exhibit pronounced immunomodulatory attributes, making them compelling candidates for managing inflammatory and autoimmune disorders. Advantages encompass expedited transplantation timelines, diminished infection risks, procedural complications, and lessened reliance on intensive immunosuppression.

One realm where the therapeutic potential of allogeneic stem cells shines is in addressing degenerative disc disease (DDD), a predominant contributor to chronic low back pain. DDD's etiology involves intervertebral disc degradation, precipitating disc herniation, spinal stenosis, and nerve entrapment. Conventional DDD interventions span medications, physical rehabilitative therapies, and surgical approaches, but their efficacy is oftentimes transient and fraught with potential risks. Research, such as the study by Pettine *et al.*, underscores the substantial efficacy and safety of MSCs in ameliorating discogenic pain and restoring function. Multiple investigations [19 - 24] corroborate the well-tolerated nature of these cells, with an absence of grave adverse outcomes, reinforcing their therapeutic promise in offering sustained respite from chronic lumbar discomfort.

Yet, navigating the therapeutic deployment of allogeneic stem cells is not devoid of challenges. Immune rejection [25], stemming from the recipient's immune defenses perceiving the introduced cells as alien, remains a concern [26]. Strategies to curb this include meticulous cell matching to the recipient's tissue. Notably, heavy immunosuppressive regimens are generally unnecessary. Nonetheless, an in-depth exploration into their clinical viability, safety contours, and economic competitiveness in juxtaposition to other regenerative modalities is imperative.

Allogenic Stem Cell Disc Therapy: A Comprehensive Analysis

A multi-site randomized trial [19] was initiated to examine the safety and efficacy of a singular intradiscal injection containing STRO-3+ allogeneic mesenchymal precursor cells (MPCs) coupled with hyaluronic acid (HA) for individuals suffering from chronic low back pain (CLBP) due to degenerative disc disease (DDD). Conducted across 13 clinical institutions, including 12 in the United States and one in Australia, the trial enrolled 100 participants with a diagnosis of CLBP and moderate DDD, based on the modified Pfirrmann score criteria. These participants, all of whom had endured CLBP for a minimum of six months, were previously unresponsive to a quarter-year of conservative treatments.

The participants were systematically divided into groups based on treatment: 6 million MPCs with HA, 18 million MPCs with HA, a HA vehicle control, and a saline control. Throughout the three-year observation period, their responses to the treatments were meticulously evaluated. Outcomes were gauged through an assortment of clinical and radiographic evaluations at specified intervals post-injection, capturing parameters like the Visual Analog Scale (VAS) and the Oswestry Disability Index (ODI). Comprehensive safety evaluations included adverse event monitoring, rigorous physical examinations, radiographic checks, and laboratory diagnostics. Efficacy was deduced by contrasting VAS, ODI, and modified Pfirrmann (MP) scores.

Conclusively, the MPC treatment groups manifested a superior trajectory in VAS and ODI enhancements in comparison to controls over various time intervals within the 36-month span. Notably, there was no detectable distinction in the modification of the MP scores from their baseline across all treatment cohorts. The entire procedure exhibited excellent tolerability, and immune responses to the allogeneic MPCs were absent. Moreover, adverse reactions were few and bore no significant difference between the MPC-treated and control groups. This comprehensive evaluation suggests that intradiscal MPC injections could be a robust, sustainable, and minimally invasive strategy for treating CLBP related to moderate DDD.

Another insightful study by Noriega *et al.* [22] delved into the feasibility, safety, and potential clinical utility of allogeneic stem cells for patients diagnosed with lumbar disc degeneration presenting with chronic back pain. In this randomized setup, 24 subjects, all of whom were refractory to conventional treatments, were equally distributed between two groups: a cohort receiving intradiscal allogeneic bone marrow mesenchymal stem cell (MSC) injections and a control group subjected to a placebo paravertebral infiltration. The monitored clinical endpoints over a year included pain perception, functional disability, life quality, and disc quality using magnetic resonance imaging.

The results from this investigation furnished initial evidence endorsing the safety and prospective efficacy of allogeneic stem cell modalities for lumbar degeneration-induced chronic back pain. Beneficiaries of MSC therapy showcased noteworthy functional improvements compared to placebo recipients. Yet, this enhancement seemed confined to a responder subset, encompassing 40% of the total participants. The MSC cohort exhibited positive disc quality changes, while controls revealed deteriorating degenerative signs. These discoveries imply allogeneic MSC therapy as a potential candidate for addressing degenerative disc pathologies, underscoring its edge over autologous MSC strategies due to logistical conveniences. The non-invasive procedure not only alleviates pain but significantly revamps the structural integrity of intervertebral discs. Further studies have validated these conclusions [26, 27].

Mesenchymal Stem Cell Harvesting and Advanced Expansion Techniques

From the umbilical cord's mononuclear cell fraction, with mothers' informed consent, allogeneic mesenchymal stem cells (MSCs) were harvested. The acquisition of umbilical cord MSCs (UC-MSC) ensued immediately postpartum. The ex-vivo amplification of these cells, specifically those derived from Wharton's Jelly (WJ-MSCs), was meticulously conducted under current good manufacturing practice (CGMP) conditions at a specialized contract manufacturing facility. The WJ-MSCs, intrinsically analogous in genetic and physiological aspects to neonates, were precisely utilized.

Aseptically harvested, 10 cm segments of the umbilical cord were immersed in a protective medium supplemented with antibiotics, stored at 4°C, and subsequently transferred to the laboratory. Thereafter, the Wharton's Jelly was sectioned into 1-2 mm fragments and situated on gelatin-coated 100 mm dishes. Each dish received 2 grams of WJ tissue and was bathed in a specialized culture medium — a concoction of low-glucose Dulbecco's Modified Eagle's Medium (DMEM-LG), fortified with fetal bovine serum (FBS) and essential antibiotics. On the eighth day, post the removal of tissue fragments, a fresh medium was introduced. Cultures, rich in WJ-MSCs, thrived at 37°C, ensconced in a controlled atmosphere with 5% CO_2. Once an 80% confluence was achieved, 0.05% Trypsin-EDTA was employed for cell dissociation, following which the cells underwent washing and centrifugation, and were systematically seeded at a density of 1×10^4 cells/cm^2.

For therapeutic applications, the cells were cultivated until the fifth passage, preserving their assumed pluripotent nature. To mitigate risks associated with cell differentiation and decreased functionality, any expansion beyond this stage was circumvented. This comprehensive cellular process, including harvesting, refinement, cryopreservation, and storage, took place at a CGMP-compliant facility certified by the Association for the Advancement of Blood & Biotherapies (AABB). The cell product's viability was scrupulously assessed using Trypan blue exclusion, human leukocyte antigen Class II (HLA-DR) expression, and thorough analysis of mesenchymal markers like CD44, CD90, CD105, and CD34 *via* flow cytometry. Rigorous tests ensured the absence of infectious agents, microbial contaminants, endotoxins, and mycoplasma. Finally, the cells, securely cryopreserved, were dispatched to clinical centers in a state primed for clinical application, ready to be administered into the target disc by proficient medical personnel.

Intervertebral Disc Inoculation

Utilizing a refined posterior-lateral technique under fluoroscopic guidance, we employed an 18-gauge needle consistent with the established procedures of provocative discography. The subjects, positioned in the prone stance and under the careful watch of monitored anesthesia care (MAC) protocols, were administered approximately 5 million allogeneic progenitor cells (APC) suspended in a 1% hyaluronic acid (HA) matrix, a widely accepted medium for human MSC injections (27,28).

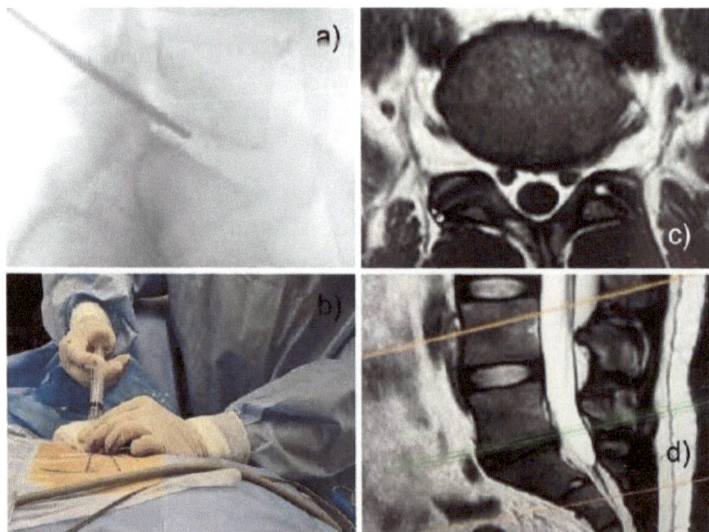

Fig. (1). A depiction of a patient undergoing intradiscal inoculation with 5 million APCs in 1% HA targeting the L5/S1 region to address intermediate degenerative disc disease, a diagnosis validated *via* provocative discography.

For prophylactic purposes, prior to and subsequent to the inoculation, patients were given oral cephalosporin or a suitable quinolone alternative in cases where second-generation cephalosporin allergies were documented. Post-inoculation, a 30-minute observation period in the recovery suite was mandated, ensuring meticulous monitoring of vital parameters to preemptively identify any anaphylactic manifestations. Pre-requisites for patient discharge encompassed stabilized vital metrics and overall well-being. Fig. (**2**): Illustration showcasing the targeted infusion of MSCs into the afflicted intervertebral disc.

Cohort-analysis

Between December 2017 and November 2018, we enrolled participants across four distinct research centers. All subjects were tracked for a minimum of 24 months, culminating in an average observation span of 26.88 months. The cohort consisted of 32 individuals, of which 14 were females and 18 were males, presenting a mean age of 47.6 years. Given the current designation of mesenchymal stem cells (MSCs) as a biological entity rather than a pharmacological agent, and their prevalent application in diverse conditions like graft *versus* host disease (GVHD) and degenerative osteoarthritis, the study proceeded without FDA endorsement or registration on clinicaltrials.gov.

Eligibility necessitated the following criteria: 1) An established diagnosis of moderate degenerative disc disease (DDD) at any segment between L1 and S1, 2) Chronic lumbar discomfort persisting over 12 months with a visual analog scale (VAS) rating exceeding 5, 3) A three-month history of refractory conservative interventions, and 4) A Pfirrmann categorization ranging between III and V. Those presenting with complicating factors like concurrent disc pathologies, infections, traumas, spondylolisthesis, radiculopathy, symptoms of stenosis in alternate zones, or neoplastic conditions were precluded. The meticulous application of these eligibility parameters culminated in a research group of 32 individuals. A preceding power analysis affirmed that this cohort size sufficiently evaluated the safety of allogeneic MSC intervertebral injections in this observational context.

To pinpoint the symptomatic disc, a composite of medical chronicles, clinical evaluations, and MRI diagnostics were employed, necessitating an initial provocative lumbar discography. Notably, the Pfirrmann classification, a tool for classifying disc degeneration *via* MRI, was not utilized for patient stratification vis-a-vis MSC treatment due to its incongruence with clinical presentations. However, this grading system was pivotal in analyzing and contrasting morphological modifications pre and post-MSC inoculation, serving as a barometer of prospective regenerative outcomes.

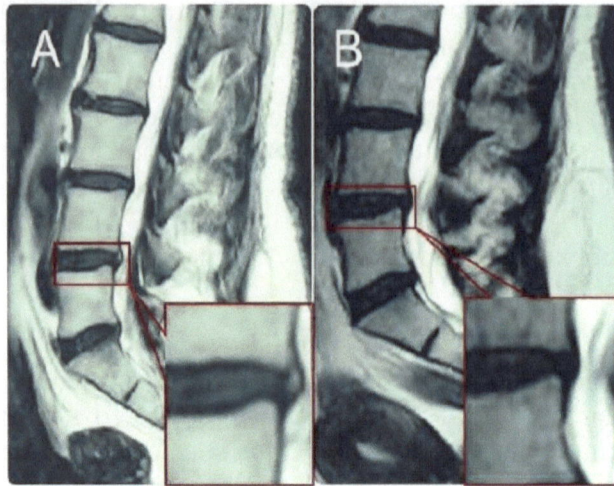

Fig. (2). In a prototypical case, an individual presenting with advanced degenerative disc disease at L4/5 received an intradiscal administration of 5 million allogeneic progenitor cells suspended in 1% hyaluronic acid. Initial sagittal T2-weighted MRI (A) depicted Pfirrmann grade III disc degeneration accompanied by an annular fissure (cutout A). Remarkably, a subsequent one-year MRI (B) intimates annular repair post-treatment (cutout B).

Our preliminary investigation found the therapeutic approach largely devoid of complications, safe for one individual who grappled with intense lumbar discomfort briefly post-procedure. Subsequent treatments specific to the MSC-injected disc level were redundant for all participants. At the two-year evaluation milestone, 22 of the initial 32 subjects remained in the follow-up. The aggregated visual analog scale (VAS) readings for lumbar pain exhibited marked declines at every standardized assessment relative to the baseline. Specifically, the VAS metrics dwindled from an initial 8.22 ± 1.43 (n = 32) to 3.31 ± 1.78 at one month, then further tapered to 2.57 ± 1.67 by the third month (n = 28), 2.03 ± 1.38 at half-year (n = 30), 1.81 ± 1.50 at the year's end (n = 27), culminating at a minuscule 1.74 ± 1.32 by the second-year's conclusion (n = 23; Table **1**). These trajectories were underpinned by robust statistical validation ($p < 0.001$) from the initial post-operative month onwards (Table **1**). By the second-year evaluation, there was a profound decrement of 6.565 ± 1.619 in the VAS metric ($p < 0.001$).

Table 1. Means and Paired Sampled T-test results of pre- and postoperative VAS scores for low back pain after allogeneic cell injections at scheduled follow-up and final visit.

VAS Back	Mean	N	Std. Deviation	Std. Error Mean
Preop VAS	8.22	32	1.431	.253
Postop VAS 1 Month	3.31	32	1.786	.316
Postop VAS 3 Months	2.57	28	1.665	.315

(Table 1) cont.....

VAS Back	Mean	N	Std. Deviation	Std. Error Mean
Postop VAS 6 Months	2.03	30	1.377	.251
Postop VAS 1 Year	1.81	27	1.495	.288
Postop VAS 2 Years	1.74	23	1.322	.276

VAS Reduction	Mean	Std. Deviation	Std. Error Mean	95% Confidence Interval of the Difference		t	df	Significance	
				Lower	Upper			One-Sided p	Two-Sided p
Preop VAS - Postop VAS 1 Month	4.906	1.990	.352	4.189	5.624	13.949	31	<.001	<.001
Preop VAS - Postop VAS 3 Months	5.500	2.134	.403	4.672	6.328	13.635	27	<.001	<.001
Preop VAS - Postop VAS 6 Months	6.167	2.001	.365	5.419	6.914	16.876	29	<.001	<.001
Preop VAS - Postop VAS 1 Year	6.370	1.644	.316	5.720	7.021	20.131	26	<.001	<.001
Preop VAS - Postop VAS 2 Years	6.565	1.619	.338	5.865	7.265	19.450	22	<.001	<.001

Evident amelioration in the Oswestry Disability Index (ODI) was observed ($p < 0.001$). From a preoperative mean of 44.81 ± 14.35 (n=32), the ODI metric systematically subsided to 19.58 ± 11.62 within a month, progressing further to 15.38 ± 12.83 at the quarter-year mark (n=29), 13.48 ± 10.16 by mid-year (n=31), 11.80 ± 10.61 after one year, and bottoming at 6.07 ± 8.34 by the second year's culmination (n=30; Table **2**). This two-year juncture marked a substantial ODI decrement of 38.333 ± 14.865 ($p < 0.001$; Table **2**). The baseline Pfirrmann grade, an MRI-based metric delineating disc degeneration, averaged 4.05 ± 0.72 but exhibited a positive shift to 3.65 ± 0.81 at the two-year assessment. This favorable trajectory in Pfirrmann gradation achieved robust statistical affirmation with a p-value of < 0.001, showcased in Fig. (**1**).

Table 2. Paired Sampled T-test of pre- and postoperative ODI scores reductions for low back pain after allogeneic cell injections and at scheduled follow-up and final visit.

	Mean	N	Std. Deviation	Std. Error Mean
Preop ODI	44.8125	32	14.34919	2.53660
Postop ODI 1 Month	19.6875	32	11.61878	2.05393
Postop ODI 3 Month	15.38	29	12.830	2.382
Postop ODI 6 Month	13.48	31	10.158	1.824
Postop ODI 1 Year	11.80	30	10.601	1.935
Postop ODI 2 Years	6.07	30	8.346	1.524

ODI Reduction	Mean	Std. Deviation	Std. Error Mean	95% Confidence Interval of the Difference		t	df	Significance	
				Lower	Upper			One-Sided p	Two-Sided p
Preop ODI – Postop ODI 1 Month	25.125	14.430	2.550	19.922	30.327	9.849	31	<.001	<.001
Preop ODI - Postop ODI 3 Months	30.137	16.448	3.054	23.881	36.394	9.867	28	<.001	<.001
Preop ODI - Postop ODI 6 Months	31.161	16.802	3.017	24.997	37.324	10.325	30	<.001	<.001
Preop ODI - Postop ODI 1 Year	33.800	15.855	2.894	27.879	39.720	11.676	29	<.001	<.001
Preop ODI - Postop ODI 2 Year	38.333	14.865	2.714	32.782	43.884	14.124	29	<.001	<.001

Post intradiscal MSC intervention, remarkable patient enhancements manifested within the initial month—a pronounced VAS dip for lumbar discomfort by 74.73%, and a 65.54% ODI alleviation were noted immediately post-operation. Macnab outcomes post-intervention were predominantly encouraging: 33.3% of patients recounted exemplary results, 57.6% acknowledged good responses, while a mere 9.1% gave a modest assessment at the terminal evaluation (Table **3**).

Table 3. Postoperative Macnab outcomes at final follow up.

	Frequency	Percent	Valid Percent	Cumulative Percent
Excellent	11	33.3	33.3	33.3
Good	19	57.6	57.6	90.9
Fair	3	9.1	9.1	100.0
Total	33	100.0	100.0	

DISCUSSION

Chronic lumbar pain (CLP), primarily attributable to intervertebral disc degeneration, is not only a leading contributor to work absenteeism but also has profound repercussions on an individual's quality of life. The economic and societal implications of degenerative lumbar disc disease are staggering and affect individuals, particularly in middle and advanced age, globally [28, 29]. Conventional therapeutic interventions range from conservative measures like anti-inflammatory medications and physiotherapy to more invasive strategies like spinal surgery. Notably, fusion surgeries can inadvertently catalyze adjacent segment degeneration due to heightened spinal stress from metal implantation. Procedures emphasizing motion preservation, such as artificial disc replacement, are not without their challenges, including implant failures and anomalous bone growth adjacent to the device [30 - 34].

Regenerative medicine is witnessing an upsurge in interest, particularly those predicated on allogeneic platforms, celebrated for their scalability, economic feasibility, and widespread availability, as underscored by the Alliance for Regenerative Medicine (ARM) [35]. ClinicalTrials.gov showcases approximately 1300 ongoing trials centered on the multifaceted therapeutic applications of mesenchymal stem cells (MSCs), with a sizable number already progressing into Phase II or III stages. A significant proportion of these investigations cater to the medical challenges predominantly faced by aging demographics [27, 36 - 38].

Annually, new clinical data burgeon the knowledge repository of regenerative medicine. The clinical endeavors thus far have vouched for the safety and efficacy of stem cell-based therapeutics [9, 22, 39 - 44]. Stem cell therapy, depending on its derivation, bifurcates into autologous or allogeneic types. The former, leveraging cells from the patients themselves, has seen application in realms like cardiac repair, cartilage regeneration, and aesthetic augmentation [14, 42, 45].

Scientific literature robustly documents the potential of platelet-rich plasma, stem cells, and other biological interventions in disc degeneration and back pain management [46]. The infancy of regulatory approvals for MSCs does not detract from their significant clinical milestones. For instance, Prochymal™ and Alofisel™ have gained regulatory nods in various countries for specific indications [52]. Recent research trajectories have shifted from MSCs to their derivatives, such as exosomes, which have demonstrated intriguing biological roles, particularly in tissue repair and immunomodulation [53 - 57]. This study delves into the potential of MSCs in managing painful degenerative disc disease, despite its inherent limitations.

Our study's findings accentuate the therapeutic potential of MSC injections in ameliorating CLP associated with lumbar disc degeneration. The study cohort evidenced consistent relief from clinical symptoms and MRI-evident enhancements over two years. While conventional back pain remedies often offer transient relief and inadvertently contribute to the opioid epidemic, our study highlights significant longitudinal benefits. Yet, the observational design, modest cohort size, and inherent clinical evidence grade call for caution against biases. Despite limitations, the discernible amelioration in clinical and radiological metrics post-MSC treatment underscores the therapeutic promise [58, 59].

CONCLUSION

Harnessing allogeneic mesenchymal stem cells (MSCs) offers an appealing alternative to autologous derivations. The readily accessible allogeneic MSCs streamline both the acquisition and expansion phases. Our preliminary data exude optimism, illustrating tangible benefits in both pain metrics and clinical functionality, corroborated by improved MRI parameters. The future will determine whether these MSC-based interventions could challenge or supersede established procedures like interbody fusion. Regardless, as the continuum of clinical evidence evolves, we stand at the cusp of potentially transformative advancements in spine care, reflective of this discipline's rapid evolution.

REFERENCES

[1] Richardson SM, Kalamegam G, Pushparaj PN, *et al.* Mesenchymal stem cells in regenerative medicine: Focus on articular cartilage and intervertebral disc regeneration. Methods 2016; 99: 69-80.
[http://dx.doi.org/10.1016/j.ymeth.2015.09.015] [PMID: 26384579]

[2] Priyadarshani P, Li Y, Yao L. Advances in biological therapy for nucleus pulposus regeneration. Osteoarthritis Cartilage 2016; 24(2): 206-12.
[http://dx.doi.org/10.1016/j.joca.2015.08.014] [PMID: 26342641]

[3] Kregar Velikonja N, Urban J, Fröhlich M, *et al.* Cell sources for nucleus pulposus regeneration. Eur Spine J 2014; 23(S3) (Suppl. 3): 364-74.
[http://dx.doi.org/10.1007/s00586-013-3106-9] [PMID: 24297331]

[4] Goldschlager T, Oehme D, Ghosh P, Zannettino A, Rosenfeld J, Jenkin G. Current and future applications for stem cell therapies in spine surgery. Curr Stem Cell Res Ther 2013; 8(5): 381-93.
[http://dx.doi.org/10.2174/1574888X113089990048] [PMID: 23971834]

[5]   Dai WL, Zhou AG, Zhang H, Zhang J. Efficacy of Platelet-Rich Plasma in the Treatment of Knee Osteoarthritis: A Meta-analysis of Randomized Controlled Trials. Arthroscopy 2017; 33(3): 659-670.e1.
[http://dx.doi.org/10.1016/j.arthro.2016.09.024] [PMID: 28012636]

[6]   Martinez-Zapata MJ, Martí-Carvajal AJ, Solà I, *et al.* Autologous platelet-rich plasma for treating chronic wounds. Cochrane Libr 2016; 2016(5): CD006899.
[http://dx.doi.org/10.1002/14651858.CD006899.pub3] [PMID: 27223580]

[7]   Harmon KG, Rao AL. The use of platelet-rich plasma in the nonsurgical management of sports injuries: hype or hope? Hematology (Am Soc Hematol Educ Program) 2013; 2013(1): 620-6.
[http://dx.doi.org/10.1182/asheducation-2013.1.620] [PMID: 24319241]

[8]   Mishra A, Harmon K, Woodall J, Vieira A. Sports medicine applications of platelet rich plasma. Curr Pharm Biotechnol 2012; 13(7): 1185-95.
[http://dx.doi.org/10.2174/138920112800624283] [PMID: 21740373]

[9]   Kim MJ, Lee JH, Kim JS, *et al.* Intervertebral Disc Regeneration Using Stem Cell/Growth Factor-Loaded Porous Particles with a Leaf-Stacked Structure. Biomacromolecules 2020; 21(12): 4795-805.
[http://dx.doi.org/10.1021/acs.biomac.0c00992] [PMID: 32955865]

[10]   Tavakoli J, Diwan AD, Tipper JL. Advanced Strategies for the Regeneration of Lumbar Disc Annulus Fibrosus. Int J Mol Sci 2020; 21(14): 4889.
[http://dx.doi.org/10.3390/ijms21144889] [PMID: 32664453]

[11]   Perez-Cruet M, Beeravolu N, McKee C, *et al.* Potential of Human Nucleus Pulposus-Like Cells Derived From Umbilical Cord to Treat Degenerative Disc Disease. Neurosurgery 2019; 84(1): 272-83.
[http://dx.doi.org/10.1093/neuros/nyy012] [PMID: 29490072]

[12]   Hwang JJ, Rim YA, Nam Y, Ju JH. Recent Developments in Clinical Applications of Mesenchymal Stem Cells in the Treatment of Rheumatoid Arthritis and Osteoarthritis. Front Immunol 2021; 12: 631291.
[http://dx.doi.org/10.3389/fimmu.2021.631291] [PMID: 33763076]

[13]   Sanapati J, Manchikanti L, Atluri S, *et al.* Do Regenerative Medicine Therapies Provide Long-Term Relief in Chronic Low Back Pain: A Systematic Review and Metaanalysis. Pain Physician 2018; 21(6): 515-40.
[PMID: 30508983]

[14]   Pettine KA, Murphy MB, Suzuki RK, Sand TT. Percutaneous injection of autologous bone marrow concentrate cells significantly reduces lumbar discogenic pain through 12 months. Stem Cells 2015; 33(1): 146-56.
[http://dx.doi.org/10.1002/stem.1845] [PMID: 25187512]

[15]   Pettine K, Suzuki R, Sand T, Murphy M. Treatment of discogenic back pain with autologous bone marrow concentrate injection with minimum two year follow-up. Int Orthop 2016; 40(1): 135-40.
[http://dx.doi.org/10.1007/s00264-015-2886-4] [PMID: 26156727]

[16]   Pettine KA, Suzuki RK, Sand TT, Murphy MB. Autologous bone marrow concentrate intradiscal injection for the treatment of degenerative disc disease with three-year follow-up. Int Orthop 2017; 41(10): 2097-103.
[http://dx.doi.org/10.1007/s00264-017-3560-9] [PMID: 28748380]

[17]   Atluri S, Murphy MB, Dragella R, *et al.* Evaluation of the Effectiveness of Autologous Bone Marrow Mesenchymal Stem Cells in the Treatment of Chronic Low Back Pain Due to Severe Lumbar Spinal Degeneration: A 12-Month, Open-Label, Prospective Controlled Trial. Pain Physician 2022; 25(2): 193-207.
[PMID: 35322978]

[18]   Discher DE, Mooney DJ, Zandstra PW. Growth factors, matrices, and forces combine and control stem cells. Science 2009; 324(5935): 1673-7.

[http://dx.doi.org/10.1126/science.1171643] [PMID: 19556500]

[19]   Sudo H, Miyakoshi T, Watanabe Y, *et al.* Protocol for treating lumbar spinal canal stenosis with a combination of ultrapurified, allogenic bone marrow-derived mesenchymal stem cells and in situ-forming gel: a multicentre, prospective, double-blind randomised controlled trial. BMJ Open 2023; 13(2): e065476.
[http://dx.doi.org/10.1136/bmjopen-2022-065476] [PMID: 36731929]

[20]   Subhan RA, Puvanan K, Murali MR, *et al.* Fluoroscopy assisted minimally invasive transplantation of allogenic mesenchymal stromal cells embedded in HyStem reduces the progression of nucleus pulposus degeneration in the damaged ntervertebral [corrected] disc: a preliminary study in rabbits. ScientificWorldJournal 2014; 2014: 818502.
[PMID: 24983002]

[21]   Sharun K, Kumar R, Chandra V, *et al.* Percutaneous transplantation of allogenic bone marrow-derived mesenchymal stem cells for the management of paraplegia secondary to Hansen type I intervertebral disc herniation in a Beagle dog. Majallah-i Tahqiqat-i Dampizishki-i Iran 2021; 22(2): 161-6.
[PMID: 34306116]

[22]   Noriega DC, Ardura F, Hernández-Ramajo R, *et al.* Intervertebral Disc Repair by Allogeneic Mesenchymal Bone Marrow Cells. Transplantation 2017; 101(8): 1945-51.
[http://dx.doi.org/10.1097/TP.0000000000001484] [PMID: 27661661]

[23]   Noriega DC, Ardura F, Hernández-Ramajo R, *et al.* Treatment of Degenerative Disc Disease With Allogeneic Mesenchymal Stem Cells: Long-term Follow-up Results. Transplantation 2021; 105(2): e25-7.
[http://dx.doi.org/10.1097/TP.0000000000003471] [PMID: 33492116]

[24]   Lewandrowski KU, Dowling A, Vera JC, Leon JFR, Telfeian AE, Lorio MP. Pain Relief After Allogenic Stem Cell Disc Therapy. Pain Physician 2023; 26(2): 197-206.
[PMID: 36988365]

[25]   Amirdelfan K, Bae H, McJunkin T, *et al.* Allogeneic mesenchymal precursor cells treatment for chronic low back pain associated with degenerative disc disease: a prospective randomized, placebo-controlled 36-month study of safety and efficacy. Spine J 2021; 21(2): 212-30.
[PMID: 33045417]

[26]   Cunha C, Almeida CR, Almeida MI, *et al.* Systemic Delivery of Bone Marrow Mesenchymal Stem Cells for In Situ Intervertebral Disc Regeneration. Stem Cells Transl Med 2017; 6(3): 1029-39.
[http://dx.doi.org/10.5966/sctm.2016-0033] [PMID: 28297581]

[27]   Freeman BJC, Kuliwaba JS, Jones CF, *et al.* Allogeneic Mesenchymal Precursor Cells Promote Healing in Postero-lateral Annular Lesions and Improve Indices of Lumbar Intervertebral Disc Degeneration in an Ovine Model. Spine 2016; 41(17): 1331-9.
[http://dx.doi.org/10.1097/BRS.0000000000001528] [PMID: 26913464]

[28]   Ravindra VM, Senglaub SS, Rattani A, *et al.* Degenerative Lumbar Spine Disease: Estimating Global Incidence and Worldwide Volume. Global Spine J 2018; 8(8): 784-94.
[http://dx.doi.org/10.1177/2192568218770769] [PMID: 30560029]

[29]   Smith JS, Shaffrey CI, Baldus CR, *et al.* Orthopedic disease burden in adult patients with symptomatic lumbar scoliosis: results from a prospective multicenter study. J Neurosurg Spine 2021; 35(6): 743-51.
[http://dx.doi.org/10.3171/2021.1.SPINE201911] [PMID: 34416734]

[30]   Leggett LE, Soril LJJ, Lorenzetti DL, *et al.* Radiofrequency ablation for chronic low back pain: a systematic review of randomized controlled trials. Pain Res Manag 2014; 19(5): e146-53.
[PMID: 25068973]

[31]   Burgstaller JM, Steurer J, Gravestock I, *et al.* Long-term Results After Surgical or Nonsurgical Treatment in Patients With Degenerative Lumbar Spinal Stenosis. Spine 2020; 45(15): 1030-8.
[http://dx.doi.org/10.1097/BRS.0000000000003457] [PMID: 32675604]

[32]   Yee TJ, Terman SW, La Marca F, Park P. Comparison of adjacent segment disease after minimally invasive or open transforaminal lumbar interbody fusion. J Clin Neurosci 2014; 21(10): 1796-801. [PMID: 24880486]

[33]   Zhu H, Wang G, Zhou Z, Fan S. Prospective Study of Long□term Effect between Multifidus Muscle Bundle and Conventional Open Approach in One□level Posterior Lumbar Interbody Fusion. Orthop Surg 2018; 10(4): 296-305. [http://dx.doi.org/10.1111/os.12402] [PMID: 30402963]

[34]   Zigler JE, Glenn J, Delamarter RB. Five-year adjacent-level degenerative changes in patients with single-level disease treated using lumbar total disc replacement with ProDisc-L *versus* circumferential fusion. J Neurosurg Spine 2012; 17(6): 504-11. [http://dx.doi.org/10.3171/2012.9.SPINE11717] [PMID: 23082849]

[35]   Alliance for Regenerative Medicine. Available from: https://alliancerm.org/publications-presentations

[36]   Fu X, Liu G, Halim A, Ju Y, Luo Q, Song AG. Mesenchymal Stem Cell Migration and Tissue Repair. Cells 2019; 8(8): 784. [http://dx.doi.org/10.3390/cells8080784] [PMID: 31357692]

[37]   Liu H, Li D, Zhang Y, Li M. Inflammation, mesenchymal stem cells and bone regeneration. Histochem Cell Biol 2018; 149(4): 393-404. [http://dx.doi.org/10.1007/s00418-018-1643-3] [PMID: 29435765]

[38]   Qian Z, Wang H, Bai Y, *et al.* Improving Chronic Diabetic Wound Healing through an Injectable and Self-Healing Hydrogel with Platelet-Rich Plasma Release. ACS Appl Mater Interfaces 2020; 12(50): 55659-74. [http://dx.doi.org/10.1021/acsami.0c17142] [PMID: 33327053]

[39]   Amirdelfan K, Bae H, McJunkin T, DePalma M, Kim K, Beckworth WJ, *et al.* Allogeneic Mesenchymal Precursor Cells Treatment for Chronic Low Back Pain Associated with Degenerative Disc Disease: A Prospective Randomized, Placebo-Controlled 36-Month Study of Safety and Efficacy. Spine J 2020. [PMID: 33045417]

[40]   Anderson DG, Markova D, An HS, *et al.* Human umbilical cord blood-derived mesenchymal stem cells in the cultured rabbit intervertebral disc: a novel cell source for disc repair. Am J Phys Med Rehabil 2013; 92(5): 420-9. [http://dx.doi.org/10.1097/PHM.0b013e31825f148a] [PMID: 23598901]

[41]   Duarte RM, Varanda P, Reis RL, Duarte ARC, Correia-Pinto J. Biomaterials and Bioactive Agents in Spinal Fusion. Tissue Eng Part B Rev 2017; 23(6): 540-51. [http://dx.doi.org/10.1089/ten.teb.2017.0072] [PMID: 28514897]

[42]   García de Frutos A, González-Tartière P, Coll Bonet R, *et al.* Randomized clinical trial: expanded autologous bone marrow mesenchymal cells combined with allogeneic bone tissue, compared with autologous iliac crest graft in lumbar fusion surgery. Spine J 2020; 20(12): 1899-910. [http://dx.doi.org/10.1016/j.spinee.2020.07.014] [PMID: 32730985]

[43]   Ishiguro H, Kaito T, Yarimitsu S, *et al.* Intervertebral disc regeneration with an adipose mesenchymal stem cell-derived tissue-engineered construct in a rat nucleotomy model. Acta Biomater 2019; 87: 118-29. [http://dx.doi.org/10.1016/j.actbio.2019.01.050] [PMID: 30690206]

[44]   Migliorini F, Rath B, Tingart M, Baroncini A, Quack V, Eschweiler J. Autogenic mesenchymal stem cells for intervertebral disc regeneration. Int Orthop 2019; 43(4): 1027-36. [http://dx.doi.org/10.1007/s00264-018-4218-y] [PMID: 30415465]

[45]   Rozier P, Maria A, Goulabchand R, Jorgensen C, Guilpain P, Noël D. Mesenchymal Stem Cells in Systemic Sclerosis: Allogenic or Autologous Approaches for Therapeutic Use? Front Immunol 2018; 9: 2938.

[http://dx.doi.org/10.3389/fimmu.2018.02938] [PMID: 30619298]

[46]   Dregalla RC, Uribe Y, Bodor M. Human mesenchymal stem cells respond differentially to platelet preparations and synthesize hyaluronic acid in nucleus pulposus extracellular matrix. Spine J 2020; 20(11): 1850-60.
[http://dx.doi.org/10.1016/j.spinee.2020.06.011] [PMID: 32565315]

[47]   Tamaki Y, Sakai T, Miyagi R, *et al.* Intradural lumbar disc herniation after percutaneous endoscopic lumbar discectomy: case report. J Neurosurg Spine 2015; 23(3): 336-9.
[http://dx.doi.org/10.3171/2014.12.SPINE14682] [PMID: 26068274]

[48]   Yurube T, Han I, Sakai D. Concepts of Regeneration for Spinal Diseases in 2021. Int J Mol Sci 2021; 22(16): 8356.
[http://dx.doi.org/10.3390/ijms22168356] [PMID: 34445063]

[49]   Hu B, He R, Ma K, *et al.* Intervertebral Disc-Derived Stem/Progenitor Cells as a Promising Cell Source for Intervertebral Disc Regeneration. Stem Cells Int 2018; 2018: 1-11.
[http://dx.doi.org/10.1155/2018/7412304] [PMID: 30662469]

[50]   Gou S, Oxentenko SC, Eldrige JS, *et al.* Stem cell therapy for intervertebral disk regeneration. Am J Phys Med Rehabil 2014; 93(11) (Suppl. 3): S122-31.
[http://dx.doi.org/10.1097/PHM.0000000000000152] [PMID: 25122106]

[51]   Pérez-Silos V, Camacho-Morales A, Fuentes-Mera L. Mesenchymal Stem Cells Subpopulations: Application for Orthopedic Regenerative Medicine. Stem Cells Int 2016; 2016: 1-9.
[http://dx.doi.org/10.1155/2016/3187491] [PMID: 27725838]

[52]   Park YB, Ha CW, Lee CH, Yoon YC, Park YG. Cartilage Regeneration in Osteoarthritic Patients by a Composite of Allogeneic Umbilical Cord Blood-Derived Mesenchymal Stem Cells and Hyaluronate Hydrogel: Results from a Clinical Trial for Safety and Proof-of-Concept with 7 Years of Extended Follow-Up. Stem Cells Transl Med 2017; 6(2): 613-21.
[http://dx.doi.org/10.5966/sctm.2016-0157] [PMID: 28191757]

[53]   Ranganath SH, Levy O, Inamdar MS, Karp JM. Harnessing the mesenchymal stem cell secretome for the treatment of cardiovascular disease. Cell Stem Cell 2012; 10(3): 244-58.
[http://dx.doi.org/10.1016/j.stem.2012.02.005] [PMID: 22385653]

[54]   Sajeesh S, Broekelman T, Mecham RP, Ramamurthi A. Stem cell derived extracellular vesicles for vascular elastic matrix regenerative repair. Acta Biomater 2020; 113: 267-78.
[http://dx.doi.org/10.1016/j.actbio.2020.07.002] [PMID: 32645438]

[55]   Wang X, Shah FA, Vazirisani F, *et al.* Exosomes influence the behavior of human mesenchymal stem cells on titanium surfaces. Biomaterials 2020; 230: 119571.
[http://dx.doi.org/10.1016/j.biomaterials.2019.119571] [PMID: 31753474]

[56]   Xia C, Zeng Z, Fang B, *et al.* Mesenchymal stem cell-derived exosomes ameliorate intervertebral disc degeneration *via* anti-oxidant and anti-inflammatory effects. Free Radic Biol Med 2019; 143: 1-15.
[http://dx.doi.org/10.1016/j.freeradbiomed.2019.07.026] [PMID: 31351174]

[57]   Yaghoubi Y, Movassaghpour A, Zamani M, Talebi M, Mehdizadeh A, Yousefi M. Human umbilical cord mesenchymal stem cells derived-exosomes in diseases treatment. Life Sci 2019; 233: 116733.
[http://dx.doi.org/10.1016/j.lfs.2019.116733] [PMID: 31394127]

[58]   Yeung AT, Lewandrowski KU. Retrospective analysis of accuracy and positive predictive value of preoperative lumbar MRI grading after successful outcome following outpatient endoscopic decompression for lumbar foraminal and lateral recess stenosis. Clin Neurol Neurosurg 2019; 181: 52.
[http://dx.doi.org/10.1016/j.clineuro.2019.03.011] [PMID: 30986727]

[59]   Lewandrowski KU. Retrospective analysis of accuracy and positive predictive value of preoperative lumbar MRI grading after successful outcome following outpatient endoscopic decompression for lumbar foraminal and lateral recess stenosis. Clin Neurol Neurosurg 2019; 179: 74-80.
[http://dx.doi.org/10.1016/j.clineuro.2019.02.019] [PMID: 30870712]

SUBJECT INDEX

A

Acid 63, 69, 83, 184, 186, 188
  hyaluronic 63, 69, 184, 186, 188
  lactic 83
  polyglycolic 63, 69
Acidic ambience 19
Activation 87, 89, 121, 127, 134
  immune system 134
  inflammatory 121
Agents 23, 63, 91, 92, 130, 156, 166, 167, 174
  anti-inflammatory 167
  biocompatible 63
  chelating 91
  enzymatic 23, 92
  hemostatic 156
  inflammation-reducing 166
  stimulate vasculogenesis 130
Aging 3, 4, 6, 7, 9, 12, 13, 20, 24, 57
  hastening 6
Allogeneic 182, 186, 188
  progenitor cells (APCs) 186, 188
  transplantation 182
Angiogenetic pathways 127
Anterior cord syndrome 118
Anti-inflammatory 45, 65, 166, 191
  cytokine 65
  drugs 45
  medications 166, 191
Assessments 76, 99, 114, 117, 127, 148, 189, 190
  electrophysiological 127
  reflexogenic 117
Astrocytes 125, 130
Atherosclerosis 7
Augmentation 69, 127, 191
  aesthetic 191
Autologous bone marrow 45, 182
  mesenchymal stem cells 45
  transplants 182
Autologous stem cells 124
Autophagy 34, 41, 42

  inhibition 42

B

Balance 6, 87, 125, 166
  chemical 125
  emotional 6
  microenvironmental 125
  osmotic 166
Biologically based polymers 67
Biomechanics 18, 94
  spinal 94
Biotechnology firms 4
Blood-spinal cord barrier (BSCB) 112, 125
Bone marrow 45, 90, 124, 126, 183
  -derived mesenchymal stem cells 126
Brain-derived neurotrophic factor (BDNF) 127
Brown-Séquard syndrome 118
Byproducts 83, 92, 170
  enzymatic 92
  metabolic 83

C

Capability 22, 23, 64, 65, 112, 122, 128, 129, 173
  anti-inflammatory 173
  augmented cellular proliferation 23
  neuronal signal transduction 112
  thermogenic 22
Cardiovascular problems 10
Chondrocytes, hypertrophic 85
Chondrogenesis 23
Chromosomal aberrations 131
Chronic lumbosacral pain 95
Coagulopathy 149
Collagen 18, 27, 41, 61, 63, 68, 69, 72, 84, 85, 88
  fiber aggregations 18
  fibers 61
  fibrils 84, 88

www.ingramcontent.com/pod-product-compliance
Lightning Source LLC
Chambersburg PA
CBHW050846220326
41598CB00006B/440